Immune Regulation

Experimental Biology and Medicine

IMMUNE REGULATION

Edited by

Marc Feldmann
and
N. A. Mitchison

Humana Press · Clifton, New Jersey

Library of Congress Cataloging in Publication Data

Main entry under title:

Immune regulation.

    (Experimental biology and medicine)
    Based on papers presented at a conference held in
1984 at Cambridge, England.
    Includes index.
    1. Immune response—Regulation—Congresses.
I. Feldmann, Marc. II. Mitchison, N. Avrion.
III. Series: Experimental biology and medicine
(Clifton, N.J.) [DNLM: 1. Cell Differentiation—
congresses. 2. Immunity, Cellular—congresses.
3. Lymphocytes—cytology—congresses. 4. Lymphocytes—
immunology—congresses. QW 568 I315 1984]
QR186.I437 1985   616.07'9   85-5786

©1985 The Humana Press Inc.
Crescent Manor
PO Box 2148
Clifton, NJ 07015

Printed in the United States of America

PREFACE

Leukocyte culture conferences have a long pedigree. This volume records some of the scientific highlights of the 16th such annual conference, and is a witness to the continuing evolution and popularity of leukocyte culture and of immunology. There is strong evidence of the widening horizons of immunology, both technically, with the obviously major impact of molecular biology into our understanding of cellular processes, and also conceptually.

Traditionally, the 'proceedings' of these conferences have been published. But have the books produced really recorded the major part of the conference, the informal, friendly, but intense and sometimes heated exchanges that take place between workers in tackling very similar problems and systems and which are at the heart of every successful conference? Unfortunately this essence cannot be incorporated by soliciting manuscripts. For this reason, we have changed the format of publication, retaining published versions of the symposium papers, but requesting the workshop chairmen to produce a summary of the major new observations and areas of controversy highlighted in their sessions, as a vehicle for defining current areas of interest and debate. Not an easy task, as the workshop topics were culled from the abstracts submitted by the participants, rather than being on predefined topics.

The unseasonal warmth in Cambridge was reflected in the atmosphere of the conference, the organization of which benefited from the administrative skills of Jean Bacon, Philippa Wells, Mr. Peter Irving, and Mrs. Jennifer Hodd (Conference Contact, Cambridge), scientific advice from: Dr. B. Askonas, Dr. P. C. L. Beverley, Dr. M. Crumpton, Dr. M. Feldmann, Dr. M. Greaves, Dr. J. Ivanyi, Dr. J. Kay, Prof. P. Lachmann, Prof. N. A. Mitchison, Dr. M. Owen, Dr. E. Simpson, Dr. R. Taylor, and Dr. T. Twose.

Financial support, without which this meeting would simply not have been possible, came from: British Society of Immunology, Cancer Research Campaign, Celltech Ltd., DNAX Research Institute, Genetic Systems Corporation, Glaxo plc, ICI Pharmaceuticals plc, Imperial Cancer Research Fund, Leukaemia Research Fund, National Institutes of Health, The Wellcome Trust, Behring Diagnostics Ltd,

Elsevier Publications, Laboratory Impex Ltd, Mercia Brocades Ltd, Nyegaard Ltd, Sera Lab Ltd, Serotec Ltd, and Seward Laboratory.
We are grateful to the above for their contributions to this conference, but in the last resort, the quality of a conference depends on the participants, and their enthusiasm was much appreciated.

Marc Feldmann
N. A. Mitchison

CONTENTS

II. GROWTH AND DIFFERENTIATION FACTORS

WORKSHOP SUMMARIES

III. LYMPHOCYTE TRANSFORMATION

IV. SELECTIVE RECOGNITION BY T AND B CELLS

WORKSHOP SUMMARIES

V. ACCESSORY CELLS AND ANTIGEN PRESENTATION

WORKSHOP SUMMARIES

PARTICIPANTS

ORESTE ACUTO · Dana-Farber Cancer Institute and Harvard Medical School, Boston, Massachusetts

PAUL M. ALLEN · Harvard Medical School, Boston, Massachusetts

AMNON ALTMAN · Scripps Clinic, La Jolla, California

JULIAN L. AMBRUS, JR. · National Institutes of Health, Bethesda, Maryland

G. L. ASHERSON · Clinical Research Center, Harrow, UK

A. BASTEN · University of Sydney, Sydney, Australia

JAY A. BERZOFSKY · National Cancer Institute, Bethesda, Maryland

P. C. L. BEVERLY · University College Hospital School of Medicine, London, UK

BEN BONAVIDA · UCLA School of Medicine, Los Angeles, California

G. FRANCO BOTTAZZO · Middlesex Hospital Medical School, London, UK

F. BROWN · Wellcome Biotechnology, Surrey, UK

G. G. BROWNLEY · John Radcliffe Hospital, Oxford, UK

R. CALLARD · Institute of Child Health, London, UK

J. -C. CEROTTINI · Ludwig Institute for Cancer Research, Lausanne, Switzerland

D. CHARMOT · Centre d'Immunologie, Marseille, France

DOMINIQUE J. CHARRON · Lab d'Immunologie, Marseille, France

EDWARD A. CLARK · Genetic Systems Corporation, Seattle, Washington

R. B. CORLEY · Duke Medical Center, Durham, North Carolina

GERALD R. CRABTREE · National Cancer Institute, Bethesda, Maryland

MICHAËL J. CRUMPTON · Imperial Cancer Research Fund, London, UK

E. CULBERT · ICI, Cheshire, UK

SUSANNA CUNNINGHAM-RUNDLES · Sloan-Kettering Cancer Center, New York, New York

MARK M. DAVIS · Stanford University, Stanford, California

JOEL M. DEPPER · National Cancer Institute, Bethesda, Maryland

T. M. DEXTER · Paterson Laboratories, Manchester, UK

KEVIN DOHERTY · Dana-Farber Cancer Institute and Harvard Medical School, Boston, Massachusetts

P. DUBREUIL · Centre d'Immunologie, Marseille, France

KLAUS EICHMANN · Max-Planck Institute für Biologie, Freiburg, Federal Republic of Germany

P. ERB · Institute für Mikrobiologie and Hygiene, Basel, Switzerland

MARINA FABBI · Dana-Farber Cancer Institute and Harvard Medical School, Boston, Massachusetts

J. FARRANT · Clinical Research Center, Harrow, UK

ANTHONY S. FAUCI · National Institute of Allergy and Infectious Diseases, Bethesda, Maryland

MARC FELDMANN · Middlesex Hospital Medical School, London, UK

GRAHAM FLANNERY · La Trobe University, Victoria, Australia

J. G. FRELINGER · University of North Carolina, Chapel Hill, North Carolina

ROBERT C. GALLO · National Cancer Institute, Bethesda, Maryland

ELIZABETH D. GETZOFF · Research Institute of Scripps Clinic, La Jolla, California

WARNER C. GREENE · National Cancer Institute, Bethesda, Maryland

BEVERLY E. GRIFFIN · Imperial Cancer Research Fund, London, UK

STEPHEN M. HEDRICK · University of California, San Diego, California

T. HIRANO · Osaka University, Osaka, Japan

NANCY HOGG · Imperial Cancer Research Fund, London, UK

T. HUFF · Johns Hopkins University, Good Samaritan Hospital, Baltimore, Maryland

J. H. HUMPHREY · Royal Postgraduate Medical School, London, UK

S. INUI · Osaka University, Osaka, Japan

K. ISHIBASHI · Osaka University, Osaka, Japan

K. ISHIZAKA · Johns Hopkins University, Good Samaritan Hospital, Baltimore, Maryland

JURAJ IVANYI · Wellcome Research Laboratories, Kent, UK

P. JARDIEU · Johns Hopkins University, Good Samaritan Hospital, Baltimore, Maryland

ELLEN E. E. JARRETT · University of Glasgow, Glasgow, UK

E. J. JENKINSON · University of Birmingham, Birmingham, UK

J. GORDIN KAPLAN · The University of Alberta, Edmonton, Canada

S. KASHIWAMURA · Osaka University, Osaka, Japan

DAVID R. KATZ · Middlesex Hospital School, London, UK

JOHN E. KAY · University of Sussex, Brighton, UK

M. KENNEDY · University of Basel, Basel, Switzerland

ROLF KIESSLING · Karolinska Institute, Stockholm, Sweden

H. KIKUTANI · Osaka University, Osaka, Japan

T. KISHIMOTO · Osaka University, Osaka, Japan

G. G. B. KLAUS · National Institute for Medical Research, London, UK

H. KISHI · Osaka University, Osaka, Japan

JAN KLEIN · Max-Planck Institut für Biologie, Tübingen, Federal Republic of Germany

MARTIN KRÖNKE · National Cancer Institute, Bethesda, Maryland

EVELYN A. KURT-JONES · Harvard Medical School, Boston, Massachusetts

J. R. LAMB · University College London, London, UK

M. -A. LANE · Dana-Farber Cancer Institute, Boston, Massachusetts

JEFFREY A. LEDBETTER · Genetic Systems, Seattle, Washington

WARREN J. LEONARD · National Institutes of Health, Bethesda, Maryland

RICHARD A. LERNER · Research Institute of Scripps Clinic, La Jolla, California

MARCO LONDEI · The Middlesex Hospital Medical School, London, UK

J. LOWENTHAL · Ludwig Institute for Cancer Research, Lausanne Branch, Epalinges, Switzerland

H. R. MACDONALD · Ludwig Institute for Cancer Research, Lausanne Branch, Epalinges, Switzerland

P. MANNONI · University of Alberta, Edmonton, Canada

PAUL J. MARTIN · Genetic Systems Corporation, Seattle, Washington

C. MARTENS · DNAX Research Institute, Palo Alto, California

K. MATSUSHIMA · Institute of Biological Chemistry, 2nd University Medical School, Napoli, Italy

C. MAWAS · Centre d'Immunologie, Marseille, France

A. J. MCMICHAEL · John Radcliffe Hospital, Oxford, UK

C. J. M. MELIEF · Cent. Laboratory of Netherlands Red Cross, Amsterdam, Netherlands

Y. MIKI · Osaka University, Osaka, Japan

K. MOORE · DNAX Research Institute of Molecular and Cellular Biology, Palo Alto, California

ALESSANDRO MORETTA · Ludwig Institute for Cancer Research, Lausanne, Switzerland

ZOLTAN A. NAGY · Max-Planck Institut für Biologie, Tübingen, Federal Republic of Germany

T. NAKAGAWA · Osaka University, Osaka, Japan

N. NAKANO · Osaka University, Osaka, Japan

VLADIMIR A. NESMEYANOV · Shemyakin Institute Bioorganic Chemistry, Moscow, USSR

RICHARD L. O'BRIEN · Creighton University, Omaha, Nebraska

D. OLIVE · Centre d'Immunologie, Marseille, France

K. ONOZAKI · Institute of Biological Chemistry, 2nd University Medical School, Napoli, Italy

J. J. OPPENHEIM · National Cancer Institute, Frederick, Maryland

JOHN ORTALDO · National Cancer Institute, Frederick, Maryland

J. J. T. OWEN · University of Birmingham Medical School, Birmingham, UK

M. J. OWEN · University College London, London, UK

NANCY J. PEFFER · National Cancer Institute, Bethesda, Maryland

FERNANDO PLATA · Institut Pasteur, Paris, France

MIKULAS POPOVIC · National Institutes of Health, Bethesda, Maryland

A. PROCOPIO · Institute for Biological Chemistry, 2nd University Medical School, Napoli, Italy

HUGH PROSS · Ontario Cancer Foundation, Ontario, Canada

RICARDO PUJOL-BORRELL · University College London, London, UK

JANET PUMPHREY · National Cancer Institute, Bethesda, Maryland

G. RAMILA · University of Basel, Basel, Switzerland

ELLIS L. REINHERZ · Dana-Farber Cancer Institute, Boston, Massachusetts

J. P. REVILLARD · Hôpital E. Herriot, Lyon, France

RICHARD J. ROBB · E. I. du Pont de Nemours & Co., Glenolden, Pennsylvania

STUART RUDIKOFF · National Cancer Institute, Bethesda, Maryland

G. SCALA · Institute of Biological Chemistry, 2nd University Medical School, Napoli, Italy

A. SCHIMPL · Institute für Virology u. Immunbiologie Würzburg, Federal Republic of Germany

ROLAND SCOLLAY · Walter and Eliza Hall Institute, Victoria, Australia

DAVID W. SCOTT · University of Rochester, Rochester, New York

J. G. SHARP · University of Nebraska Medical Center, Omaha, Nebraska

K. SHIMIZU · Osaka Univeristy, Osaka, Japan

R. SHIMONKEVITZ · Ludwig Institute for Cancer Research, Lausanne Branch, Epalinges, Switzerland

ELIZABETH SIMPSON · Clinical Research Centre, Middlesex, UK

I. SKLENAR · Institute for Microbiology, University of Basel, Basel, Switzerland

H. A. F. STEPHENS · Dana-Farber Cancer Institute and Harvard Medical School, Boston, Massachusetts

PENNY B. SVETLIK · National Cancer Institute, Bethesda, Maryland

T. TAGA · Osaka University, Osaka, Japan

JOHN A. TAINER · Scripps Clinic, La Jolla, California

R. B. TAYLOR · University of Bristol, Bristol, UK

M. B. TOBIN · Dana-Farber Cancer Institute, Boston, Massachusetts

IAN TODD · University College London, London, UK

A. R. M. TOWNSEND · John Radcliffe Hospital, Oxford, UK

EMIL R. UNANUE · Harvard Medical School, Boston, Massachusetts

B. M. VOSE · ICI Pharmaceutical, Cheshire, UK

PETER WALDEN · Max-Planck Institut für Biologie, Tübingen, Federal Republic of Germany

THOMAS A. WALDMANN · National Cancer Institute, Bethesda, Maryland

A. D. WHETTON · Paterson Laboratories, Christie Hospital & Radium Institute, Manchester, UK

KOZO YOKOMURA · Nippon Medical School, Tokyo, Japan

E. D. ZANDERS · University College London, London, UK

SECTION I

T CELL RECEPTORS

MOLECULAR AND FUNCTIONAL ANALYSIS OF THE HUMAN T CELL ANTIGEN/MHC RECEPTOR

Oreste Acuto, Marina Fabbi & Ellis L. Reinherz

Dana-Farber Cancer Institute and Harvard Medical School
44 Binney Street, Boston, MA   02115

INTRODUCTION

T lymphocytes, unlike B lymphocytes, predominantly recognize antigen when it is associated with membrane-bound products of the major histocompatibility complex (MHC)(1-4). This "dual" recognition is important for activation of both cytotoxic effector T cells and immunoregulatory T cells. T cells act as inducers or suppressors for interactions between T cells, B cells, macrophages and other cells (8-13).

The specificity of T cells is determined by their cell surface receptors, and therefore, knowledge of these receptors is particularly useful in understanding the cellular interactions that underlie the different activities of T cells. Because T lymphocytes recognize antigen in a precise fashion, certain receptors on their surface were thought to be specific to single T cell clones (i.e. clonotypic). The ability to propagate human T lymphocyte clones in vitro (14-18) has made it possible to identify these clonotypic recognition determinants. Using T cell clones as immunogens, murine monoclonal antibodies specific to single clones have been generated and used to define a novel class of clonotypic molecules found on the surface of all T cells (19,20).

3

FUNCTIONAL EFFECTS OF ANTI-Ti MONOCLONAL ANTIBODIES

Earlier studies indicated that the human T3 molecule present on all peripheral T cells and mature thymocytes played an important role in immune recognition (21-26). Specifically, anti-T3 monoclonal antibodies were able to inhibit T cell function at the effector and induction phase and in the presence of macrophages to provide a mitogenic stimulus for resting T cells. Biochemical analysis of the T3 molecule showed that it was comprised of at least three subunits (27-29)(25-28KD, 21-23KD and 19KD, respectively) without detectable "variability" in subunits of T3 molecules derived from different T cell lines. Since the latter is an essential prerequisite for an antigen/MHC receptor molecule, it was concluded that T3, although intimately linked to the antigen recognition process, did not itself contain the Ag/MHC binding site.

To identify "clonotypic" molecules in the initial studies, we produced monoclonal antibodies against two distinct human T cell cytotoxic clones (CT8$_{III}$ and CT4$_{II}$) derived from the same individual and developed a screening strategy that selects for anticlonotypic antibodies. In this way, a series of non-crossreactive monoclonal antibodies that reacted only with the respective immunizing clone but not with a large number of additional T cell clones or peripheral T cells from the same donor were generated (19,20). These were termed anti-Ti.

Since the unique reactivities of anti-Ti monoclonals suggested that the surface structures defined were involved in the individual clonal specificity, it was determined whether these antibodies in soluble form could block recognition of antigen. To this end, effector cells were incubated with one or another monoclonal antibody for varying periods prior to assay of the clones' cytolytic and proliferative capacities. It was shown that cytolytic activity and the proliferative response of such clones were affected only by their respective anticlonotypic antibodies (19). That these effects were not simply due to an inactivation of the clones as a result of antibody treatment was clear from the fact that the same anti-Ti treatment augmented proliferation to IL-2 (20).

If anti-Ti monoclonal antibodies defined variable regions of the T cell receptor, then we reasoned that under

the appropriate conditions, anti-Ti antibodies might induce
clonal T cell activation in a fashion analogous to that of
antigen itself. Because the alloantigens that serve as
receptor ligands are membrane bound and likely interact via
multi-point surface attachment, and because anticlonotypic
monoclonal antibodies, by themselves, were not mitogenic,
the functional effects of purified monoclonal antibodies
bound to a solid surface support (Sepharose beads) was investigated (30). A number of important points emerged from
these experiments: a) Sepharose linked anti-Ti and Sepharose linked anti-T3 caused very similar functional effects,
initiating clonal proliferation and secretion of lymphokines including IL-2; b) triggering of a single clonally
unique epitope appears to be sufficient to induce antigen
specific functions and to substitute for antigen plus MHC
determinant; c) multimeric interactions between ligand and
antigen receptor was an essential requirement for the initiation of clonal T cell responses; and d) these clones produced and responded to IL-2. In addition, immunofluorescence studies showed that T3 modulation was accompanied by
loss of anti-Ti reactivity (20). These data imply that both
T3 and Ti have a role in antigen recognition and suggest a
relation between the cell surface structures defined by
these two antibodies.

Ti: A 90,000 DALTON DISULFIDE LINKED HETERODIMER

Because all studies described above demonstrated a
close functional and phenotypic relation between T3 glycoproteins and the Ti clonotype, it was important to biochemically define the surface molecules detected by clonotypic
antibodies. Therefore we selected two effector clones,
CT4$_{II}$ and CT8$_{III}$, for which we had specific monoclonal
anti-Ti antibodies (anti-Ti$_{1B}$ and anti-Ti$_{2A}$, respectively)
and surface labelled cells from these clones with ^{125}I Na.
Cell membranes were solubilized, immunoprecipitated with
the appropriate anticlonotypic antibody and electropheresed
to enable protein bands to be visualized (Fig. 1)(19).

The two anticlonotypic antibodies were noncrossreac-
tive by immunofluorescent studies and specifically precipitated material only from the clone to which they were directed (Fig. 1). Furthermore, neither antibody reacted
with peripheral T cells or with a total of 80 other clones
derived from the same donor. Immunoprecipitated CT8$_{III}$ mem-

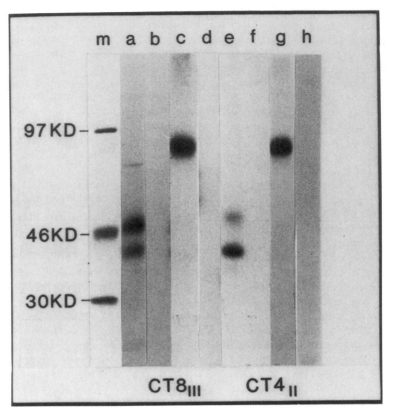

FIG. 1. SDS-PAGE analysis of anti-Ti immune precipitates from ^{125}I surface labelled CT8$_{III}$ and CT4$_{II}$. Lanes a to d depict immunoprecipitated proteins from CT8$_{III}$ membranes with anti-Ti$_{1B}$ antibody (a and c) and anti-Ti$_{2A}$ antibody (b and d) under reducing (a and b) and nonreducing conditions (c and d). Lanes e to h depict proteins immunoprecipitated from CT4$_{II}$ with anti-Ti$_{1B}$ antibody (e and g) and anti-Ti$_{2A}$ antibody (f and h) under reducing (e and f) and nonreducing conditions (g and h).

branes yielded two specific bands when electropheresed under reducing conditions (conditions that break disulfide bonds)(Fig. 1): a 49KD α chain and a 43KD β chain (lane a). Under nonreducing conditions (lane c) this structure appears as a single band at approximately 90KD. Anti-Ti$_{2A}$ antibody precipitates a similar molecule from ^{125}I labelled CT4$_{II}$ with subunits of 51KD and 49KD under reducing conditions,

and 90KD under nonreducing conditions. Thus, although the
Ti_1 and Ti_2 antigens can be defined by non-crossreactive
monoclonal antibodies, they both appear to be disulfide
linked heterodimers with distinct structural similarities.

The receptor for antigen on inducer and suppressor
clones is also a T3 associated disulfide linked heterodimer. Moreover, when anti-T3 antibody was used to precipitate surface antigens from these effector or regulatory
clones, electropheresis (reducing) produced four bands: a
major protein band at 20KD, a band at 25KD and two higher
molecular weight (41-43KD and 49-52KD) bands identical to
those precipitated by anti-Ti antibody. Under nonreducing
conditions, the latter two bands migrated as a single band
at 90KD and the smaller molecular weight bands were unchanged. These results suggested that anti-T3 antibody
precipitated a T3-Ti complex, whereas clonotypic antibodies
disassociated the T3 subunits from the Ti structure. Together, these data show that each functional T cell population (cytotoxic, suppressor or inducer) expresses a T3-Ti
complex.

PEPTIDE VARIABILITY IN Ti MOLECULES

Ti_1 molecules immunoprecipitated from $CT4_{II}$ and subjected to two dimensional gel electropheresis migrated at
pI 4.4 (α subunit) and pI 6.0 (β subunit). In contrast, Ti_2
α and β subunits from $CT8_{III}$ migrated at pI 4.7 and 6.2,
respectively (32). However, in both clones each subunit
migrated as a tight cluster of spots. To determine if the
microheterogeneity we observed within an individual clone
represented actual peptide differences, we pretreated the
Ti molecules with neuraminidase. After such treatment,
subunits from both Ti molecules resolved into single distinct spots, implying that the slight intraclonal microheterogeneity represented different degrees of sialylation,
whereas the intraclonal differences in isoelectric point
resulted from actual peptide differences.

These data suggested to us that like the immunoglobulin molecule, Ti molecules might be composed of constant
and variable domains. To test this hypothesis, we compared
peptide maps obtained from isolated ^{125}I labelled subunits
after digesting them with proteolytic enzymes (32). The
tryptic peptide maps of the α chains from clones $CT4_{II}$ and

and CT8$_{III}$ were similar yet distinct, and at least one minor and one major peptide were clearly identical in both
clones. Of the remaining peptides, a group of six migrated
minimally in both directions and although distinct,appeared
to be related. All other peptides were clearly different.

The β subunits were not well digested with trypsin and
therefore proteolysis with pepsin was required. Out of 11
to 13 peptides, two were identical and the rest migrated as
a single large cluster. These data may indicate that variability in the β subunit is confined to a single region.
Note that when peptides from both subunits were compared,
no similarities were found (unpublished data), indicating
that they are products of different genes without homology.
These peptide map studies show unequivocally that Ti structures are analogs, and support the notion that both α and β
·subunits of Ti have constant and variable domains.

PARTIAL N-TERMINAL AMINO ACID SEQUENCING OF THE Ti β SUBUNIT

To study the amino acid sequence of the β subunit of
Ti protein, we isolated microgram amounts of this structure
from the REX thymic tumor cell line using immune affinity
chromatography and polyacrylamide gel electropheresis. Because the peptide analysis showed that the β subunit was
highly variable, we chose this subunit for sequencing (33).
Using a gas-liquid-solid phase protein sequenator, we obtained unambiguous amino acid analysis on 17 out of 20 residues in the N-terminal sequence of this subunit. A synthetic peptide with a sequence identical to that postulated
for residues 2-11 was created, and used to produce a rabbit
antiserum. This antiserum immunoprecipitated the isolated
denatured β subunit of REX Ti, confirming that the postulated protein sequence was indeed that of the Ti β subunit.

To determine if homologies existed between this N-
terminal sequence (residues 2-11 and 2-20) and known proteins, we did a computer search using the Dayhoff protein
data bank. As shown with the representative amino acid
sequence in Table 1, homologies with the first framework of
the variable region of the immunoglobulin λ and κ light
chains were found. Lambda homology was evident with the
shorter 2-11 peptide, and κ homology was obvious with residues 2-20. In total, 44 of 60 matches were made with
human and mouse light chain framework.

TABLE 1. Ti β AND IMMUNOGLOBULIN LIGHT CHAINS ARE HOMOLOGOUS IN PORTIONS OF THEIR N-TERMINAL AMINO ACID SEQUENCES

Protein	1				5					10					15						
Ti	X	V* (10)	I	Q	S	P	R	H	E	V	T	E	X	X	G	X	E	V	T	L	R
Bvr: VλII		V	S	G	S	P	G	H	S	V	T										
Tro: VλII		V	S	G	S	P	G	Q	S	V	T										
Nig48: λV VI		V* (4)	S	E	S	P	G	K	T	V	T										
Ag: VκI		M	T	Q	S	P	S	S	L	S	A	S	V	G	D	R	V	T	I		
Ni: VκI		M	T	Q	S	P	S	S	L	S	A	T	V	G	D	R	V	T	L		
Pom: VκIV		M	T	Q	S	P	V	T	L	S	V	P	G	E	R	A	A	T	L	S	
MOPC21: Vκ		M	T	Q	S	P	K	S	M	S	M	S	V	G	E	R	V	T	L	T	

Note that all protein homologies shown are with human immunoglobulin except for MOPC21 (mouse). Single amino acid nomenclature is utilized with bound areas showing homology. *Denotes amino acid positions corresponding to start of sequence homology in the immunoglobulin proteins.

GENES ENCODING THE T CELL RECEPTOR

By using a novel technique of complementary DNA cloning known as subtractive hybridization, two groups recently isolated complementary DNA clones encoding putative membrane proteins that are expressed uniquely in human and murine T cell clones. Genes that rearranged in these cells
were also identified (34-36). The N-terminus of the gene
product predicted by the complementary human DNA clones was
completely consistent with the 17 amino acids we had identified unambiguously in the N-terminal sequence of the human Ti β subunit. This predicted N-terminal sequence began
at residue 22, identifying the first 21 residues as the
leader signal peptide. In addition, the gene product predicted by subtractive hybridization is remarkably homologous to the human immunoglobulin chain in both N-terminal
and C-terminal regions, particularly in the location of
cysteine residues. These results also agree with our study
of the N-terminal sequence of the Ti β subunit.

The correspondence of sequence data obtained by two
different methods, and the additional fact that the molecular weight of the polypeptide predicted by the complementary DNA studies (35KD) corresponded closely with that of the
membrane form of Ti (43KD) strongly suggest that this DNA
clone is the gene for the β subunit of the human Ti molecule. Differences in the molecular weight of the predicted
and observed protein can be explained by glycosylation; Ti
is known to be a glycoprotein and at least two potential
glycosylation sites for complex oligosaccarides have been
identified on the cloned DNA product.

Based on NH_2-terminal amino acid determinations and
the predicted protein sequence, the 291 amino acid human Ti
β subunit appears to contain two extracellular domains,
each with a disulfide loop and a carboxyterminal hydrophobic transmembrane region followed by a cytoplasmic tail.
This overall structure is reminiscent of both immunoglobulin
light chains and major histocompatibility gene products,
suggesting that all three evolved from the same supergene
family. The similarity of Ti β with immunoglobulin also
places constraints on the structure of the Ti α subunit of
the heterodimer, making it likely that it will be immuno-
globulin-like as well.

     The N-terminal variable-like and C-terminal constant-
like regions of the putative protein encoded by the murine
T cell complementary murine DNA clone also corroborated the
peptide map data. The high degree of homology between the
3' regions in the human and mouse complementary DNA clones
(80% between residues 134-306), and the lack of homology
between the α and β subunits at the protein level indicates that this putative protein is the mouse equivalent
of the Ti β subunit. Based on the similarities between
mouse and human proteins, we would predict that the T cell
receptor in both species will consist of a T3-Ti complex
as shown in Fig. 2.

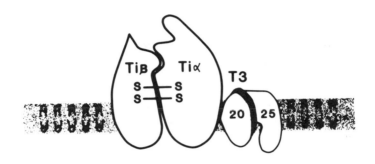

FIG. 2.   The human T cell receptor complex.

ACKNOWLEDGEMENTS

     This work was supported by NIH grants AI 19807, AIGM
21226, and AI 12069-11.

REFERENCES

1. Benacerraf, B. & McDevitt, H. Science 175, 273 (1979).
2. Schlossman, S.F. Transplant. Rev. 10, 97 (1972).
3. Zinkernagel, R.M. & Doherty, P.C. J. Exp. Med. 141,
    1427 (1975).
4. Corradin, G. & Chiller, J.M. J. Exp. Med. 149, 436
    (1979).

5. Hunig, T. & Bevan, M. Nature 294, 460 (1981).
6. Cerottini, J.C. Prog. Immunol. 4, 622 (1980).
7. Doherty P.C. Prog. Immunol. 4, 563 (1980).
8. Quinnan, G.V. et al. N. Engl. J. Med. 307, 7 (1982).
9. Wallace, L.E., Rickinson, A.B., Rose, M. & Epstein, M.A. Nature 297, 413 (1982).
10. Meuer, S.C. et al. J. Immunol. 131, 186 (1983).
11. Gershon, R.K. Contemp. Top. Immunol. 3, 1 (1974).
12. Cantor, H. & Boyse, E.A. Cold Spring Harbor Symp. Quant. Biol. 41, 23 (1977).
13. Cohen, S., Pick, E. & Oppenheim, J.J. In: Biology of the Lymphokines (Oppenheim, J.J. ed), Academic Press, New York, pp. 179-195.
14. Morgan, D.A., Ruscetti, R.W. & Gallo, R.C. Science 193, 1007 (1976).
15. Kurnick, J.T. et al. J. Immunol. 122, 255 (1979).
16. Bonnard, G.D., Yasaka, K. and Maca, R.D. Cell. Immunol. 51, 390 (1980).
17. Sredni, B., Tse, H.Y. & Schwartz, R.H. Nature 283, 581 (1980).
18. Meuer, S.C., Schlossman, S.F. & Reinherz, E.L. Proc. Natl. Acad. Sci. USA 79, 4395 (1982).
19. Meuer, S.C. et al. Nature 303, 808 (1983).
20. Meuer, S.C. et al. J. Exp. Med. 157, 705 (1983).
21. Reinherz, E.L., Hussey, R.E. & Schlossman, S.F. Eur. J. Immunol. 10, 758 (1980).
22. van Wauwe, F.P., DeMay, J.R. & Goossener, J.G. J. Immunol. 124, 2708 (1980).
23. Chang, T.W., Kung, P.C., Gingras, S.P. & Goldstein, G. Proc. Natl. Acad. Sci. USA 78, 1805 (1981).
24. Burns, G.F., Boyd, A.E. & Beverley, P.C.I. J. Immunol. 124, 1451 (1982).
25. Reinherz, E.L. et al. Cell 30, 735 (1982).
26. Umiel, T. et al. J. Immunol. 129, 1054 (1982).
27. Borst, J., Prendiville, M.A. & Terhorst, C. J. Immunol. 128, 1560 (1982).
28. Borst, J., Alexander, S., Elder, J. & Terhorst, C. J. Biol. Chem. 258, 5135 (1982).
29. Kannelloplos, J.M., Wigglesworth, N.M., Owen, M.J. & Crumpton, M.J. Embo. J. 2, 1807 (1983).
30. Meuer, S.C. et al. J. Exp. Med. 158, 988 (1983).
31. Meuer, S.C. et al. Science 218, 471 (1982).
32. Acuto, O. et al. J. Exp. Med. 158, 1368 (1983).
33. Acuto, O. et al. Proc. Natl. Acad. Sci. USA 81, 3851 (1984)
34. Yanagi, Y. et al. Nature 308, 145 (1984).

36. Hedrick, S.M., Cohen, D.I., Nielsen, E.A. & Davis, M.M.
    Nature 308, 153 (1984).
37. Meuer, S.C. et al. Science 222, 1239 (1983).

EXPRESSION PATTERNS OF THE BETA CHAIN

OF THE T CELL RECEPTOR FOR ANTIGEN

Stephen M. Hedrick and Mark M. Davis[*]

University of California, San Diego
La Jolla, California   92093

[*]Stanford, University
Stanford, California 94305

INTRODUCTION

With the isolation of recombinant clones encoding the beta chain of the T cell receptor[1-3], the similarity of expression patterns in functionally and developmentally distinct T cell subsets can be determined. In this report, we present the transcriptional patterns of the beta chain in thymocytes and peripheral T cells, and the expression of the beta chain in functionally defined T cells. Special interest is directed at the abundance and size of transcripts in immature vs. mature T cells, and at the structure of transcripts found in different tissues, i.e., message transcribed from aberrant or productively rearranged genes. Further attention is paid to the expression of the beta chain in helper, cytotoxic, and suppressor T cells as a reflection of the nature of the antigen-specific receptor in these cell types.

BETA CHAIN GENE EXPRESSION IN MATURE VS. IMMATURE T CELLS

T cells are known to arise from stem cells in the bone marrow, and differentiate in the thymus into immature T cells, and finally into functionally mature regulatory or effector T cells. The somatic processes thought to occur during this differentiation scheme include a selection for tolerance to self components, and for preferential reactivity to antigens in association with major histocompatibility complex (MHC) molecules expressed in the thymus[4-8]

15

(MHC restriction). Superimposed on these functionally
defined selection steps is a tremendous proliferation of
thymocytes followed by the expiration of all but a small
percentage of cells. The cells targeted for demise could be
those that are autoreactive, those that lack an ability to
react with antigen in the context of self MHC molecules,
those that have been unsuccessful in achieving appropriately
rearranged receptor genes, or none of the above. With
molecular probes for the receptor genes, some of these
facets of T maturation can be approached.

One scheme put forth to explain the somatic selection
events posit a differential level of receptor expression at
various stages of maturation which would thus have the
effect making T cells sensitive to differing levels of
liquid stimulation[9]. For example, high levels of receptor
expression in the thymus might increase the sensitivity of
the T cells such that reaction with MHC molecules in the
absence of antigen molecules would occur. Upon maturation
and migration from the thymus, the peripheral T cells might
decrease the level of receptor expression such that they no
longer react to MHC molecules alone, but only in the context
of another ligand (such as antigen). Such a scheme would
predict that thymocytes would express substantially more
receptor than mature peripheral T cells.

The first experiments presented allowed us to determine
the level of receptor message expressed in different populations of T cells. The level of expression was determined by
screening cDNA libraries made using RNA extracted from thymocytes, Con A activated spleen cells, and a T cell hybridoma. In the absence of secondary structure in the message,
the percentage of positive clones in the library is a direct
measure of message abundance. The data presented in Table 1
shows the frequency of clones in each of the three
libraries.

Table 1. Frequency of Beta Chain Clones in cDNA Libraries

	Positives	Frequencies
Thymocyte*	170/100,000	0.17%
Con A-spleen*	41/100,000	0.04%
T Cell Hybridoma[1]	10/5,000	0.01%
(T-B subtrated 20-fold enriched)		

* cDNA libraries generously provided by Dr. C. Benoiste.

As shown, the level of receptor in the thymus greater
than 4-fold higher than Con A-activated spleen cells, and
almost 20-fold higher than the T cell hybridoma. Of course,
not all of the cells in a Con A activated spleen population
are T cells, but clearly a majority of the cells are. These
data appear to indicate that the level of beta chain message
(and perhaps expressed receptor) is higher in immature T
cells (thymocytes) than in mature periphera T cells. How
the level of receptor message in hybridomas correlates to
that of functional T cells is presently not known exactly,
however, comparisons made between RNA from hybridomas and IL
2-dependent cytotoxic T cells indicate that there is no sys-
tematic difference[10]. The fact that thymocytes express significantly higher levels of message is consistent with the
notion that they may also express greater amounts of receptor on their surface and are correspondingly more sensitive
to stimulation by MHC molecules in the absence of antigen[9].

One of the possibility for the high turnover of cells
in the thymus is that many cells have aberrantly rearranged
chromosomes, and are thus expendible to the immune system.
We were therefore interested in the size and structure of
the transcripts originating from the thymus as compared to
other sources of T cells. The first and simplest experiment
was to examine message from different sources on Northern
blots for size. Since the translatable message is 1,300
nucleotides, any short messages almost certainly could not
contain the entire complement of v-,d-,j-, and c-exons.
Results of such experiments (Table 2) indicate that T cell
hybridomas and clones express message at 1,300, 1,000, and
sometimes 650 nucleotides. The amount of the smaller messages varies between cell lines, but these differences
appear to be random. Not surprisingly, therefore, thymocytes express both the 1,300 and 1,000 nucleotide messages,
and these appear to be reproducibly expressed in equal
amounts (Table 2). Although we have not seen 650 nucleotide
messages in thymocyte RNA, we feel that this reflects a
difference in the sensitivity of the experiments, and not a
real difference in the expression patterns. T cells, therefore, in general express what appears to be aberrant message, perhaps off of a chromosome inappropriately rearranged.

Table 2. Message Sizes in T Cell Lymphomas and Thymocytes

	Message Sizes
T cell hybridomas:	
C 10	1,300
2B4	1,300, 1,000, 650
T cell lymphomas:	
BW 5147	1,300, 1,000
BAL 9	1,300, 1,000, 650
BAL 13	1,300
BAL 4	1,300, 1,000
Thymocytes	1,300, 1,000

The next question we addressed concerned the structure of the different transcripts found in thymocytes, i.e., what is the origin of the sequences comprising the short messages in terms of coding or noncoding elements encoded in the genome. In order to address this question, we compared the sequence of cDNA clones isolated from the thymocyte library with the sequences of the rearranged and germline beta chain genes[11-13]. In Fig. 1 we have schematized the genomic organization of the beta chain genes in three configurations: unrearranged (top), a rearrangement involving only d and j regions (middle), and a productive rearrangement involving v, d, and j elements (bottom). In comparing the sequences of these genes versus the cDNA clones we have isolated and sequenced, we have find cDNA clones representing three different patterns. The clone 86T3 (top) has 5' sequences identical to the intervening sequence just upstream from the $C_T 1$ exon indicating that the transcription initiated in the intervening sequence, and proceded into the coding regions. Since the remainder of the cDNA clone had only the appropriate coding sequences, the other intervening sequences were appropriately spliced out. We have pictured this transcript as originating from an unrearranged chromosome, since we assume strong promoters would be available and thus used in the rearranged configuration. Clearly, this is an assumption, and there is no way of knowing exactly what the chromosmal configuration was that gave rise to the 86T3 transcript. From the size of the 86T3 cDNA clone, the message size of this sort of aberrant transcript would be greater than 1,200 nucleotides, and therefore indistinguishable from the translatable message on a Northern blot. Therefore, of the message in the 1,300 nucleotide band, some of the transcripts are aberrant.

Figure 1.

Alternate Gene Rearrangements and
Transcription in Thymocytes

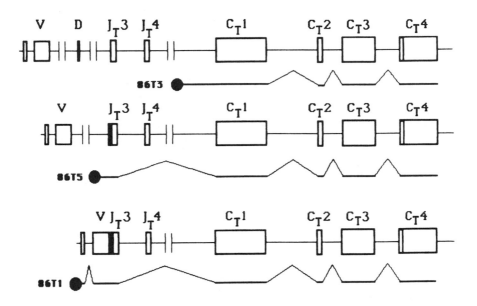

The clone 86T5 has the exact nucleotide sequence of the constant region C_T and the joining region J_T3. The sequence 5' to the j region shows the rearrangement repeat sequences followed by nine nucleotides presumably encoding a d region. This transcript, therefore, originated from a d-j rearrangement as pictured (Fig. 1, middle), and would correspond to the ubiquitous 1,000 nucleotide message band. Finally, a productively rearranged chromosome with v, d, and j regions rearranged in frame is pictured at the bottom, and such a chromosome gives rise to a transcript such as that of 86T1. Presumbly, this transcription is initiated at the appropriate promoter 5' to the exon encoding the leader sequence, and has been shown to give rise to the 1,300 nucleotide message. The origin of the 650 nucleotide messages is not clear, and may in fact not be a discrete message but result from a limited message degradation. In addition, as discussed below, 1,000 nucleotide messages are seen at very low

levels in NK lymphomas in the absence of detectable gene
rearrangements. The aberrant d-j rearrangement is therefore
not the only source of the 1,000 nucleotide messages.

The clones isolated from the Con A-activated splenocyte
cDNA library have not been as extensively characterized as
those from the thymocyte cDNA library, but a group of clones
were characterized with respect to size and found to be
comprised of short clones at least as frequently as the
group isolated from the thymocyte library. The sequence of
one of these clones showed that in fact there were aberrant
transcripts expressed. The implications of these data are
that aberrant transcripts are present in thymus, but also in
peripheral T cells, and these transcripts probably come from
the many cells that have one aberrantly rearranged chromosome and one productively rearranged chromosome. We thus
far cannot say whether the aberrant transcripts occur more
frequently in thymocytes than in peripheral T cells, and
therefore cannot say whether the aberrant rearrangements are
involved in the high turnover of T cells in the thymus.

BETA CHAIN EXPRESSION IN FUNCTIONALLY DEFINED T CELL SUBSETS

The cDNA clone TM86 that encodes the putative beta
chain of the T cell receptor was isolated from T cell hybridomas that are of the helper cell lineage. Of importance in
understanding T cell recognition of antigen is whether different functional T cells use the same, similar, or different versions of the beta chain as part of their receptor.
Perhaps the crucial distinctions concern the specificity for
MHC molecule recognition. Cytotoxic T cells recognize
antigen in association with Class I molecules, helper T
cells recognize antigen in association with Class II
molecules and suppresor T cells appear to bind and recognize
antigen in the absence of MHC molecules. A further class of
recognition is by natural killer cells that are thought to
be close to, or part of the T cell lineage, and have an
uninducible reactivity to certain tumor cells. Various
examples of each of these types of cells were examined in
two ways. First, productive gene expression, as described
above, requires that the beta chain locus undergo rearrangements to juxtapose v, d, and j elements into an active gene.
Therefore, any cell with the potential for beta chain gene
expression must exhibit beta chain gene element rearrangements which can be determined by genomic Southern blots.
Second, transcription of translatable mRNA requires that
cells express a 1,300 nucleotide message seen on Northern

blots. Parenthetically, as described above, some messages
of this approximate size (86T3) are not translatable, but
most appear to be. A compilation of a large number of
experiments is presented in Table 3. The data indicate that
T helper cells all show beta gene rearrangements and express
a message long enough to encode a v-, d-, j-, and c-region[1].
Further we have isolated cDNA clones from several helper
cells, and found in each case a complete transcript. We
would tentatively conclude from this sampling that all T
helper cells express the beta chain as part of the receptor.
In the case of T killer cells again all of the cell lines
examine showed gene rearrangements, and message expression
of the appropriate length[10]. Also consistent with these
data we have cloned and isolated a beta chain cDNA from an
alloreactive cytotoxic T cell, and found the sequence to be
that of a complete transcript including v-, d-, j-, and c-
region gene elements (Staerz, Bevan, and Hedrick, unpublished observation). We would therefore tentatively conclude that cytotoxic T cells also express the beta chain as
part of the antigen-specific receptor, notwithstanding the
dichotomy between Class II MHC-specific helper cells, and
Class I-specific cytotoxic cells.

Table 3. Beta Chain Expression in Functionally Distinct
T Cell Subsets

	Gene Rearrange- ments Detected	Message Expression 1,200-1,300 nucleotides
Helper T cells:		
Hybridoma clones	12/12	6/6
IL 2-dependent	2/2	n.d.
Cytotoxic T cells:		
Hybridoma clones	2/2	2/2
IL 2-dependent	4/4	3/3
Suppressor T cells:		
Hybridoma clones	2/14	n.d.
Natural killer cells:		
Spontaneous lymphomas	0/6	0/2

* n.d.: not done

The expression of the beta chain in T suppressor cells would not necessarily be predicted since they do not recognize antigen in association with MHC moleculs, and their specificity appears to be in the form of a secreted factor, and not a membrane bound receptor. The suppressor cell clones we examined[10] were hybridomas made between BW5147 and spleen cells from immunized mice, and were selected for the ability to suppress the immune response in the appropriate manner. The cell lines tested were representative of all of the suppressor cell phenotypes including Ts1, Ts2, Ts3, idiotype-specific suppressors, suppressor inducers, and suppressor acceptors. One of the fourteen clones tested, only two exhibited gene rearrangements different from those of BW5147. One of these clones was a Ts2 cell, and one was a Ts3, however, neither phenotype showed consistent gene rearrangements. The conclusion from these experiments is that suppressor T cells can mediate antigen-specific suppression without beta chain expression. The beta chain is thus not part of the antigen-specific secreted suppressor factor, and these data are consistent with the structure of the beta chain which includes a transmembrane polypeptide sequence not compatible with a soluble protein.

Finally, the beta chain genes were examined in spontaneous rat lymphomas that mediate natural killer activity[11]. The simple result was that in all cases the genes were unrearranged, and the cells did not express a transcript long enough to be translated into a functional beta chain. Message expression was seen at 1,000 nucleotides, but even this was at least 40-fold less abundant than the message in rat and mouse T cell lymphomas. Again these results strongly suggest that natural killer activity is not a function that is mediated by a receptor partly comprised of the beta chain. Although some in vitro natural killer lines may express the beta chain, the above data suggest that such expression is irrelevant to the functional activity.

DISCUSSION

As discussed above, T cells appear to be selected for the recognition of antigen preferentially in association with the allelic form of the MHC molecules expressed in the thymus. A difficulty in explaining thymic selection of the T cell repertoire is that the receptor would be selected for reactivity to MHC molecules in the absence of antigen and yet only manifest immune reactivity to MHC molecules in the

presence of antigen. The dichotomy of these two specificities required of the same T cell receptor poses an enigma.
One way of dealing with such an enigma has been to postulate
the existence of two receptors or two distinct receptor combining sites. Under such a model, the T cell would be
selected in the thymus by binding to MHC molecules via the
MHC-specific portion of the receptor, but only react in an
immune response when both the MHC-specific and the antigen-
specific portions of thhe receptor(s) were bound. The hallmark of such a model for the T cell receptor is that there
are separate recognition sites for antigen and MHC
molecules. Although consistent with much of the functional
data regarding the selection and specificity of T cells,
such a model is not consistent with experiments showing that
the specificity of antigen recognition by the T cell is
highly dependent on the structure of the MHC molecules
simultaneously bound (indicating a three-way interaction
between the receptor, MHC molecules, and antigen). This
model is also not consistent with the structure of the
receptor as currently known, that is, a single disulfide
bonded protein heterodimer analogous in structure to immunoglobulin. If we accept the idea (or fact) that the T cell
receptor binds a complex determinant formed from an interaction between antigen and MHC molecules, then there is the
above stated difficulty in explaining the selection of the T
cell population based on binding to thymic MHC molecules in
the absence of antigen. In order to explain such a system
based on a single receptor-combining site, we propose that
the sensitivity of T cells to stimulation with MHC molecules
is significantly higher than the sensitivity exhibited by
peripheral T cells. One simple mechanism that would account
for a difference in sensitivity would be a difference in the
number of receptors expressed per cell. For instance, if
thymocytes expressed ten-fold more receptors than peripheral
T cells, they would be sensitive to stimulation by MHC
molecules of a ten-fold lower concentration than that
required in the periphery. Such a difference in sensitivity
could easily explain the requirement for an additional
ligand (antigen) in an immune response, and the absence of
such requirement for stimulation in the thymus.

The expression patterns of the beta chain in thymocytes
and peripheral T cells suggests that there are significantly
higher levels of expression in thymuc T cells than in peripheral T cells. Further experiments in progress (Fink,
Bevan, and Hedrick, unpublished data) indicate that immature

thymocytes express an even higher level of message than that
of the average thymocyte. These data would be consistent
with the notion that immature T cells express high levels of
receptor during maturation in the thymus. Furthermore, we
speculate that this difference in the receptor levels has a
significant physiological basis, and may explain the enigma
of thymus selection and MHC restriction.

   We have presented evidence that T cell lines, thymocytes, and peripheral T cells express a number of transcripts that are not translatable, and by DNA sequence
analysis these transcripts were shown to arise from aberrantly rearranged chromosome, e.g., d-j rearrangements with
no v-region. Because rearrangements appear to take appear
to take place on both chromosomes in most cells we cannot
currently determine what percentage of thymocytes have both
chromosomes aberrantly rearranged, and what percentage of
cells have one chromosome aberrantly rearranged. Thus far,
there do not appear to be a preference for aberrant transcripts in thymocytes compared with peripheral T cells, and
so the nature of the high cell turnover in the thymus cannot
be addressed.

BIBLIOGRAPHY

1. Hedrick, S.M., Cohen, D.I., Nielsen, E.A. and Davis,
       M.M. 1984. Nature 308:149.
2. Hedrick, S.M., Nielsen, E.A., Kavaler, J., Cohen, D.I.
       and Davis, M.M. 1984. Nature 308:153.
3. Yanagi, Y., Yoshikai, Y., Leggett, K., Clark, S.P.,
       Aleksander, I. and Mak, T.W. 1984. Nature 308:145.
4. Zinkernagel, R.M., Callahan, G.N., Althage, A., Cooper,
       J., Klein, P.A. and Klein, J. 1978. J. Exp. Med.
       147:882.
5. Bevan, M.J. and Fink, P.J. 1978. Immunological Rev.
       42:3.
6. Waldmann, H., Pope, H., Pettls, C. and Davies, A.J.S.
       1978. Nature 277:137.
7. Doherty, P.C. and Bennink, J.R. 1979. J. Exp. Med.
       150:1187.
8. Hedrick, S.M. and Watson, J. 1980. J. Immunol.
       125:1782.
9. Hedrick, S.M., Ashwell, J.D. and Matis, L.A. 1984. In:
       Recognition and Regulation in Cell-Mediated Immunity,
       eds. J. Marbrook and J.D. Watson. Marcel Dekker, New
       York. (In press).

10. Hedrick, S.M., Germain, R.N., Bevan, M.J., et al.
       (1984). Proc. Natl. Acad. Sci. USA (In press).
11. Chien, Y.-H., Gascoigne, N.R.J., Lee, N., Kavaler, J.,
       Davis, M.M. 1984. Nature 309:322.
12. Gascoigne, N.R.J., Chien, Y.-H., Becker, D.M., Kavaler,
       J. and Davis, M.M. 1984. Nature 310:387.
13. Malissen, M., Minard, K., Mjolsness, S. et al. 1984.
       Cell 37:1101.
14. Hedrick, S.M., Bonyhadi, M., Hunig, H., Reynolds, C.
       1984. Manuscript in preparation.

This work is supported in part by grants from USPHS
AI-21372, AI-20302, AI-19512; and ACS IN 93L.

NON ANTIGEN-SPECIFIC SURFACE MOLECULES INVOLVED IN T LYMPHOCYTE FUNCTION

J.-C. Cerottini, H.R. MacDonald,
J. Lowenthal and R. Shimonkevitz

Ludwig Institute for Cancer Research,
Lausanne Branch, Epalinges, Switzerland

I.   INTRODUCTION

Until recently, it was generally assumed that cell surface structures other than antigen-specific receptors were not involved in T cell function. However, the reports in 1979 by Nakayama et al.[1] and Shinohara and Sachs[2] that antibodies to the Lyt-2/3 antigenic complex inhibited the specific cytolytic activity of murine cytolytic T lymphocytes (CTL) suggested that differentiation antigens expressed on the surface membrane of T cells may have functional importance in T cell immune responses. Since these early reports, a great many studies have been devoted to the identification of functionally important surface structures in murine, rat and human T lymphocytes. As a result of these studies, which have been greatly facilitated by the use of cloned T cell populations and monoclonal antibodies (MAbs), it has been proposed that several surface protein molecules that are clearly distinct from antigen receptors participate in antigen-dependent interactions between T lymphocytes and antigen-bearing cells, and/or may be involved in T cell activation. Moreover, comparative biochemical and functional analyses of murine and human T cells have indicated a remarkable degree of phylogenetic conservation of some of these molecules. As shown in Table I, these surface structures include both those which are expressed on all peripheral T cells (such as Thy-1, T11, T3 and LFA-1) and those which

27

TABLE I
Functional Effect(s) of Individual MAbs to T-Cell
Surface Antigens

Antigen		Inhibition	Stimulation	Heterogeneity
Murine	Human			
LFA-1	LFA-1	+	−	No
Lyt-2,3	T8	+	−	Yes
L3T4	T4	+	−	Yes
Thy-1		−	+	N.D.
	T11	+ (−)	− (+)	No
	T3	+	+	Yes

are specific to a particular T cell subset (such as
Lyt-2,3/T8 and L3T4/T4). It is also noteworthy that several
of these structures (i.e. Thy-1, LFA-1 and T4) are not
restricted to T lymphocytes.

The identification of functionally important
structures on T lymphocytes has generally been based on the
ability of the corresponding antibodies to inhibit
antigen-driven functions such as cytolytic activity,
lymphokine production or proliferation. Alternatively,
antibodies have been tested for their ability to stimulate
proliferation and/or lymphokine production in the absence
of antigen. In most cases studied so far, it appears that a
given MAb can not display both inhibitory and stimulatory
activities (Table I). While this may reflect the role
played by the corresponding molecules, studies on the
properties of anti-T11 MAbs indicate that the functional
effect (inhibition or stimulation) of such antibodies may
be related to the epitope they recognize. Moreover, in the
case of anti-T3 MAbs, there is evidence that some
antibodies exhibit inhibitory activities when used in
solution, whereas they have stimulating properties when
coupled to a solid support or bound to the Fc receptors of
monocytes. Finally, it should be stressed that analysis of
cloned T cell populations has revealed in several instances
a clear heterogeneity in the susceptibility of T cells to
functional inhibition by MAbs. This heterogeneity which has
been observed with antibodies to Lyt-2,3, L3T4, T8, T4 and

T3, is not related to the level of expression of the corresponding antigens.

In this paper, we focus our attention on the role of the Lyt-2,3 molecular complex. Further discussion of the functional role of T-cell surface structures can be found in recent articles[3-22].

II.   INHIBITORY ACTIVITY OF ANTI-LYT-2,3 MAbs ON CTL FUNCTIONS

Lyt-2,3 antigens are expressed on thymocytes as well as a subset of peripheral T lymphocytes in the mouse. Biochemical analysis of these molecules has revealed that they consist, at least in thymocytes, of three disulfide-linked subunits of 37,000, 32,000 and 28,000 apparent mol. wts, respectively[10]. All three subunits are surface-expressed glycopeptides possessing hydrophobic regions residing within the lipid bilayer[23]. From a recent analysis of the tryptic peptides derived from each of these subunits, it appears that the 37,000 and 32,000 mol. wt components have a similar polypeptide structure, whereas the 28,000 mol. wt is structurally different[24]. While the three subunits are co-precipitated by either anti-Lyt-2 or anti-Lyt-3 antibodies, there is still some controversy as to the precise location of the corresponding epitopes on these subunits. Of practical interest is the fact that Lyt-2,3 molecules are relatively sensitive to proteolytic digestion by trypsin, the Lyt-3 epitopes being considerably more trypsin-sensitive than the Lyt-2 epitopes.

Studies by several groups indicate that MAbs directed against different determinants of the Lyt-2,3 molecular complex all display inhibitory activities on antigen-driven T cell functions. In contrast, there is no report that such MAbs can have T cell activating properties.

The inhibitory activity of anti-Lyt-2,3 antibodies on CTL activity appears to be related to inhibition of antigen recognition, and not to interference with the cytolytic process per se. In addition, studies in our laboratory showed that a number of antigen-dependent, although mechanistically distinct, functions of CTL clones, including specific target cell lysis, lymphokine production and cellular proliferation, were inhibited in parallel by

anti-Lyt-2,3 MAbs[25] . In contrast, IL-2 induced
proliferation or mitogen-induced lymphokine production by
these clones were not inhibited by anti-Lyt-2,3 MAbs.
Collectively, these results suggest that anti-Lyt-2,3 MAbs
are inhibiting a common event, presumably antigen
recognition, which is required for the initiation of all
the various functions exhibited by CTL clones. Moreover,
additional experiments have showed that such antibodies are
able to inhibit the antigen-dependent activation of normal
Lyt-2,3$^+$ CTL precursors (CTL-P) in limiting dilution
microcultures[26]. Since addition of interleukin 2 (IL-2) in
excess could not overcome the inhibition, it was suggested
that anti-Lyt-2,3 antibodies interfered with antigen
recognition by CTL-P, thus preventing the expression of
surface receptors for IL-2 and, hence, responsiveness to
IL-2. Recently, this hypothesis has been directly tested in
our laboratory by using a CTL clone, Bl.8, whose growth was
strictly dependent on periodic exposure to antigen and
IL-2. While the cloned cells grown for 3 days in the
presence of antigen and IL-2 expressed an average of 7000
IL-2 receptors per cell, this number was drastically
reduced after 7 days, so that Bl.8 cells responded very
poorly to IL-2 alone. Expression of IL-2 receptors (and
IL-2 responsiveness) was rapidly induced by re-exposure to
antigen. However, the induction of IL-2 responsiveness was
totally inhibited by anti-Lyt-2 MAb when the antibodies
were added before or at the time of antigen addition[27].
Susceptibility to such inhibition declined rapidly after
antigen addition, and completely disappeared within 3
hours. It is of interest that a similar pattern of
responsiveness (or lack thereof) to IL-2 was observed when
Bl.8 cells were re-exposed to antigen (i.e. K alloantigen)
in the presence of anti-K MAb. These results thus confirm,
at the clonal level, that anti-Lyt-2 MAb can inhibit the
antigen-induced acquisition of IL-2 responsiveness by
resting T cells, and that a few hours exposure to antigen
is sufficient to induce such responsiveness[28].

III. HETEROGENEITY OF INHIBITION OF CTL FUNCTIONS BY
      ANTI-LYT-2,3 MAbs

     Early studies of inhibition of CTL activity by
anti-Lyt-2,3 MAbs at the population level revealed a
striking degree of heterogeneity which correlated with in
vivo priming[6,29] . Analysis of the cellular basis for this

heterogeneity at the clonal level indicated that CTL clones derived from a single source of lymphoid cells were heterogeneous in terms of their susceptibility to inhibition of cytolytic activity by anti-Lyt-2,3 MAbs, and that the degree of inhibition in individual clones were distributed in a continous (rather than "all or none") fashion. An example of such a distribution is shown in Fig.1.

Further analysis of clonal heterogeneity in the degree of inhibition by anti-Lyt-2,3 MAbs showed that it was not related to the level of expression of the Lyt-2,3 molecules. In contrast, susceptibility (or resistance) of CTL clones to inhibition by anti-Lyt-2,3 MAbs was found to correlate with loss (or persistence) of cytolytic activity after treatment with low doses of trypsin (which selectively cleaved Lyt-2,3 antigenic determinants from the cell surface)[30]. It is noteworthy that inhibition of cytolytic activity by MAbs directed against another cell surface structure expressed by CTL, i.e. LFA-1, does not display clonal heterogeneity, thus arguing in favor of a unique mechanism governing anti-Lyt-2,3 inhibition.

Subsequent studies showed that inhibition of antigen-dependent proliferation or lymphokine production by anti-Lyt-2,3 MAbs was also heterogeneous at the clonal level and correlated directly with inhibition of specific cytolytic activity[25]. Based on these findings, it has been proposed that the observed heterogeneity among CTL clones in the degree of inhibition of antigen-dependent functions by anti-Lyt-2,3 molecules could reflect heterogeneity in the functional requirement for Lyt-2,3 molecules in antigen recognition and, consequently, could be related to variations in the number and/or affinity of CTL antigen receptors rather than variations in the structure or function of Lyt-2,3 molecules per se[6]. According to this model, the role of Lyt-2,3 molecules is to facilitate and/or stabilize the interaction between the CTL antigen receptors and the corresponding determinants on antiben-bearing cells. Such an effect is only required by CTL that possess few and/or low affinity receptors.

Although the available data do not allow definitive conclusions as to the validity of this model, there is a set of observations which are compatible with this hypothesis. For example, experiments on CTL clones which

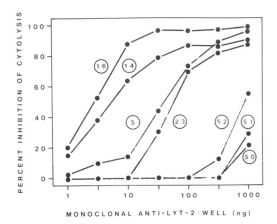

MONOCLONAL ANTI-LYT-2/WELL (ng)

Figure 1.   Susceptibility   of   individual   CTL   clones   to
inhibition of cytolytic activity by anti-Lyt-2 monoclonal
antibodies.   A total   of   23 clones   derived from   a single
alloimmune   (C57BL/6   anti-P815)   peritoneal   exudate
lymphocyte population were assayed for cytolytic activity
against P815 target cells at a 2:1 effector:target cell
ratio in the presence of increasing amounts of anti-Lyt-2
monoclonal antibodies.   For simplicity, data from only 7
representative   clones   are   shown.   For   purposes   of
comparison, these data are expressed as percent inhibition
relative to control lysis in the absence of antibody (40 to
80% according to the clone tested).

had been primed in vivo against Moloney leukemia virus-
associated   antigens   and   exhibited   cross-reactivity   with
uninfected allogeneic target cells revealed a differential
effect of anti-Lyt-2 MAb and trypsin treatment on the
cytolytic activity of these clones according to the target
cells used.   Lysis of target cells bearing the original
antigen was resistant to such treatment, whereas that of
target cells bearing the cross-reactive alloantigen was
susceptible[30].   Also consistent with the model mentioned
above is the finding that CTL clones which do not require
Lyt-2,3 molecules (i.e. are not inhibited by anti-Lyt-2,3
MAbs) are able to react to "suboptimal" antigenic stimuli,
whereas CTL clones susceptible to inhibition do not.   For

example, we found recently that, although CTL clones that widely differed in their requirement for Lyt-2,3 molecules for their function produced comparable amount of macrophage activating factor upon stimulation with living cells bearing the appropriate antigen, only those which were Lyt-2,3-independent were capable of producing this lymphokine upon stimulation with the same target cells fixed with gluteraldehyde.

In addition to qualitative changes, quantitative changes in antigenic determinants on the target cells appear to influence the dependence or independence of individual CTL clones on Lyt-2,3 molecules for their cytolytic activity. For example, we observed recently that H-2K^d specific CTL clones which were relatively resistant to anti-Lyt-2 inhibition were highly susceptible to inhibition by the same antibodies when their activity was assayed on target cells coated with anti-K^d MAb (at a concentration which was hardly inhibitory by itself). Lyt-2,3 independence was not affected by using target cells coated with anti-D^d MAb (Fig. 2), thus indicating that nonspecific effects of MAbs were not involved in the observed change of Lyt-2,3 requirement.

An alternative means of testing the role of antigen density in the requirement for Lyt-2,3 molecules would be to use target cells in which the number of antigenic molecules expressed on the cell surface can be selectively altered without significant modification in the expression of other surface structures. Recent work from our laboratory indicates that such an approach is feasible. During the course of a study on the expression of various surface markers on murine leukemia or lymphoma lines, it was found that the BALB/c thymoma SP-4.5 had a very low basal expression of H-2K^d antigens (as well as undetectable levels of D^d and L^d antigens). After two days of culture in the presence of interferon gamma, however, the level of K^d expression by ST-4.5 cells increased approximately six-fold (D^d expression also increased, whereas L^d remained undetectable). Untreated and interferon-treated ST-4.5 cells were used as target cells to measure the cytolytic activities of two H-2K^d specific CTL clones, 3 and 4, which widely differed in their requirement for Lyt-2,3 molecules (as assessed by inhibition of cytolysis of the standard, high H-2K^d positive P815 target cells). As shown in Table 2, both clones lysed the interferon-treated ST-4.5 cells

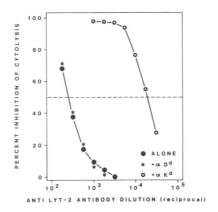

<u>Figure 2.</u> Differential susceptibility of a single clone to
inhibition of cytolytic activity by anti-Lyt-2 monoclonal
antibodies according to the amount of antigen available on
the target cell. A H-2K^d specific CTL clone which was
relatively resistant to anti-Lyt-2 inhibition was assayed
for cytolytic activity against P815 target cells at a 2:1
effector:target cell ratio in the presence of various
dilutions of anti-Lyt-2 monoclonal antibodies. The target
cells were either untreated (•——•), or treated with
anti-H-2D^d (✼——✼) or anti-H-2K^d (o——o) monoclonal
antibodies (at a dilution which was not inhibitory by
itself). For purposes of comparison, the data are expressed
as percent inhibition relative to control lysis in the
absence of antibody (62%).

(as well as P815 cells) with the same efficiency. In
contrast, untreated ST-4.5 cells were only lysed by clone
4. Moreover, while the lytic activity of this clone on P815
and interferon-treated ST-4.5 cells was relatively
resistant to inhibition by anti-Lyt-2 MAb, it was highly
susceptible when tested on untreated ST-4.5 cells. It thus
appears that the ability of CTL clones to lyse target cells
expressing low levels of antigen can vary according to
their Lyt-2,3 dependence. Moreover, the requirement for
Lyt-2,3 molecules in the activity of single CTL clones may
greatly vary according to the density of the corresponding
antigen on the target cells.

TABLE II

Effect of Antigen Density on the Requirement for
Lyt-2,3 Molecules in CTL Activity[a]

K^d-specific CTL clone	Lytic activity (susceptibility to inhibition)[b]		
	P815	ST-4	ST-4/IFN
≠ 3	1:1 (1:12'800)	100:1 (N.D.)	2:1 (1:6'400)
≠ 4	1:1 (1:200)	2:1 (1:12'800)	2:1 (1:800)

[a]The indicated anti-H-2K[d] CTL clones were assayed for cytolytic activity against P815, untreated ST-4 and interferon-gamma treated ST-4 target cells at various effector:target cell ratios in the presence or absence of various dilutions of anti-Lyt-2 monoclonal antibodies.
[b]Effector:target cell ratio required for 50% lysis of target cells as assessed in a 3 hour ^{51}Cr release assay (dilution of anti-Lyt-2 antibodies required for 50% inhibition of cytolytic activity).

IV.   CONCLUDING REMARKS

Based on the experimental observations summarized in the preceding sections, it can be tentatively concluded that the Lyt-2,3 molecular complex expressed on a distinct subset of T lymphocytes may be involved in antigen recognition by these cells both at the induction and effector phases. It has been proposed that the function of Lyt-2,3 molecules is to facilitate and/or stabilize the interaction between T-cell antigen receptors and the corresponding determinants on antigen-bearing cells[6,13,14]. Two models, which are not mutually exclusive, could account for this function. First, Lyt-2,3 molecules may be involved in an antigen-nonspecific "adhesive strenghtening" process which accompanies antigen-specific recognition. This process may include a functional association between Lyt-2,3 molecules and antigen receptors and/or other CTL membrane constituents required for the formation of stable cell-cell interactions. In this context, it is noteworthy that electron microscopic examination of conjugates between CTL and target cells showed the existence of restricted contact zones between the cells, with extensive interdigitation of the plasma membranes and accumulation of actin in the CTL (but not the target cell) contact

area[31-33]. While the mechanism of formation of stable
intercellular contacts is unknown, it may depend on an
uneven distribution of several membrane structures,
including Lyt-2,3 molecules.

In a second model, the Lyt-2,3 molecular complex may
serve as an "associative recognition" unit by interacting
with surface structures on the target cells. Since most T
lymphocytes bearing the Lyt-2,3 marker recognize antigen in
association with class I MHC antigens, it has been proposed
that Lyt-2,3 molecules interact with nonpolymorphic
determinants of class I MHC on antigen-bearing cells[14]. As
a corollary, the L3T4 surface structure expressed on the
subset of T lymphocytes which are primarily reactive with
(or restricted by) class II MHC molecules has been
postulated to interact with nonpolymorphic determinants of
these molecules on antigen-bearing cells[12]. Given the
similarities between Lyt-2,3 and T8 molecules, on the one
hand, and L3T4 and T4 molecules, on the other, it is
evident that such an hypothesis would apply to human T-cell
surface structures as well[13,15].

Whatever the actual mechanism might be, there is
suggestive evidence that the degree of Lyt-2,3 involvement
in antigen recognition by a given CTL (or its precursor)
may be inversely proportional to the affinity of its
antigen receptors. In addition, the continuous distribution
observed in terms of Lyt-2,3 dependence of individual
clones is consistent with the concept of a wide range of
receptor affinities. Furthermore, the correlation between
Lyt-2,3 independence and in vivo priming suggests a
mechanism of selection in vivo for CTL precursors of high
affinity. Finally, the possibility should be considered
that the Lyt-2,3 molecular complex plays a role even in CTL
with high affinity receptors when the amount of antigen on
target cells becomes limiting. Since antibody inhibition
experiments suggest that other molecules may also be
involved in the early phase of T lymphocyte interaction
with antigen-bearing cells, it thus appears that several
non antigen-specific cell surface structures on T
lymphocytes may play an important functional role in
antigen recognition.

REFERENCES

1. Nakayama, E., Shiku, H., Stockert, E., Oettgen, H.F. & Old, L.J. Proc. natl. Acad. Sci. U.S.A. 76, 1977-1981 (1979).
2. Shinohara, N. & Sachs, D.H. J. exp. Med. 150, 432-444 (1979).
3. Golstein, P. et al. Immunological Rev. 68, 5-42 (1982).
4. Hollander, N. Immunological Rev. 68, 43-66 (1982).
5. Larsson, E.L., Gullberg, M., Beretta, A. & Coutinho, A. Immunological Rev. 68, 67-88 (1982).
6. MacDonald, H.R., Glasebrook, A.L., Bron, C., Kelso, A. & Cerottini, J.-C. Immunological Rev. 68, 89-115 (1982).
7. Nakayama, E. Immunological Rev. 68, 117-134 (1982).
8. Sarmiento, M. et al. Immunological Rev. 68, 135-169 (1982).
9. Springer, T.A. et al. Immunological Rev. 68, 170-195 (1982).
10. Ledbetter, J.A. & Seaman, W.E. Immunological Rev. 68, 197-218 (1982).
11. Martz, E., Heagy, W. & Gromkowski, S.H. Immunological Rev. 72, 73-96 (1983).
12. Dialynas, D.P. et al. Immunological Rev. 74, 29-56 (1983).
13. Reinherz, E.L., Meuer, S.C. & Schlossman, S.F. Immunological Rev. 74, 83-112 (1983).
14. Swain, S.L. Immunological Rev. 74, 129-142 (1983).
15. Biddison, W.E., Rao, P.E., Talle, M.A., Goldstein, G. & Shaw, S. J. exp. Med. 159, 783-797 (1984).
16. Meuer, S.C. et al. Proc. natl. Acad. Sci. U.S.A. 81, 1509-1513 (1984).
17. Swain, S.L., Dialynas, D.P., Fitch, F.W. & English, M. J. Immunol. 132, 1118-1123 (1984).
18. Moretta, A., Pantaleo, G., Mingari, M.C., Moretta, L. & Cerottini, J.-C. J. exp. Med. 159, 921-934 (1984).
19. Meuer, S.C. et al. Cell. 36, 397-406 (1984).
20. Greenstein, J.L., Kappler, J., Marrack, P., & Burakoff, S.J. J. exp. Med. 159, 1213-1224 (1984).
21. Platsoucas, C.D. Eur. J. Immunol. 14, 566-577 (1984).
22. Gunter, K.C., Malek, T.R. & Shevach, E.M. J. exp. Med. 159, 716-730 (1984).
23. Luescher, B., Naim, H.Y., MacDonald, H.R. & Bron, C. Molecular Immunology 21, 329-336 (1984).

24. Naim, H.Y., Luescher, B., Corradin, G. & Bron, C. Molecular Immunology 21, 337-341 (1984).
25. Glasebrook, A.L., Kelso, A. & MacDonald, H.R. J. Immunol. 130, 1545-1551 (1983).
26. Glasebrook, A.L. & MacDonald, H.R. J. Immunol. 130, 1552-1555 (1983).
27. Lowenthal, J.W., Tougne, C., MacDonald, H.R., Smith, K.A. & Nabholz, M. Submitted for publication.
28. Gullberg, M. & Larsson, E.-L. Eur. J. Immunol. 12, 1006-1011 (1982).
29. MacDonald, H.R., Thiernesse, N. & Cerottini, J.-C. J. Immunol. 126, 1671-1675 (1981).
30. MacDonald, H.R., Glasebrook, A.L. & Cerottini, J.-C. J. exp. Med. 1156, 1711-1722 (1982).
31. Kalina, M. & Berke, G. Cell. Immunol. 25, 41-51 (1976).
32. Ryser, J.-E., Sordat, B., Cerottini, J.-C. & Brunner, K.T. Eur. J. Immunol. 7, 110-117 (1977).
33. Ryser, J.-E., Rungger-Brandle, E., Chaponnier, C., Gabbiani, G. & Vassalli, P. J. Immunol. 128, 1159-1162 (1982).

T CELL ACTIVATION ANTIGENS : KINETICS, TISSUE

DISTRIBUTION, MOLECULAR WEIGHTS, AND FUNCTIONS ;

INDUCTION ON NON T CELL LINES BY LYMPHOKINES

D. OLIVE[1], P. DUBREUIL[1], D. CHARMOT[1],
C. MAWAS[1] and P. MANNONI[2]
1. Centre d'Immunologie INSERM-CNRS de
Marseille- Luminy, Case 906, 13288 Marseille
Cedex 9 - France.
2. University of Alberta, Edmonton, Canada.

Among the first activation antigens defined on human T cells, some were thought to be T cell specific like the Il-2 receptor (1, 2) or the T200 family (2) while others were not T specific like the transferrin receptor (3) or class II antigens (4). Operationally such antigens were classified as early or late onset activation antigens (5). Depending upon their kinetics, one could further discriminate those in plateau from those back to background expression at day 7 (5).

Many mAbs defining such antigens but not all were found to be interfering with in vitro T cell functions. MAbs raises against T cell clones or lectin activated T cells have allowed to define a new set of activation antigens, the kinetics of which are very early with peaks around 12 hours. At the moment most of these antigens are not T cell specific, except for a few of them. Their functions are still unknown, although some preliminary biochemical data will be presented.

Finally we shall report that many of the T cell activation antigens (or T cell markers in general) absent from myeloid cell lines can be induced through cytokines, the most surprising being the induction of the Il-2 receptor on such cell lines. We shall review some of our recent data in this report.

MATERIALS AND METHODS

— MAbs used in this study were derived, for the essential, by one fusion where rats were immunized by lectin activated T cell lines and fused with the myeloma X63AG8.653. MAbs made following the immunization of mice by T cell clones were also used (2).

— Screening was initially done using the immunizing cells and EBV B cell lines followed by a tissue distribution analysis using a variety of cell lines.

— Functional studies included MLR, Il-2-dependent growth of T cell lines, anti-class I and class II CTL clones as well as NK lysis using K562 as a target.

Cytofluorographic studies were performed using an Epics V cell sorter (Coultronics, Hialeah, Florida), with indirect labelling using Cappel's F(ab')2 FITC mixture of anti-murine and rat Igs.

— Biochemical studies were performed as previously described (2).

— Induction using cloned γ interferon (kindly provided by E. Falcoff through M. Fellous) was performed and the induced cells assayed on day 3 for phenotypic studies and biochemical studies performed on day 4 following the induction.

RESULTS AND DISCUSSION

Kinetics of expression of T cell activation antigens and tissue distribution

Most activation antigens described on T cells following mitogen or antigenic stimulation fell in three categories :

I, early peak (before day 1) ; II, peak on day 3-4 ; III, plateau from day 4 to 7 : some of those included here are staining a small percent of resting T cells. Examples from each category are given, in Table 1, together with the appropriate controls. Ficoll-Hypaque peripheral blood lymphoblasts (PBLs) stimulated by phytohemagglutinin (PHA) were tested from day 0 to day 7.

Among the T.Ac. group 1, or early activation antigens, all are absent from resting T cells, but one is clearly present on resting B cells. They are all negative on thymocytes but positive on some T cell lines, some myeloid cell lines or acute myeloid leukemias (AML).

Among the T.Ac group 2, the Il-2 receptor is not detectable on resting T, B and thymus cells and among the

Table 1 : Activation antigens, Kinetics,

	Day 0	Day 1	Day 4	Day 7	MW
T.Ac I					
13G10.1	9	16	10	6	–
36F1.23	8	14	5	5	60K
15H10.1	8	13	5	4	–
12A1.9	6	18	4	5	100K
T.Ac II					
TAC	16	61	84	22	55K
B1.49.9	12	52	78	29	"
11H2.1	3	18	74	17	"
27E4.6	3	18	72	22	"
36A1.2	3	22	68	17	"
18E6.11	4	27	73	22	"
22D6.11	6	44	73	18	"
33B3.1	3	23	68	18	"
33B7.3	6	26	76	8	"
39C6.5	8	27	68	36	"
T.AcIII					
B1.19.2	7	6	21	40	220K
39C818	24	56.5	87	89	20K
39H73	19	53	88.5	93	50K
39B2.1	26	70	92.5	94	70K
Controls					
irrelevant mAb	7	6	7	5	
35A1.6 (class I)	75	88	97.5	99	
Leu 4 (CD3)	54	21	56	79	
9.6 (CD2)	62	66	92	98	
BL4 (CD4)	52	20	60	89	
B9.8 (CD8)	24	27	32	31	
BK19 (Transfer. Rec.)	8	33	60	35	
B3.15 (class II)	26	26.5	41	36	

myeloid or monocytic cell lines ; some of the 10
different anti-Il-2 mAbs tested do react weakly either
with MOLT4, HPB-ALL or ICHIGAWA. On EBV transformed B
cell lines, weak reactions were also seen on some but not
all the cell lines tested (data not shown).

The T.Ac group 3 is peculiar : except for Bl.19.2
antigenic determinant most mAb defined antigens are found
on a proportion of resting T cells and are strongly
expressed on thymocytes. Their membrane expression
increases dramatically as soon as 24 hours following
culture and a stable plateau is reached by day 4 and
remains stable until day 7. These determinants are
strongly positive on HPB-ALL, RPMI 8402 and ICHIGAWA and
not infrequently on AML cells. Although some of their
features do not correspond stricto sensu to activation
antigens, we included them in this review since their
membrane expression changed drastically with culture
and/or stimulation.

Preliminary biochemical characterization and functions

Table 3 summarizes some of the molecular weights
observed for these surface antigens.

Table 4 summarizes some of the functional
interferences observed in the in vitro assays tested
using such mAbs. Group 1 mAbs have no detectable effect
on the in vitro assays used.

Group 2 mAbs have profound effects on some of the
assays ; however among a panel of mAbs recognizing the
Il-2 receptor molecule, the functional effects are
heterogenous.

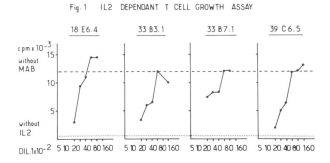

Fig. 1   IL2 DEPENDANT T CELL GROWTH ASSAY

As shown in Fig. 1, the ability to inhibit the Il-2

Table 2 : Tissue distribution of T activation antigens

	T	B	RPMI 8402	CEM	Molt4	1301	HPBALL	ICHI. ⊖	HL60	KG1	AML	U937	Mono	PMN
TAC I														
13G10.1	7[1]	55	4	9	7	21	80	11	2.5	7	19	33	7	30	6
36F1.2	6	12	6	6	9	5	62	12	3	6	5	35	5	20	3
15H10.1	8	12	4	5	9	6	26	8	3	6	1.5	28	5	20	4
12A1.9	5	15	NT	NT	NT	NT	NT	NT	NT	4	3	8	5	20	3
TAC II														
18E6.11	3	9	4	5	30	7	35	12	4	4	13	2	5	3	6
22D6.11	3	12	8	5	6	6	21	32	4	3	10	1.5	4	2	5
TAC III														
39C8.18	24	10	40	4	11	8	48	54	80	6	3	34	7	14	3
39H7.3	19	12	42	6	14	6	64	60	57	6	3	27	18	16	4
39B2.1	26	10	41	4	11	11	55	61	81	4	4	8	5	12	4
Controls														
Leu 4 (CD3)	78	8	83	23	53	6	93	0	40	4	5	25	4	10	4
BL4 (CD4)	53	11	5	92	52	97	94	51	66	20	NT	10	31	15	4
B9.8 (CD8)	32	5	4	6	28	6	96	15	67	4	NT	18	4	14	3
BK19 (Transf. Rec.)	9	5	99	97	98	86	89	64	12	86	99	82	NT	22	5
9.6 (CD2)	70	7	84	80	58	14	96	NT	81	6	7	8	6	12	4

[1] Results are expressed as percent of specifically stained cells.

Table 3 : M.W. of some the activation antigens

T.Ac 1	15H10.1	60K
	12A1.9	100K
T.Ac 2	Il-2 receptor	55K (PHA blasts)
T.Ac 3	31C8.18	20K
	39B2.1	70K
	39H7.3	50K

Table 4 : Summary of the functional interferences observed in in vitro assays with these m.Abs

MAbs defining :	Il-2 growth	MLR	CML I (CTL clone)	CML II (CTL) clone)	NK (population)
T.Ac group 1	$-^1$	$-^1$	$-^2$	$-^2$	$-^2$
T.Ac group 2	$++^1$	$++$	$-$	$-$	$+^3$
T.Ac group 3	$+$	$++$	$++$	$++$	$++$

[1]. The mAbs were present in these assays from the start to the end of the culture period.

[2]. The mAbs were present in the CML assay itself only.

[3]. Clear inhibition seen with one mAb out of 10 tested (18E6.4).

dependent growth of a human T cell line varies from
antibody to antibody ; mAb B1.49.9 has almost no
inhibitory activity despite the fact that cold inhibition
of radiolabelled B1.49.9* is observed with the four mAbs
used in this inhibition assay (Table 5). MAb 27E4.6 does
not compete with B1.49.9 and does not block Il-2
dependent T cell growth. All mAbs immunoprecipitated a
55 K band on reducing conditions from day 4 PHA blasts
solubilized membranes (Fig. 2).

Two anti-Il-2 receptor when added during the 4 hours
assay mAbs were reproducibly able to inhibit the NK lysis
of the target cell K562 by its effector cells (day 6
allogeneic primed responder cells) : mAbs 18E1.4 and
27E4.6. These mAbs were unable to inhibit the CML lysis
of two T cell clones respectively anti-class I and
anti-class II specific (data not shown).

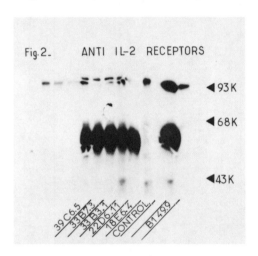

Fig. 2.   ANTI IL-2 RECEPTORS

Among the TAc group III, if B1.19.2 has no effect,
the other mAbs have pleiotropic functional effects in in
vitro assays. These mAbs affect mainly the primary MLR
and block anti-class I, anti-class II and NK cytolysis at
the effector level. Many features of their functional
effects resemble those found with the anti-CD2 mAbs (E
rosette receptors). However, such mAbs as 30H7.3 do not
stain 100% resting T cells but only a fraction varying
from 10 to 30% ; following T cell activation, they tend
to label the T cells as mAb 9.6, the reference anti-E

Table 5 : Cold inhibition by anti-Il-2 receptor mAbs of the reference
            radiolabelled mAb Bl.49.9

	Cold mAbs	Cross-binding on day 4 PHA blasts
	LFA-1 (25.3)	14500[1]
	Bl.49.9	6500
	33.B3.1	4500
Anti-Il-2	33B7.1	7400
	39C6.5	5620
Receptor	18E1.4	6635
	22D6.11	8200
	27E4.6	14900
	39C1.5 (E rosette)	17900

[1] Results are expressed as cpm - 2.5×10^5 cells per well and 3×10^5 cpm (labelled Bl.49.9) were applied per well.

Table 6 : "T" activation antigens induced on HL-60
following γ interferon treatment

		untreated HL-60	γIFN HL-60[1]
T.Ac I	13G10.1	9^2	25
	36F1.2	7	65
	15H10.1	8	52
	12A1.9	4	6
T.Ac II	TAC	10	80
	B149.9	8	97
I1-2	11H2.16	4	6
Receptor	27E4.6	2.5	6
	36A1.2	2.5	6
	18E6.11	2.5	5
	22D6.11	4	8.5
	33B3.1	3	31
	39C6.5	2.5	88
Transferrin receptor	BK19	44	21
T.Ac III	B1.19.2	59	97
	39C8.18	8.5	63
	39H7.3	9	70
	39B2.1	8	7
Controls	anti-HLA I (B9.12)	90	↗↗
	anti-HLA II (B3.15)	5	80

[1] HL-60 cells were treated for four days with 500 U/ml IFNγ.

[2] Results are expressed as % of positive cells, using a cytofluorograph analyser.

rosette receptor, and have similar tissue distribution.
By immunoprecipitation, a 50K band on reduced gel is
observed, parallel to the 50K band immunoprecipitated by
mAb 9.6 (data not shown).

The two other types of antigens recognized by mAb
39C8.18 (20K) and 39B2.1 (70K) are not respectively
indentical to CD3 (T3) or CD5 (T1).

Expression of the T Ac. antigens on a myeloid cell line, HL-60, following induction by recombinant γ interferon

Four days γ interferon (γIFN) treated HL-60 (6), a
myeloid leukemia line derived in 1977 from a
promyelocytic leukemia, was shown to express more HLA
class I at the membrane than the untreated cell line but
also to express class II antigens, undetectable on the
membrane of untreated HL-60 cells (P.M., unpublished
data). Since the expression of HLA class II is induced on
T cells following activation (antigenic or mitogenic), we
were interested to screen on HL-60 untreated and γIFN
treated the expression of the activation antigens
described in this report. Table 6 summarizes the data
obtained with the mAbs selected for this report. Among
T.Ac group 1, 3 out 4 are induced on HL-60. Among the
T.Ac group 2, results concerning the Il-2 receptor were
unexpected : 1) clearly, the Il-2 receptor is induced on
most HL-60 γIFN treated cells as shown by the clearcut
reactivity with the three following mAbs (out of 10
tested) : TAC, B1.49.9 and 39C6.5, the cytofluorographic
patterns (Fig. 3) and the immunoprecipiation data (Fig.
4). 2) Many Il-2 receptor specific mAbs are not able to
bind to the HL-60 induced Il-2 receptor, thus
demonstrating serological heterogeneity among the mAbs as
well as heterogeneity between the Il-2 receptors detected
on PHA blasts versus HL-60 γIFN induced.

The significance of the induction of the Il-2
receptor on a myeloid cell line following γIFN treatment
remains unknown, and a physiological role must await
confirmation using normal bone marrow stem cells. In
parallel, the transferrin receptor which is
constitutively expressed on HL-60 cells sees its
expression decrease following γIFN treatment. Finally,
among the T.Ac group III, B1.19.2 is expressed on the
untreated HL-60 cells but both 39C8.18 and 39H7.3 but not
39B2.1 are induced following γIFN.

That most T.Ac antigens can be induced on HL-60, a
myeloid cell line came as a surprise, but all T cell
markers (CD1 to CD8) are inducible as will be reported
elsewhere. We anticipate therefore that the relationships
between γIFN and pluripotential haematopoietic stem cells
in T cell differentiation could be very close.

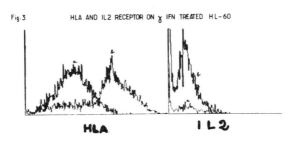

Fig:3   HLA AND IL2 RECEPTOR ON γ IFN TREATED HL-60

HLA   IL2

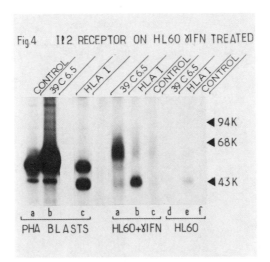

Fig4   I L2 RECEPTOR ON HL60 γIFN TREATED

◀94K
◀68K
◀43K

a   b   c   a   b c   d e f
PHA BLASTS   HL60+γIFN HL60

REFERENCES

1. Leonard, W.J., Depper, J.M., Uchiyama, T., Smith,
    K.A., Waldmann, T.A. and Greene, W.C. Nature 300,
    267-269 (1982).
2. Hemler, M.E., Malissen, B., Rebai, N., Liabeuf, A.,
    Mawas, C., Kourilsky, F.M. and Strominger, J.L.
    Human Immunol. 8, 153-159 (1983).

3. Haynes, B.F., Hemler, M., Cotner, T., Mann, D.L.,
    Eisenbarth, G.S., Strominger, J.L. and Fauci, A.S.
    J. Immunol. 127, 347-352 (1981).
4. Ko, H., Fu, S.M., Winchester, R.J., Yu, D.T., and
    Kunkel, H.G. J. Exp. Med. 150, 246-252 (1979).
5. Cotner, T., Williams, J.M., Christenson, L.,
    Shapiro, H.M., Strom, T.B. and Strominger, J.L. J.
    Exp. Med. 157, 461-472 (1983).
6. Collins, S.J., Gallo, R.J. and Gallagher, R.E.
    Nature 270, 347-349 (1967).

THE INDUCTION OF ANTIGEN SPECIFIC UNRESPONSIVENESS

IN CLONED T LYMPHOCTYES

J.R. Lamb and E.D. Zanders

Imperial Cancer Research Fund
Tumour Immunology Unit, Department of Zoology
University College London
Gower Street, London WC1E 6BT.

INTRODUCTION

The recognition that T lymphocytes can be maintained in long term culture has allowed the isolation of mono-clonal populations of antigen specific T lymphocytes. Such reagents have facilitated the analysis of the T cell reper-toire, the genetic restriction of lymphoid cell inter-actions and receptor structure[1,2]. Additionally, T cell clones have been useful for the analysis of mechanisms regulating the activation[3] and induction of unresponsive-ness[4] in T cells. In the regulation of T cell unrespons-iveness, antigen is also of importance since administered in vivo in either supraoptimal or repeated suboptimal concentrations antigen induces specific unresponsiveness termed immunological tolerance[5,6]. In contrast to B cell tolerance[7,8] the in vitro investigation of the cellular mechanism of T cell tolerance generally has been lacking. Recently, however, we have isolated T lymphocyte clones reactive with a defined peptide (p20) located at the carboxyl terminus (306-329) of the HA-1 molecule of influenza haemagglutinin (HA)[9] that can be rendered unresponsive by supraimmunogenic concentrations of that peptide in the absence of other lymphoid cells[4]. The present report reviews the antigen specificity, requirement for MHC recognition, phenotypic and biochemical changes occurring during antigen induced T cell unresponsiveness.

MATERIALS AND METHODS

The isolation and characterisation of HA peptide specific T cell clones (TLC) have been described in detail elsewhere[9], as have the methods for the in vitro induction of T cell unresponsiveness[4].

RESULTS AND DISCUSSION

Antigen Induced Unresponsiveness

Cloned T cells[9] were preincubated for 16 hrs with differing concentrations of p20 (0.3-100µg/ml) in the absence of any other lymphoid cells, and then stimulated with irradiated autologous E⁻ cells (as a source of antigen presenting cells, APC) pulsed with an immunogenic concentration of p20[4]. The cloned T cells incubated with p20 at concentrations > 10 µg/ml failed to proliferate in response to the immunogenic challenge (Fig. 1). However, the IL-2 responsivenss of the TLC cells remained intact after the pretreatment, confirming that antigen specific unresponsiveness was not the result of toxicity. These results demonstrate that T cells can be inactivated by direct exposure to antigen, implying that in certain circumstances T cell tolerance may occur independently of suppressor T cells[10]. In addition, the induction of unresponsiveness was more efficient in the absence of presenting cells[4].

Antigen Specificity of T Cell Inactivation

A fundamental requirement of T cell tolerance is that it is induced by antigen and specific for that antigen, therefore it was important to determine the antigen specificity of peptide induced T cell unresponsiveness[11]. TLC cells reactive with p11[12] (residues 105-140; Tp11) or p20 (Tp20) were preincubated alone or together with supraimmunogenic concentrations of p11 and/or p20, the challenged with an immunogenic dose of p11, p20 or p11 and p20 together in the presence of APCs[4]. The clones, as individual populations or a cell mixture, were inactivated by only the relevant peptide (Table 1).

Figure 1

Antigen dose dependency of the induction of T cell unresponsiveness. After antigen pretreatment response to IL-2 (□) or to p20 in the presence of antigen presenting cells (■).

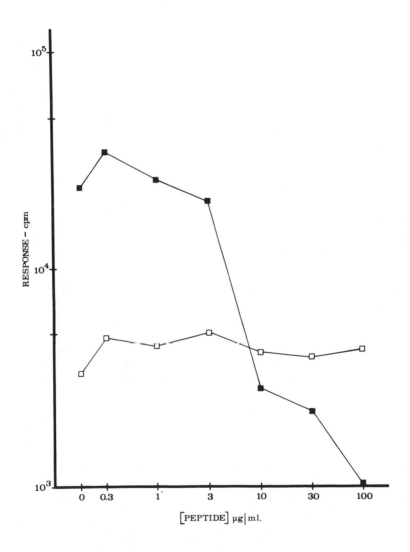

Table 1
Antigen Specificity of T Cell Inactivation

Ind^n of Unresponsiveness		Response			
Cloned T cells	Antigen	p11	p20	p11 + p20	IL-2
Tp11	0	+	−	+	+
+	p11	−	−	−	+
+	p20	+	−	+	+
Tp20	0	−	+	+	+
+	p11	−	+	+	+
+	p20	−	−	−	+
Tp11 + Tp20	0	+	+	+	+
+	p11	−	+	+	+
+	p20	+	−	+	+
+	p11 + p20	−	−	−	+

Thus the induction of unresponsiveness is antigen specific and is not mediated by the presence of diffusible non specific inhibitors from the T cells themselves following exposure to antigen.

The Requirement for MHC Recognition in the Induction of T Cell Unresponsiveness

The activation of regulatory T cells involves the recognition of extrinsic antigen in association with Class II MHC gene products expressed on the presenting cell population[13,14]. Since, human TLC express MHC Class II antigens[15] it was possible that in the induction of tolerance that antigen was recognized in association with T cell Class II determinants. To test this hypothesis, T cells were pretreated with anti-Class II antibodies before exposure to antigen[16]. It was observed that antibodies to monomorphic Class II antigens, in contrast to anti-Class I antibodies inhibited the induction of T cell tolerance (Table 2). The pattern of blockade of T cell activation was identical mapping to the DQ determinants[16,17].

Recent studies on T cell tolerance in vivo also demonstrate that the induction is MHC restricted[18]. Both of these observations that T cell tolerance is MHC restricted

Table 2
Requirements For MHC Recognition in T Cell Activation and
the Induction of Unresponsiveness

| | Inhibition of | |
Antibody Specificity	Activation	Unresponsiveness
MHC Class I		
(i) anti-HLA,A,B,C	−	−
(ii) anti-β_2M	−	−
MHC Class II		
(i) anti-Ia	++	++
(ii) anti-DQ	++	++
(iii) anti-DR	+/−	+/−

argue against the hypothesis of Cohn and Epstein[19] which
suggests that T cell tolerance involves the recognition of
antigen alone, whereas the recognition of antigen is
associated with MHC results in activation.

Phenotypic Modulation of Helper T Cells After Exposure
To Supraimmunogenic Doses of Antigen

Recent experiments have revealed that antibody
reactive with idiotypic determinants on human T cell clones
will comodulate the receptor (Ti)/T3 complex from the cell
surface[20]. It was proposed that the interaction of ligand
(p20) with receptor in the induction of unresponsiveness
may mimic this phenomenon. Indeed a supraimmunogenic
concentration of p20 induces the loss of the Ti/T3 receptor
complex from the cell surface that is accompanied by
functional unresponsiveness[21]. Additionally, the T1
antigen was weakly down regulated (Table 3). Both MHC
Class II and T4 determinants were unaffected by antigen
treatment. As regards the up regulation of surface
phenotype, the IL-2 receptor expression increased in
parallel with the decrease in T3, both dependent on antigen
concentration. A marginal increase in the sheep E rosette
receptor was also sometimes observed. Thus, it appears
that a tolerizing concentration of antigen induces a down

Table 3

Effect of Supraimmunogenic Concentrations of Peptide
On Surface Phenotype of Cloned Helper T Cells

Helper T Cell Surface Phenotype Expression

Decreased	No Change	Increased
T3	MHC Class II	IL-2 receptor
TR constant	T4	E rosette receptor
region[a]	Transferrin receptor	
T1	heat shock antigen	
	common leucocyte	
	MHC Class I	

[a] Ti/T3 complex as recognized by WT31, an anti-receptor
          constant region antibody[22].
   [b] Marginal increase sometimes observed.

regulation of the Ti/T3 complex in association with an
increase of the IL-2 receptor. This phenotypic modulation
provides an explanation for the loss of antigen specific
but not IL-2 responsiveness after antigen treatment. The E
rosette receptor has been associated with non specific T
cell activation[23] and this possibly may be reciprocally
linked to the Ti/T3 receptor in a similar way to the IL-2
receptor. Since complex phenotypic changes occur after
exposure to antigen it suggests that the mechanism of
unresponsiveness is not simply receptor blockade.

Biochemical Events During the Induction of Unresponsiveness

     Biochemical analysis of the cellular metabolism after
incubation with supraimmunogenic concentrations of p20
induced mRNA synthesis although the overall protein
synthesis remained unaltered (Table 4). Following surface
iodination or biosynthetic labelling changes in certain
proteins were observed, however, from analysis of their
behaviour on reduced and non reduced gels none of these
proteins corresponded to the Ti/T3 complex (Zanders, E.D.,
Feldmann, M. and Lamb, J.R., manuscript submitted). The
enhancement of a biosynthetically labelled protein of 60 Kd

Table 4
Biochemical Events in the Induction of T Cell
Unresponsiveness

Metabolic and Biochemical Changes			
Changes in Protein Expressed (kd)			
Surface labelling (^{125}I)		Biosynthetic (^{35}S)	
Enhanced	Diminished	Enhanced	Diminished
50		24	42
83		29	92
87		44	
		47	
		60	
		70	
		135	

Macromolecular synthesis: DNA and protein, no change;
RNA increased.

may correspond to the Il-2 receptor, which by FACS analysis
is observed to increase in expression after tolerance
induction. However, as yet these problems remain to be
identified and one can only speculate as to their nature
and fornetin such as cytoskeletal or stress antigens.

CONCLUSIONS

The results reported here demonstrate that in the
absence of accessory cells or suppressor T cells, peptide
antigen alone at supraimmunogenic concentrations can render
T cells unresponsive to an immunogenic challenge, while the
IL-2 response remains intact. This unresponsiveness is
antigen specific and dependent upon the recognition of MHC
Class II determinants expressed on the T cells themselves.
Analysis of the surface phenotype of the T cells after
tolerance induction revealed complex changes. The Ti/T3
receptor complex was modulated from the cell surface as was
T1 to a lesser extent. Paralleling the decrease in T3,

there was an increased expression of the IL-2 receptor, and less markedly the E rosette receptor. This result suggests that the antigen specific receptor on T cells may be reciprocally linked to receptors that can mediate non specific T cell proliferation. Investigation of the biochemical events during the induction of T cell unresponsiveness revealed changes in the synthesis of certain proteins. However, none of these proteins could be identified as the Ti/T3 complex and as yet remain to be determined. The resolution of the cellular mechanisms in the induction of T cell unresponsiveness may depend upon molecular genetics and investigation of changes in the level of mRNA for the antigen specific receptor have begun using a cDNA clone that encodes for the β chain (Collins, M.K.L. and Owen, M.J.).

ACKNOWLEDGEMENTS

We thank Drs P. Beverley, M. Collins, M. Contreras, M. Feldmann, N. Green, R. Lerner and M. Owen for their invaluable contributions to this project. These studies were supported by the Imperial Cancer Research Fund, National Institutes of Health and Arthritis and Rheumatism Council.

REFERENCES

1. Fathman, C.G. and Fitch, F.W. (eds) Isolation, Characterisation and Utilization of T Lymphocyte Clones (Academic Press, Inc., New York, 1982).
2. Saito, H. et al. Nature **309**, 757-762 (1984).
3. Meuer, S.C. et al. Proc. Natl. Acad. Sci (USA) **81**, 1509-1513 (1984).
4. Lamb, J.R., Skidmore, B.J., Green, N., Chiller, J.M. and Feldmann, M. J. Exp. Med. **157**, 1434-1447 (1983).
5. Mitchison, N.A. Proc. R. Soc. Lond. B. Biol. Sci. **161**, 275-292 (1964).
6. Chiller, J.M. and Weigle, W.O. Contemp. Top. Immunobiol. **1**, 199-142 (1972).
7. Diener, E. and Feldmann, M. Transplant. Rev. **8**, 76-103 (1972).
8. Feldmann, M. J. Exp. Med. **135**, 735-753 (1972).
9. Lamb, J.R., Eckels, D.D., Lake, P., Woody, J.N. and Green, N. Nature **300**, 66-69 (1982).

10. Gershon, R.K. Contemp. Top. Immunobiol. **3,** 1-40.
11. Green, N. et al. Cell **28,** 477-487 (1982).
12. Howard, J.G. and Mitchison, N.A. Prog. Allergy **18,** 43-96. (1975).
13. Rosenthal, A.S. and Shevach, E.M. J. Exp. Med. **138,** 1194-1212 (1973).
14. Klein, J. and Nagy, Z.A. Adv. Cancer Res. **37,** - 233-317 (1982).
15. Lamb, J.R. et al. J. Immunol. **128,** 233-238 (1982).
16. Lamb, J.R. and Feldmann, M. Nature **308,** 72-74 (1984).
17. Eckels, D.D. et al. Immunogenetics **19,** 409-423 (1984).
18. Groves, E.S. and Singer, A. J. Exp. Med. **158,** 1483-1497 (1983).
19. Cohn, M. and Epstein, R. Cell. Immunol. **39,** 125-153 (1978).
20. Meuer, S.C. et al. J. Exp. Med. **157,** 705-719 (1983).
21. Zanders, E.D., Lamb, J.R., Feldmann, M., Green, N. and Beverley, P.C.L. Nature **303,** 625-627 (1983).
22. Tax, W.J.M., Willems, H.W., Reckers, P.P.M., Capel, P.J.A. and Koene, R.A.P. Nature. **304,** 445-448 (1983).
23. Meuer, S.C. et al. Cell **36,** 897-906 (1984).

SIGNALS IN B CELL ACTIVATION

A. Schimpl
University of Würzburg, FRG

R. B. Corley

Duke University, North Carolina, USA

The discussion in the workshop focussed on three topics a) requirements for excitation of resting B cells to an activated state, b) growth factors and c) the controversial issue of specific mitogen receptors for lipopolysaccharide (LPS) on B cells.

Addressing themselves to the requirement for excitation of B cells, Finnegan & Hodes and Corley et al. investigated the effect of helper T cells directly recognizing class II-MHC molecules either by virtue of being auto-CL II-reactive or by seeing alloantigens. Not surprisingly, auto-reactive T cells behave very much like alloreactive T cells. Thus, Finnegan & Hodes showed that such auto-Cl II-reactive cells can act as helper cells for polyclonal B cell activation or for antigen-specific responses in the presence of antigen bound to the B cells. In their experiments, only the IgG but not the IgM responses required direct MHC controlled T - B interaction. This view was challenged from the audience, from where experiments were reported indicating that both IgG and IgM responses required direct T - B interaction. This may well reflect a difference in the degree of "restingness" of precursors of IgM producing cells. The experiments reported by Corley et al. seemed to bear out this point. The authors have established a B cell line, CH12, specific for an antigen on sheep red blood cells, which although a lymphoma seems to behave like a resting B cell in its requirements for activation to IgM secretion.

CH12 could only be activated by helper T cells recognizing IE of class II but not by those specific for IA, even though both IE and IA are expressed by CH12 and both IE and IA-specific T cells can be activated by CH12. The latter experiment clearly seems to place the defect in responsiveness to IA restricted T cells to the B cell line CH12. This was further supported by experiments by LoCascio et al. who could activate CH12 by mcl antibodies to IE (in the presence of specific antigen, SRBC) but not to IA, even though both mcl antibodies did bind to CH12. As with all of the studies mentioned above, these data make it clear that T and B cells need not be "linked" by a hapten-carrier conjugate (although this may be the normal mechanism in vivo), but that independent occupation of surface immunoglobulin and Ia molecules can lead to successful B cell triggering.

These experiments raised several points: 1) Can individual B-cells under physiological conditions only be "helped" by either IA + X or IE + X - specific T cells? An exclusive role of IE in mediating help seem unlikely in view of the normal response in various strains not expressing IE. 2) Can antibodies to IA or IE induce normal B cells? While antibody mediated activation has clearly been shown by LoCascios using the B lymphom CH12, a general survey conducted during the workshop indicated that most investigators failed to so activate normal B cells using a panel of mcl antibodies. Indeed, the same monoclonal antibodies that stimulated CH12 were ineffective when tested on normal B cells from the CH12 donor strain. Since CH12 does not bear Fc-receptors the failure to activate the FcR$^+$ normal B cells might be due to FcR mediated inhibition a point easily to be clarified by using F(ab')$_2$ fragments of the various anti Cl II antibodies. Alternatively, CH 12 as a representative of the Ly 1$^+$ subset of B cells may be more easily activated than the much more frequent Ly 1$^-$ B cells.

A different way of stimulating B cells - possibly via anti-MHC molecules - was suggested by work of Seman et al. This group reported on a factor derived from Ag-activated T cell lines or clones which can stimulate Percoll fractionated resting B cells to proliferate. The factor is Ia restricted in action and does not act on LPS blasts. The authors suggest that the growth factor was an autoreactive molecule acting via recognition of Cl II structures on B cells activating a subset to proliferate. Ig secretion induced in so activated cells was reported to be poor and probably due to contamination of the restricted growth factors by B cell differentiation factors. Cl II-restricted T cell derived factors acting in B cell induction have of course been reported previously but have usually not stood up well to further scrutiny and one hopes that Seman et al. will finally sort out this issue.

Several papers presented settled another long disputed point, i. e. involvement of Ag receptors in B cells in actual triggering rather than just binding and thereby focussing T cell help. Finnegan's, Corley's and LoCacio's contributions clearly showed that occupation of the Ag-receptor lead to a synergism with Cl II mediated help by auto- or alloreactive T cells, especially when lower numbers of T cells were used. Taking these data together with those on activation of B cells by antibodies to the Ag receptor (see abstracts by Bijsterbosch & Klaus and Chen et al.) it seems that at very high signal densities either cross linking of the Ag receptor or engangement of Cl II by Cl II restricted T cells can alone activate B cells. At the physiologically "more relevant" lower signal densities, activation will, however, be optimal only if both these structures are involved.

Further evidence for a signalling function (in this case a negative one) of the surface immunoglobulin molecule came from Chen et al., who showed that cross-linking of Ig on the B cell membrane inhibited LPS-mediated differentiation of B cells. Inhibition was shown to be a direct result of reduction in mRNA for secretory μ chains. These data suggest that the relative degree of replication vs. differentiation of a B cell clone is regulated in part by the occupancy and cross-linking of the antigen receptor on B cells.

The absolute need for engagement of either Ag receptor or Cl II on B cells to obtain a response was apparently challenged by Leclercq et al. These authors presented data showing that "resting B cells" could be polyclonally activated to both proliferation and Ig secretion by super-natants derived from (Ag + MHC)-activated helper T cells. Contrary to Seman's factor, the onese reported here were not MHC restricted. Some more trivial explanations such as myco-plasma derived mitogens contained in the supernatants seemed to be ruled out. It was not quite clear what proportion of B cells responded but the data would indicate that at least some "resting" B cells already express receptors for growth factors.

There was little discussion in the workshop on the biochemical characterization of growth factors but a report by Erdei et al. implicated a well known molecule, i.e. C3, probably C3d. Sepharose-bound or crosslinked C3 was shown to be able to stimulate further DNA synthesis in LPS blasts while being inactive on resting B cells. Soluble C3 was inactive. The very important point to be answered is whether C3 activated within the complement cascade by antigen antibody complexes will behave like crosslinked or Sepharose bound C3.

The final discussion of the workshop focussed on the long debated LPS-receptors on B cells. Jacob's et al., using a sensitive hapten-sandwich immunofluorescence technique, showed that the vast majority of LPS binding cells were also μ^-, although some Thy 1^- or μ^- Thy 1^- - LPS binding cells were found. The number of LPS binding cells in the LPS non-responder strain C3H/HeJ was identical to that in the LPS responsive C3H/St. Jacobs et al. interpret their data as indicating that an LPS binding protein, mostly expressed on B cells, helps to dissociate LPS-micelles, thereby facilitating LPS interaction with the lipid bilayer of the cell membrane. This latter interaction would then eventually lead to signalling to the cell. The binding protein would still be present in LPS non-responder C3H/HeJ B cells, but signal transmission might be faulty. If so, experiments reported by Kleine et al. will have to be viewed in a different light. Kleine reported that the B lymphoma line WEHI279.1 is inhibited in its growth by the addition of LPS. Resistant variants were obtained and their ^{35}S labelled membrane proteins were compared in 2 D gels with those of the LPS sensitive wild type cells. It was hoped that consistently different protein pattern could be found and the putative LPS receptor be thus identified. So far differences which were found were, however, not consistent. In view of Jacobs' data this might be expected since LPS non-reactivity could either be due to the loss of expression of the LPS binding protein but also be brought about by an alteration of loss of some signal transmitting structure(s).

MOLECULAR EVENTS IN T LYMPHOCYTE ACTIVATION

J. Gordin Kaplan[*] and John E. Kay[+]

*Department of Biochemistry, University of
Alberta, Edmonton, Alberta, Canada.

+Biochemistry Laboratory & Centre for
Medical Research, University of Sussex,
Brighton, U.K.

The central question to which the research described
and discussed in this workshop was directed may be put as
follows: what is the train of biochemical events that
causally links the initial triggering of T-cells (and
B-cells, since some papers dealing with these were also
included in this session by the conference organizers) to
the DNA synthesis and mitosis that ensue 24 hr and more
later? In other words, which of the molecular events that
follow antigen recognition by the T-cell (and B-cell)
receptor are essential for activation of the subsequent
events leading to proliferation and expansion of the clone
displaying the appropriate receptor? And which are merely
epiphenomena?

We arbitrarily divided the some 20 communications into
two groups, those dealing with early events at the lymphocyte membrane and those occurring, usually somewhat later,
in the nucleus; we shall observe this grouping in the
following summary.

Early Events at the Lymphocyte Membrane

Let us begin this brief account somewhat perversely by
mentioning some topics of current interest that were not
discussed. There was but one paper that dealt, somewhat
indirectly indeed, with the role of calcium in lymphocyte

activation (Quastel et al., No.93, Immunobiology vol.167, p.60). This showed that calmodulin inhibitors such as trifluoperazine (TFP) prevent subsequent entry of treated, mitogen-activated lymphocytes into S phase, provided that the drugs were present during the few hours immediately following addition of the mitogen. There was also a marked secondary inhibition of K^+ uphill transport, suggesting a point of contact of the metabolic pathways involving the monovalent and divalent cations. Only a single paper (Bonnafous et al., no.82, p.53) made reference to cyclic AMP, and this only to report studies with a new unusually powerful adenylate cyclase stimulant, forskolin, that proved a correspondingly powerful inhibitor of Con A-induced lymphokine production and proliferation.

Another topic that we would have wished to have discussed was the role of the Ca^{++}- and phospholipid-dependent kinase which is linked to the formation in the plasma membrane of diacylglycerol from its substrate phosphatidylinositol. This was the subject of a communication that was published with the abstracts (no.85, p.55) but not presented. Some characterization of the tyrosine kinases present in resting lymphocytes was reported by Linna (no.92, p.60), but these studies have not yet been extended to include their role, or changes in their activities, during the stimulation process.

Another abstract (no.98, p.63) was the subject of some controversy, even in the unfortunate absence of its authors. Szamel and Resch claimed that a subfraction of purified calf lymphocyte plasma membranes (described at previous meetings) contained enzymes, including the $[Na^+K^+]$ATPase, whose specific activity was "several-fold enriched and preferentially stimulated upon Con A treatment". In the oral presentation of his poster (no.97, p.63), Severini came to a diametrically opposite conclusion. In the case of pig lymphocytes, assay of the $[Na^+K^+]$ATPase of permeabilized cells of membrane fragments (operationally defined as the ouabain-sensitive hydrolysis of ATP) showed that the specific activity of this enzyme measured in vitro remained unchanged after Con A-stimulation. The increased uphill transport of monovalent cations that follows mitogen treatment (and noted in this system within 5 min) was attributed to in situ enhanced activity of the enzyme caused by a transient increase in intracellular Na^+ due to a mitogen-induced leakiness in this ion. In other words,

Severini maintains that mitogen causes neither the appearance of new pump sites in the membrane (confirmed by ^{3}H-ouabain binding studies) nor greater activity per site in isolated membrane fractions where the activity is no longer governed by internal levels of Na^+.

There was a vigorous discussion of the significance to lymphocyte activation of the sharply increased monovalent cation fluxes that follow triggering of lymphocytes by T-cell and B-cell mitogens. Severini pointed out that the increased fluxes are observed only when purified T-cell suspensions are treated with Con A and B-cells with LPS but not vice-versa, although T-cells can bind LPS and B-cells Con A. An interesting study of the murine mixed lymphocyte reaction (MLR) by Roy (no.94, p.61) showed that the increased cation flux, as well as the other early events observed in induction of proliferation by T-cell mitogens, must also occur in the T-cells of the stimulating population, even when the latter had been treated with mitomycin C. Thus a subpopulation of the stimulating population must itself undergo the early events of activation in order for this population to be capable of causing a maximal stimulation.

Another controversial subject was the putative transient decrease in membrane potential reported at previous meetings to occur in lymphocytes following mitogen treatment (Kiefer and Gerson, I.L.C.C. 1979, 1981 & 1982). Careful studies by Wilson et al. (no.100, p.64) in which membrane potentials were measured by computer-aided flow cytometry utilizing fluorescent membrane-potential probes, showed that cell activation by a variety of T- and B-cell mitogens did not alter the membrane potential of mitogen-treated cells, at least within the first 6 hr of activation. The increased ionic fluxes that are essential to maintenance of the activated state seen not to be accompanied by a membrane depolarization. Wilson attributed the contrary results of others to technical artefacts.

Suggested evidence that an early step in activation involves cross-linking of membrane molecules (same cell and/or different cells) was presented by the Montepellier group (Favero et al. no.86, p.55). The non-mitogenic peanut agglutinin caused enhancement of the blastogenic response and of IL-2 production in thymocytes activated by neuraminidase followed either by Con A or by galactose

oxidase treatment. Soybean agglutinin produced the same
effect; these data favour, but do not prove, the hypothesis
that molecular crosslinking and cell aggregation may be
important early events in the activation sequence.

Changes in DNA Metabolism and Gene Expression

There were two communications dealing with novel
methods for the study of lymphocyte radiosensitivity. The
first by Barth et al. (no.81, p.52) showed that the
particles produced in response to capture of thermal
neutrons by boron (^{10}B) caused extensive inhibition of
subsequent incorporation of ^{3}H-thymidine into DNA. An
interesting technique, involving clonal outgrowth from
limiting dilution culture, was used to measure the radiosensitivity of long-term T-cell cultures (James et al.
no.89, p.57); this method should be useful for studying
DNA repair and its deficiency in certain disease states.

Greer and Kaplan (no.88, p.57) confirmed and extended
recent reports from their own and other laboratories that
unstimulated lymphocytes contain several thousand DNA strand
breaks that are repaired early in the activation process.
This repair is an essential process mediated by the ADP
ribosyl transferase system, as inhibitors of this system
prevented not only the DNA repair, but also the initiation
of DNA synthesis. Both the production and repair of strand
breaks were shown to occur continuously in resting and
stimulated cells, but Greer presented evidence that the
repair activity of the resting lymphocytes was restricted by
the low intracellular concentration of NAD^{+}, the substrate
of ADP ribosyl transferase. Reduction in the number of
strand breaks in resting lymphocytes could be achieved when
nicotinamide was supplied to increase the intracellular
NAD^{+} concentration, but this did not of itself initiate
proliferation, indicating that the repair process was
necessary but not sufficient for this purpose.

An interesting group of five posters addressed the
regulation of lymphocyte gene expression. Two presentations
from Schäfer's laboratory (nos.90 and 99, pp.58 & 64)
concerned the regulation of mRNA availability during
stimulation by Con A. They showed that the complexity of
the mRNA present decreased after activation, the proportion
of abundant mRNA species present in the cytoplasm being
increased, and individual species became even more abundant,

at the expense of the rare mRNA species, which were actually
reduced in number. The percentage of mRNA molecules bearing
a 5' cap increased from 24% in resting lymphocytes to 37%
(still well below the HeLa cell level) after 40 hr Con A.
Investigation of the factors responsible for the alteration
in cytoplasmic mRNA was focussed on the HnRNA processing
step, and in particular on the part played by HnRNA-
associated proteins. Analysis of these showed that one
HnRNP core protein, protein A1, was almost entirely absent
from resting lymphocytes, but appeared progressively after
Con A addition. All the core proteins occurred as multiple
charge isomers, the proportions again being changed after
activation. It was proposed that these changes may account
for at least some of the increased HnRNA-processing
efficiency reported after activation.

Brown and Swanson Beck (no.83, p.53) also addressed
the increase in total lymphocyte RNA, in this case
primarily ribosomal RNA, in individual cells after activation by PHA, in the course of an attempt to develop a
mathematical model to measure lymphocyte activation. One
conclusion of their study was that, by this criterion, the
proportion of peripheral blood lymphocytes responding to
PHA by an increase in cytoplasmic RNA content was very high
- much higher than the proportion that would subsequently
progress to DNA synthesis. Forsdyke (no.87, p.56) noted
that lymphocyte mRNA patterns could also be changed by
addition of the protein synthesis inhibitor, cycloheximide.
A prominent group of new mRNAs appeared in response to this
treatment, but it was not yet established whether transcriptional mechanisms were responsible.

Two further presentations, by Wecker et al. (no.92,
p.62) and Kikatuni et al. (no.91, p.59) concentrated on the
expression of one specific gene, the cellular homologue of
the myc oncogene. Both groups agreed that the transcription
of this gene increased dramatically very early after the
polyclonal activation of either B or T lymphocytes. The
c-myc RNA sequences were most abundant in the period 2-8 hr
after polyclonal activation, and declined in number
considerably at later times. Wecker's group had also
studied the expression of the cellular homologues of several
other oncogenes: they found increased expression of
c-Ha-ras about 20 hr after stimulation, but no expression
of the other genes studied.

Finally, Sahai and Kaplan drew attention to the spontaneous activation that is observed on prolonged culture of human lymphocytes (no.95, p.61). Although part of this effect may be in response to fetal calf serum, as previously noted, a significant proliferation remained even when strenuous efforts were made to remove all known mitogenic substances from the culture medium.

HUMAN REGULATORY CELL INTERACTIONS

Nancy Hogg and J. Farrant

ICRF, London and CRC, Harrow

This workshop concentrated on characteristics of the cells associated with accessory functions in immune response rather than with functional mechanisms. Three new monoclonal antibodies specific for mononuclear phagocytes were described by Hogg (London), one being a long sought after pan-human monocyte/macrophage marker and another two, defining two tissue macrophage subsets. Rosenberg (Rehovot) outlined the usefulness of peanut agglutinin for selectively identifying circulating monocytes. Another monocyte product, alpha-1-antitrypsin (AAT) is normally synthesised by monocytes and hepatocytes. Jones (Southampton) described AAT deficient individuals whose hepatocytes fail to secrete AAT but whose monocytes behave normally, raising interesting questions about handling of this molecule by two different cell populations. An example of altered antigen expression by myeloid cells is provided by the LFA/C3biR/150, 95 family of molecules which bear distinctive α chains but share the 95 kd β chain. MAbs specific for LFA molecules block many leukocyte functions and Melief (Amsterdam) added to the information about these molecules by showing that the blocking of K cell activity was independent of the Fc receptor and that myeloid cells from the small group of patients suffering from bacterial infections who have previously been shown to lack the phagocytic C3bi receptor, CR3, are also missing LFA molecules. This suggests that the lesion is at the level of the β chain. Phenotypic characteristics of dendritic cells remained elusive except for the stable expression of high levels of Class II

71

molecules (McDowell, London).

The function of dendritic cells as antigen presenters of PPD and mitogen and in MLC was reported. Forre (Oslo) showed that synovial tissue dendritic cells were more potent than those from synovial fluid or peripheral blood. Interestingly, he also reported that dendritic cells are powerful secretors of IL-1, which suggests that they may be 'self sufficient' in their interactions with T cells. Farrant (Harrow) reported a defect in the presentation of PWM on dendritic cells from hypogammaglobulinaemic patients. This may be the first reported lesion in this cell type.

Abnormal expression of HLA-DR by endocrine epithelium was discussed in the context of the possible role this phenomenon might play in autoimmune disease. Todd (London) showed evidence that γ interferon but not α interferon or IL-2 was capable of inducing HLA.DR on normal thyroid cells. As γ lFN would appear to be a physiological inducer of HLA.DR, this suggests that in vivo, an immune response, possibly of viral origin triggers HLA.DR expression on thyrocytes and subsequent ability to present self antigen in some susceptible individuals. Bottazzo (London) hypothesised that the reason why certain haplotypes e.g. HLA.DR3 appeared more frequently in autoimmune disease could be explained by the deletion of regulatory anti-idiotypic clones which shared cross reactivity with the particular HLA-DR haplotype. Davies (New York) showed that thyrocytes induced by lectin to express HLA.DR could prime naive T cells to self thyroid antigen suggesting that these cells do have the capacity for accessory cell function. The question remains as to whether this is, in vivo, a primary or subsequent event in tissue immune responses.

Two novel forms of immune modulation were discussed. Antigen-specific suppression by high doses of influenza strain A was demonstrated not to be due to conventional suppressor cells or monocytes but to a direct interaction of antigen and the T cell (either T4 or T8) membrane affecting the B cells and decreasing immunoglobulin production. Using a B cell line, the requirement for T cells could be overcome and antibody synthesis could be abrogated, by antigen overload alone (McCaughan, Sydney). In the streptococcal antigen activation system a novel T8+ adherent and antigen binding cell was shown both to help and to have contrasuppressor activity (Lehner, London). These observations suggest that possible cellular interactions in human immune responses will not be less complex than those already described in the mouse.

Our discussion ended with a report of transfection of L cells with SB(DP) genes which were demonstrated to be successful presenters of influenza virus to T cell clones (Trowsdale, ICRF, London). This approach to analysing the molecular aspects of cell interactions is obviously one important way to our future understanding of the regulation of the immune system.

HUMAN NATURAL KILLER CELLS

Rolf Kiessling[*] and Hugh Pross[**]

[*] Department of Immunology, Karolinska Institute
S-10401 Stockholm 60 Sweden

[**] Departments of Radiation Oncology and
Microbiology and Immunology, Queen's University
Kingston, Ontario, Canada   K7L 3N6

The workshop on human natural killer (NK) cells was one of two NK workshops held at the 16th Leukocyte Culture Conference and consisted of discussion of several issues relevant to human NK cells, primarily as they related to the papers and posters presented at the session. These presentations have been published as Abstracts numbered 251-271 (Immunobiology <u>167</u>, 166-179, 1984) and will not be reviewed individually here.

The following topics were discussed in some detail by the participants: the nature and significance of lymphokines produced by purified large granular lymphocytes (LGL) or NK clones, phenotypic characteristics and cytotoxic function of LGL clones, the importance of NK activity against non-malignant target cells and the role of carbohydrate moieties in NK-target interaction and target lysis.

Several presentations at the workshop dealt with lymphokine production by LGL-enriched peripheral blood cells (PBL)[1,2] or by LGL clones [3]. The data suggest that LGL can produce gamma interferon (IFN)[1,3], interleukins 1[3] and 2[1,3], B cell growth factor [1,3] and burst promoting activity[1]. Furthermore, Leu-M1⁻OKT3⁻ Percoll-enriched LGL were shown to be capable of acting as antigen-presenting cells (APC) for T cell responses to Staphylococcus aureus protein A, Streptolysin O, and surface antigens in both allogeneic and autologous mixed lymphocyte reactions[2]. The

75

active cells had high NK activity and were in the HLA-DR$^+$
subpopulation. These results have profound implications
for establishing a role for NK cells as a regulatory cell.
The discussion consisted of fairly detailed technical
questions as to the methods of purification and cloning
which were used in these studies. There are two basic
questions in the interpretation of these data – what
constitutes adequate purity in the LGL enriched
preparations, and can the clones really be considered to be
NK cells? The questions of cell purity is obviously
fundamental to the interpretation of the results. The
presence of even a low percentage of contaminating
monocytes may be sufficient to cause the results obtained
in spite of several consecutive nylon wool or plastic
adherent steps. It was pointed out by one of the
participants that 1% contamination by monocytes still
leaves an appreciable number of these cells present in the
assay. It was also suggested that a functional assay such
as chemiluminescence was the best way to detect such
contamination. The chemiluminescence assay detects
activated oxygen species produced by stimulated monocytes
and is extremely sensitive and reliable, providing that
proper instrumentation is available and adequate care is
taken to avoid pH shifts during the assay. The corollary
to this statement is, of course, that LGL themselves are
not capable of oxygen radical formation. This has been a
controversial issue recently and it was agreed that the
weight of evidence overwhelmingly suggests that any
chemiluminescence detected in LGL-tumour target
combinations is due to monocyte contamination. A
presentation relevant to this question by Ernst et al.[4]
demonstrated that the degree of chemiluminescence obtained
from monocytes triggered by tumour cells could be increased
by the presence of NK cells in the assay system, i.e. there
is a synergistic effect. This interesting result explains,
to some extent, published observations by others showing a
correlation between the level of NK activity and the
chemiluminescence of monocyte-contaminated NK preparations.
In the discussion of monocyte contamination, the point was
also made that negative in vitro reconstitution
experiments, in which an attempt is made to mimic monocyte
contamination, do not necessarily serve as adequate
controls to demonstrate the purity of LGL preparations. It
is theoretically possible that the monocytes used for
reconstitution may not be similar in function to the
contaminating cells, because of the manipulations involved.

In conclusion, it was noted that it may be necessary to discard "purified" LGL preparations which are monocyte-contaminated, rather than produce erroneus results.

The discussion of LGL clones and their functions and phenotype[5-7] also involved a number of technical questions. The importance of cloning at 0.5-1 cell per well or less was stressed, since the universally-observed limited generation number (50 at best) of these clones makes recloning difficult. As can be seen from the abstracts, there is marked heterogeneity on the phenotype of clones having NK function and it is still by no means clear whether these cells are derived from the same precursor cell as the fresh PBL NK cell. Very few NK clones have exactly the same phenotype as fresh PBL NK cells which are T3 negative and B73.1 (anti-Fc receptor) positive. It was also pointed out that even the in vivo lymphoproliferative disorders of Tgamma cells with NK function[5] involved cells which had more T cell characteristics than the usual NK cell population. The relationship between all of these phenotypically different NK cells has still to be resolved. In contrast to this heterogeneity in the surface phenotype among various clones, most of them showed a very similar specificity when tested on a panel of NK sensitive and resistant tumor targets. Thus no evidence was presented supporting any extensive heterogeneity at the clonal level as regards the "NK receptor", a structure which still remains as enigmatic as the "NK target structure".

Although research into NK cell function has been primarily concerned with the role of these cells in malignant disease, considerable evidence has accumulated recently that they are involved in regulatory activities and NK-mediated effects can be shown in a number of "normal" situations against non-malignant cells. Lately much interest has been focused around a possible role of NK cells as suppressor cells for B-cells, and the suppression of antibody production by NK cells activated by the complement fragment C3a was discussed[8]. The action of NK cells may not always be beneficial to the host, as is illustrated by the fact that NK-Tgamma lymphocytosis[5] is a disease frequently associated with neutropenia and occasionally anemia, which may be caused by the abnormal NK cells. The frequency of this comparatively benign condition was discussed and it was concluded that subclinical NK lymphocytosis may be commoner than is realized, simply because it is not looked for.

Finally, the role of carbohydrate moieties in NK-target interactions was briefly discussed. Three abstracts were presented on this topic [9-11], but the discussion centred around the importance of the mannose-6-phosphate moiety in particular. It is apparent that NK function is independent both of mannose-6-phosphate as a ligand and of the mannose-6-phosphate-dependent packaging of lysosomal enzymes.

In conclusion, the field of natural killer cells continues to present fascinating and perplexing problems which are gradually but certainly being solved. As more and more investigators examine these cells in the context of their own particular interests, the function and potential role of these cells is becoming more and more complex. Future work in this field must attempt to place these cells in their appropriate place in the lymphocyte hierarchy and establish their role in vivo.

References

1. Pistoia, V., Cozzolino, F. & Ferrarini, M. Abst. 261. Immunobiology, 167, 172, 1984.
2. Scala, G., Allavena, P. Djeu, J., Ortaldo, J., Herberman, R.B. & Oppenheim J.J. Abst. 266. Immunobiology, 167, 175-176, 1984.
3. Allavena, P., Scala, G., Djeu, J., Procopio, A., Oppenheim, J.J., Herberman, R.B. & Ortaldo, J.R. Abst. 251. Immunobiology, 167, 166, 1984.
4. Ernst, M., Havel, A. & Flad, H.-D. Abst. 253. Immunobiology, 167, 167-168, 1984.
5. Van De Friend, R.J., Smeekens, F. & Bolhuis, R.L.H. Abst. 270. Immunobiology 167, 178-179, 1984.
6. Bolhuis, R.L.H. & Van De Griend, R.J. Abst. 252. Immunobiology, 167, 166-167, 1984.
7. Roberts, K. & Moore, M. Abst. 263. Immunobiology, 167, 173-174, 1984.
8. Fox, R.I., Hugli, T., Howell, F. & Morgan, E. Abst. 254. Immunobiology, 167, 168-169, 1984.
9. Pross, H., Werkmeister, J. & Partington, M. Abst. 262. Immunobiology, 167, 173, 1984.
10. Haubeck, H.-D., Kolsch, E., Imort, M., Hasilik, A. & Von Figura, K. Abst. 256. Immunobiology, 167, 169-170, 1984.
11. Stankova, J. & Rola-Pleszczynski, M. Abst. 269. Immunobiology, 167, 177-178, 1984.

CONTROL OF MHC GENE EXPRESSION

J.G. Frelinger and M.J. Owen

University of N. Carolina at Chapel Hill and
Imperial Cancer Research Fund, University College London

The overall organization of the MHC has become clear during the last few years. The molecular genetic organization of both Class I and Class II genes have revealed unsuspected complexity. The number of Class I sequences ($\sim$ 30) were a surprise. The number of Iaα and β chains while fewer, (5 α and 7 β genes in man) are still considerable. The central questions of MHC genetics have changed from the number and structure of genes to their regulation. A number of systems have been defined to examine changes in Class II gene expression. Among the best examined so far are the effects of IFγ on Class II antigen expression. Here it is clear that IFγ causes an increase in the expression of Class II products on the membrane by increasing the mRNA levels of the cytoplasm. The mechanism of this increase is not known, although simple models, such as regulation by limiting the amount of invariant chain have been excluded. More importantly, the mechanism of coordinate or lack of coordinate regulation of the Ia genes is not yet known. The mechanics of Ia regulation both at the DNA and protein levels remain to be elucidated.

In addition to the question of control in a single cell over a short time following an inductive signal, the question of regulation of Class II (and Class I molecules) in different tissues remains. Ia differences either in gene expression (i.e. DR vs. DC) or posttranslational differences involving glycosylation resulting in differences of Ia derived from B cells/macrophage and T

cells have been described. Experiments to examine the
effects of these differences and their functional
consequences on the immunologic function of Ia molecules
have been inconclusive, but suggest that the changes may
result in differences of the efficacy of antigen
presentation by macrophages to T cells.

A considerable amount of information describing the
mapping of epitopes on the surface of both Class I and
Class II molecules using both monoclonal antibodies and
molecular genetic approaches was presented. These data
together reveal little evidence for functional
differentiation of the protein domains of either Class I or
Class II MHC molecules. This seems to be the case for
both epitopes detected by monoclonal antibodies and by H-2
restricted cytolytic T cells.

In summary, the field is in a period of consolidation,
which has followed a rapid expansion. Promising systems to
address the next set of questions are being developed, and
considerable progress will be seen by the next LCC.

SECTION II

GROWTH AND
DIFFERENTIATION FACTORS

HAEMOPOIETIC CELL GROWTH FACTOR: CHARACTERISATION AND MODE OF ACTION

A.D. WHETTON & T.M. DEXTER

Paterson Laboratories, Christie Hospital & Holt

Radium Institute, Manchester M20 9BX, U.K.

The process of haemopoiesis provides a heterogenous population of peripheral blood cells with diverse morphological characteristics and functions. The site of production of these cells is mainly the bone marrow in the adult animal. In the marrow resides a population of pluripotent stem cells which give rise to the mature blood cells (see 1). These stem cells can either self-renew (that is, form exact copies of themselves) or differentiate depending on the needs of the organism, in this way the stem cell population can be maintained throughout a life-time (and in fact could be maintained throughout several lifetimes[2]). A stem cell can also give rise to a series of progenitor cells upon division that are the precursor cells of the different lineages or blood cell types found in the circulation (see 3). The progeny of a pluripotential stem cell are committed to a defined differentiation pathway whereby there is a restriction as to which mature blood cell type they will be able to yield[4].

The committed progenitor cell populations (still found in the bone marrow) can undergo extensive proliferation and whilst doing so mature into functional "end" cell populations prior to release into the bloodstream. Under normal circumstances haemopoiesis provides mature blood cells (which have a naturally short lifetime) in balance with the loss of these cells. However, in certain stress situations, such as bleeding or infection, the production of

83

cells of specific types can be enlarged to meet increased demand.

To control the production of mature blood cells a series of stimulatory polypeptide growth factors are apparently required which can promote proliferation and allow the maturation of progenitor cell populations. Examples of such factors include erythropoietin[5] (which can promote the production of cells in the erythroid compartment) and CSF-1 (Colony Stimulating Factor-1 or Macrophage-CSF [6] (which promotes macrophage production) These and other stimulatory factors play an important role in the haemopoietic process, a great deal of which has been demonstrated by the use of colony assay systems.

Studies using the *in vitro* colony assays for bone marrow haemopoietic progenitor cells have revealed that the presence of the appropriate regulatory factor is essential for the survival of specific haemopoietic progenitor cells as well as their proliferation and maturation to "end" (fully differentiated) cells[7]. When these growth regulators are absent, progenitor cells are steadily lost from culture; there is apparently no quiescent state in the absence of these factors but only a steady deterioration[8]. Also the stimulatory factor(s) must be provided throughout the developmental process. Survival, proliferation and maturation are not dependent on a short-term ("hit-and-run") addition of regulatory molecules but their constant presence[5,7,8]. There is now evidence from studies of haemopoiesis *in vivo* and *in vitro* that the stimulatory factors that regulate the growth and differentiation of progenitor cells are normally supplied by the surrounding stromal cell milieu in the marrow. This ensures a strict and local control of haemopoietic cell development[9,10].

Although some haemopoietic regulatory molecules show a lineage restriction in their ability to promote survival, proliferation and maturation, the description and purification of a multilineage stimulatory factor has also been achieved. Because of its broad range of activities we have named this important regulatory molecule haemopoietic cell growth factor (HCGF)[11]. Briefly HCGF (a glycoprotein of molecular weight 28,500 with a basic peptide molecular weight of 15,000) can allow the self-renewal of stem cells, and also stimulates the haemopoietic progenitor cells of granulocyte, macrophage, megakaryocyte and erythroid

lineages to proliferate and develop[11]. This molecule
therefore acts on the very earliest haemopoietic cell
types and as such can be considered to be a key regulatory
factor in the control of haemopoiesis. Other multi-lineage
stimulatory factors have also been characterised, and it is
probable that multi-CSF[8], Burst-Promoting Activity[12],
Interleukin-3[13], Mast Cell Growth Factor[14], Persisting Cell
Stimulating Factor[15] and HCGF are the same molecular entity.

Another important characteristic of HCGF is that it
can support the continuous growth of non-leukaemic
granulocyte precursor cell lines[16]. These factor dependent
cells (FDC-P cells) will survive and proliferate in the
presence of HCGF; in its absence they die within 48 hours.
Other similar cell lines with an absolute dependence on
multilineage stimulatory factors have also been
established[13,15,17]. Of some importance is that the FDC-P
cells can be produced in sufficient numbers to allow a
biochemical characterisation of growth factor mediated
survival and proliferation. FDC-P cells therefore represent
an important tool in the study of the mechanisms underlying
the absolute requirement of haemopoietic progenitor cells
for specific regulatory molecules to enable them to survive
and proliferate.

Attempts to replace HCGF with other defined growth
factors proved to be unsuccessful in maintaining the
viability of FDC-P cells, these agents included Epidermal
Growth Factor, Fibroblast Growth Factor, Macrophage-CSF,
Granulocyte-Macrophage CSF, and Insulin. To date, no other
protein factor we have used can replace HCGF, thus the
maintenance, survival and growth of these cells is
specifically associated with HCGF. However, one other agent
has been able to maintain FDC-P2 cells in culture for up to
48 hours, an ATP regenerating system consisting of ATP,
creatine phosphate and creatine phosphokinase (or
alternatively phosphoenolpyruvate and pyruvate kinase)[18].
The ATP present was found to be the active constituent for
cellular survival. This implied some role for HCGF in the
maintenance of energy levels within the cells. We
investigated this and found that the removal of HCGF from
FDC-P2 cells does lead to a rapid and steady depletion of
the intracellular ATP levels after as little as 1.5 hours in
the absence of the factor. The ATP regenerating system we
employed maintained the intracellular ATP levels at values
found in FDC-P2 cells which had been grown in the presence

of HCGF. Furthermore, when FDC-P2 cells were cultured in
the absence of HCGF for 5 hours (leading to a depleted
intracellular ATP level) then supplemented with HCGF the
ATP levels increased within 10 minutes. The short time
interval necessary for this increase would argue that the
ability of HCGF to modulate cellular ATP levels is
essential for the survival and proliferation of FDC-P2
cells.

How are the ATP levels maintained by the (necessarily
constant) presence of HCGF in the growth medium of these
cells? Also by what mechanism can the cells respond to the
readdition of HCGF with such a large increase in ATP
synthesis? The generation of ATP is associated with two
major pathways in the cell. Firstly, the Embden-Meyerhof or
glycolytic pathway which converts glucose to pyruvate (and
finally pyruvate to lactate as the end product of anaerobic
respiration). Secondly, pyruvate or other 2 to 4 carbon
molecules can yield substrates for the mitochondrial
(aerobic) respiration process. We have found that factor-
dependent cells are not killed when grown in the presence
of mitochondrial poisons which argues against mitochondrial
respiration *per se* being central to cellular survival. This
infers that the HCGF acts to maintain ATP levels via its
effect on the glycolytic pathway. To assess the rate of
glycolysis in the absence and presence of HCGF we assayed
lactate production. This was found to be greatly reduced in
the absence of HCGF, an effect which was observable after as
little as 0.5 hours in the absence of the growth factor.
However, the activities of the key regulatory enzymes of
glycolysis was unaltered after as much as 5 hours in the
absence of HCGF. The rate of glycolysis is therefore not
modulated by the regulation of the bulk level of
glycolytic enzymes, but a rapid fall in glycolytic activity
is observed. This indicates that the provision of glucose
(the "raw" material of glycolysis) for this pathway may be
the site where HCGF acts to maintain FDC-P cell respiration,
thereby maintaining cellular viability. This possibility was
strongly underlined by our observations that HCGF can
activate a specific D-hexose transport protein in the factor
dependent cells in a dose dependent fashion, thereby,
permitting the uptake of hexose-sugars into the cell. This
dose-dependent increase in the uptake of hexose-sugars
mirrors the effect of HCGF on cell viability and
proliferation. Our model for factor-dependence in FDC-P
cells would then be that when HCGF is removed from the cells

glucose uptake rapidly falls, leading to a decreased glycolytic flux and a lack of ability to maintain ATP levels within the cell[19]. This fall in the cellular energy charge then leads to the ultimate death of the cell.

These data provide some ideas of the nature of haemopoietic progenitor cell factor-dependence and the mechanism underlying the apparent need for the continuous presence of the haemopoietic growth factors for the maintenance of cell viability. It is well documented that stimulatory factors are required for survival and proliferation of progenitor cell populations *in vitro*.There is also an increasingly large body of evidence to implicate these factors in the *in vivo* production of mature blood cells. These factors are probably produced by the stromal elements of the bone marrow and "presented" to haemopoietic progenitor cells facilitating their self-renewal and/or development. Thus should a progenitor cell be removed from the source of the specific regulatory molecule(s) required for its maintenance and development it would die. Our experiments suggest that this would be as a consequence of the lack of factor leading to a fall in hexose uptake and a failure to maintain intracellular energy levels. An escaped progenitor cell (with a large proliferative potential) is programmed to die when released from the permissive environment provided for its development, an obvious benefit to the maintenance of a controlled haemopoietic system.

However, leukaemic cells are distinctly different from normal haemopoietic cells in this respect, for they can survive and proliferate in environments which are not normally associated with haemopoietic cell proliferation. This is possibly because leukaemic cells have by-passed the requirement for factors or are themselves constitutive producers of these factors. If this is indeed correct, then an important feature of the leukaemic transformation process may be the loosening of growth factor mediated-mechanism associated with survival (such as hexose uptake) leading to a cell capable of autonomous (survival and) proliferation. Our observations on the nature of HCGF-dependence in haemopoietic progenitor cells and the ability of HCGF to modulate hexose transport provide some indications of the nature of haemopoietic cell regulation and the possible aberrations that occur in leukaemia.

REFERENCES

1. Metcalf, D. and Moore, M.A.S. in Haemopoietic cells
    550pp (Amsterdam North Holland, 1971).
2. Harrison, D.E. Proc.Natl.Acad.Sci., U.S.A. 70, 3184-
    3188 (1973).
3. Till, J.E. and McCulloch, E.A. Biochim. Biophys. Acta.
    605, 431-459 (1980)
4. Metcalf, D. in Hemopoietic Colonies in vitro. Cloning
    of Normal and Leukemic Cells, 227pp. (Springer Verlag,
    1977).
5. Miyake, T., Kung, C.K.H. and Goldwasser, E. J. Biol.
    Chem. 252, 5558-5564 (1977).
6. Stanley, E.R. et al. J. Cell Biochem. 21, 151-159
    (1983).
7. Metcalf, D. in Tissue Growth Factors (ed. Baserga, R)
    343-384 (Springer-Verlag, 1981).
8. Burgess, A.W.et al. Biochem. J. 185, 301-314 (1982).
9. Allen, T.D. and Dexter, T.M. Differentiation, 6, 191-
    194 (1976).
10. Dexter, T.M. et al. J. Supramol. Struct. 13, 513-524
    (1980).
11. Bazill, G.W. et al. Biochem. J. 210, 747-759 (1983).
12. Iscove, N.N. et al. J. Cell Physiol. (suppl) 1, 65-78
    (1982).
13. Ihle, J. et al. Immunol. Rev. 63, 532-549 (1982).
14. Tokota T. et al. Proc. Natl. Acad. Sci., U.S.A. 81,
    1070-1074 (1984).
15. Schrader, J.W. Crit. Rev. Immunol. 4, 197-277 (1983).
16. Dexter T.M. et al. J. Exp. Med. 152, 1036-1047 (1980).
17. Greenberger, J.S. J. Supramol. Struct. 13, 501-514
    (1982).
18. Whetton, A.D. and Dexter, T.M. Nature (London) 303,
    629-631 (1983).
19. Whetton, A.D., Bazill, G.W. and Dexter, T.M. EMBO J.
    3, 409-413 (1984).

Regulation of human B lymphocytes differentiation:

Characterization of B cell stimulatory factors

T. Hirano, H. Kikutani, K. Shimizu, H. Kishi, T. Taga, K. Ishibashi, S. Inui, S. Kashiwamura, N. Nakano, Y. Miki, T. Nakagawa and T. Kishimoto

Institute for Molecular and Cellular Biology, Osaka University, 1-3, Yamada-Oka, Suita city, Osaka

Introduction:
B lymphocytes originate from pluripotent hematopoietic stem cells and differentiate into antibody producing cells through several distinct differentiation stages. Commitment of the antigen specificity in each B cell clone occurs at the stage of pre B cells by two step DNA rearrangements including V,D and J segments, i.e. from DJ joining to the functional VDJ formation (1). Following the rearrangement of heavy chain genes, light chain gene rearrangements occur (2) and 7S IgM molecules are expressed as antigen receptors on the surface of mature B cells. A given antigen selects a B cell clone with a matched receptor and activates this clone into antibody producing cells under the influence of helper T cells.

Since the discovery of T and B cell interactions in the antibody response, mechanism of B cell activation has been one of the area for the most extensive studies. Dutton and his colleagues (3) originally proposed the presence of soluble mediators responsible for T and B cell interactions. Schimpl and Wecker (4) and several other investigators (5-7) also demonstrated that T cell-derived soluble factors could reconstitute the function of helper T cells. Kishimoto and Ishizaka (8) and Kishimoto et al. (9) succeeded in the induction of polyclonal immunoglobulin (Ig) secretion in B cells with anti-Ig and T cell-derived helper factors, suggesting that two signals, crosslinkage of Ig-receptors and T

89

cell-derived helper factors, are essential for the activation of B cells into Ig-secreting cells. The result was confirmed by Parker and his colleagues (10) with murine B cells and a culture supernatant of Con A-stimulated T cells.

Further studies with more homogeneous B tumor cells as target cells were carried out and it was shown that T cell-derived helper factors could be devided into growth and differentiation factors (11). Establishment of human T hybridomas clearly demonstrated the presence of B cell specific growth factor (BCGF) and B cell specific differentiation factor (BCDF) (12-14). In vitro IgM secretion could be induced in anti-Ig-stimulated leukemic B cells by the addition of hybridoma-derived BCGF and BCDF. All of these results have indicated that process of B cell activation into Ig-secreting cells can be devided into three steps, i.e. activation with anti-Ig, proliferation with BCGF and differentiation with BCDF.

Isolation and characterization of human BCDF:

As the concentration of T cell-derived immuno-regulatory molecules in a culture supernatant of mitogen-stimulated T cells is extremely low, isolation and purification of such molecules are almost impossible without the establishment of T cell lines secreting a relatively large amount of factors. It is also essential to establish a simple and quantitative method for the measurement of the activity of B cell stimulatory factors. As has been reported, T hybridomas are suitable for obtaining homogeneous factors. However, they usually are not stable and do not secrete a large amount of factors. Therefore, we attempted to transform T cells with HTLV (Human T cell Leukemia Virus) and to establish T cell lines secreting a relatively large amount of factors. As an assay system for BCDF, we employed an EBV-transformed B cell line, CESS, which expressed BCDF receptors and was responsive to BCDF (15). Incubation of 6×10^3 CESS cells with varing concentrations of conventional T cell factors including BCDF activity for 48 hr induced IgG secretion in their culture supernatants, which could easily be measured by ELISA assay, and the amount of IgG induced was proportional to the concentration of BCDF. The activity of human BCGF-II, which will be described in the next section, was measured by the induction of proliferation of murine leukemic B cells, BCL_1.

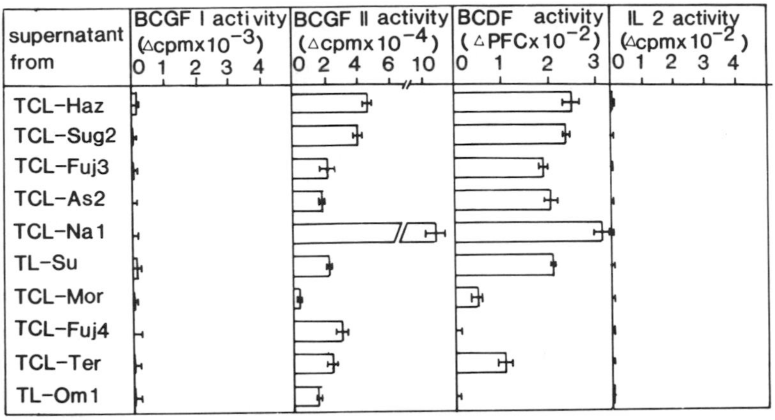

supernatant from	BCGF I activity (Δcpmx10^{-3}) 0 1 2 3 4	BCGF II activity (Δcpmx10^{-4}) 0 2 4 6 10	BCDF activity (ΔPFCx10^{-2}) 0 1 2 3	IL 2 activity (Δcpmx10^{-2}) 0 1 2 3 4
TCL–Haz				
TCL–Sug2				
TCL–Fuj3				
TCL–As2				
TCL–Na1				
TL–Su				
TCL–Mor				
TCL–Fuj4				
TCL–Ter				
TL–Om1				

Fig.1   Establishment of HTLV-transformed human T cell lines secreting B cell stimulatory factors.

As described in Fig.1, many HTLV-transformed T cell clones were established and their culture supernatants were tested for the activities of BCGF-I, BCGF-II and BCDF. Several clones secreted a relatively large amount of BCGF-II and almost all T cell clones except 2 clones secreted BCDF. It is noteworthy that no clones secreted any BCGF-I nor IL-2 and mRNA for IL-2 could not be detected. As a clone, TCL-Na1, secreted a relatively large amount of both BCGF-II and BCDF, we employed this clone for isolation and characterization of BCDF and BCGF-II. A culture supernatant of this clone could induce IgG secretion in CESS cells even when it was 1,800 fold diluted and the concentration of BCDF in the supernatant was approximately 900 fold as much as that in a supernatant of PHA-stimulated normal T cells. For the purification of BCDF, a serum free culture supernatant was concentrated, ultracentrifuged to remove HTLV particles and then sequentially applied to gel filtration on AcA 34, and mono P column with FPLC. The active fraction was further applied to reverse phase column on HPLC and BCDF activity was eluted with 50 to 55% of

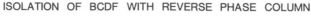

ISOLATION OF BCDF WITH REVERSE PHASE COLUMN

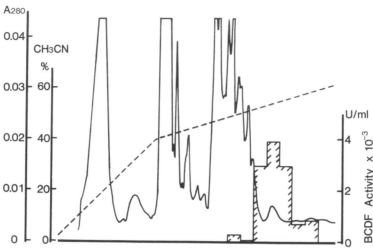

Fig.2   Isolation of BCDF by HPLC-reverse phase column.
Highly purified sample was applied to a reverse phase
column and eluted with the gradient of acetonitrile from
0 to 70% in the presence of 0.1% TFA.   BCDF activity was
shown by hatched column.

acetonitrile (Fig.2).   This active fraction was iodinated
with Bolton-Hunter reagents and a radiolabelled material
was further fractionated on the column of G2,000SW with
HPLC.   The radioactivity was eluted as a single peak with
a molecular weight of approximately 30-35K and BCDF
activity was detected only in the radioactive fraction.
Therefore, the result strongly suggests that BCDF has
been highly purified to an apparent homogeneity.   When
CESS   cells   were   incubated   with   the   radiolabelled
material, binding of radioactivity to CESS cells was
detected, while it did not bind with T cell lines or
BCDF-non-responsive B cell lines, further confirming that
the   radiolabelled material is BCDF.

Mechanism of the transduction of BCDF-mediated signals:
In   order   to   analyse   the   mechanism   of   the   signal
transmission,   a   BCDF-reactive   cell   line,   CESS,   was

employed. As described, incubation of CESS cells with BCDF induced IgG secretion in a dose-dependent manner without any effect on cell proliferation and inhibition of cell division with hydroxyurea did not affect the induction of IgG, showing that CESS cells could maturate into IgG secreting cells without any requirement of cell division when BCDF was provided. Metabolical labelling of CESS cells with ^{35}S-methionine in the presence or absence of BCDF showed that BCDF stimulation induced an increase in biosynthesis of secretory type of γ chains. Northern blot analysis of mRNA from BCDF-stimulated or non-stimulated cells also showed that BCDF stimulation induced an increase in mRNA for secretory type γ chains and no increase or rather decrease in mRNA for membrane type γ chains. All of these results indicate that BCDF is responsible for the final maturation of B cells to a high rate of Igs secretion by increasing a transcription of mRNA for secretory type heavy chains.

By employing CESS cells, the biochemical process involved in BCDF-induced IgG secretion was studied. Incubation of CESS cells with BCDF induced an increase in phospholipid methylation within 15 min and two-dimensional thin-layer chromatography demonstrated the methylation of phosphatidylethanolamine into phos-phatidylcholine. BCDF-stimulation also induced an increase of ^{3}H-DFP binding to CESS cells within 2 h, suggesting an activation of serine esterase. Several organophosphorous inhibitors, such as DFP (diiso-propylfluorophosphate) and P-NPEPP (P-nitrophenyl ethylpenthylphosphate) showed a dose dependent inhibitory effect on BCDF-induced IgG secretion. DMP (di-isopropylmethylphosphate, non-phosphorylating analogue of DFP) did not show any inhibitory effect. Pretreatment of cells with DFP in the absence of BCDF was also ineffective, indicating that stimulus-activable serine esterase was involved in the activation process of CESS cells with BCDF. As shown in Table I, DFP inhibited BCDF-induced IgG secretion but not BCDF-induced methylation of phospholipids. On the other hand, IBDA (isobutyldeoxyadenosin), inhibitors of transmethylation, inhibited phospholipid methylation, serine esterase activation and IgG induction. The result suggest that binding of BCDF with its receptors induces phospholipid methylation which may be required for the activation of serine esterase and activated serine esterase may be involved in the generation of the active cytoplasmic

Table I
Effect of inhibitors of serine esterase and
transmethylation on IgG induction, serine esterase
activation and phospholipid methylation[a]

CESS cells cultured with	IgG-PFC	methylation (cpm)	DFP-binding (cpm)
-	46 ± 5	782 ± 76	193 ± 9
BCDF	314 ± 63	2,316 ± 52	428 ± 15
BCDF+IBDA(2x10^{-4})	96 ± 15	695 ± 14	174 ± 3
BCDF+DFP(1x10^{-3})	44 ± 8	2,149 ± 34	
BCDF+P-NPEPP(1x10^{4})	55 ± 13		
BCDF+DMP(1x10^{-3})	310 ± 13		

a)   Details of the experiments were described in the
     previous papers (Miki et al. 1982, Kishi et al.
     1983).

substance responsible for signal transmission by limited
proteolysis (16,17). If this is the case, injection of
the cytoplasm from BCDF-stimulated CESS cells into B
cells may activate B cells into IgG-producing cells.
Therefore, an attempt was made to transfer cytoplasm from
CESS cells into SAC-stimulated normal B cells by red
cell-mediated microinjection. Transfer of cytoplasm from
BCDF-stimulated CESS cells into SAC-stimulated B cells
induced a comparable number of IgG-producing cells to
those observed by stimulation of the same cells with
BCDF. Injection of cytoplasm from non-stimulated CESS
cells or from a T cell line did not induce IgG secretion
in SAC-stimulated B cells, suggesting that a certain
substance involved in signal transmission may be
generated in cytoplasm by limited proteolysis with BCDF-
activated serine esterase (18).

Physicochemical and immunological properties of BCGF-II:
     The presence of two distinct kinds of BCGFs was
first demonstrated by the establishment of an IL-2
dependent alloantigen-specific human T cell clone, d4

BCGF II (BGDF) induces proliferation as well as IgM secretion in BCL$_1$ cells

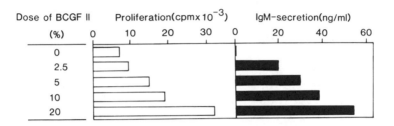

Fig.3   Induction of proliferation as well as IgM secretion in BCL$_1$ cells with partially purified human BCGF-II.

(19).   BCGF activity from this particular cell line (d4) was eluted in the fraction with the molecular weight of 50K, which showed a marked contrast to BCGF-I (BSFp$_1$) with the molecular weight of 20K (20).   A similar high molecular weight BCGF was also observed in murine system by Swain and Dutton (21).   Both human and murine BCGF-II did not induce proliferation of anti-μ or SAC-(Staphy-lococcus aureus strain Cowan I)-stimulated B cells, but induced proliferation of murine B leukemic cells, BCL$_1$ or DXS (dextran sulfate)-stimulated murine B cells.

An interesting finding is that BCGF-II is able to induce proliferation as well as IgM secretion in BCL$_1$ cells as well as DXS-stimulated B cells (Fig.3).   As described, some of HTLV-transformed T cell lines secreted a relatively large amount of BCGF-II.   Therefore, BCGF-II was partially purified from a culture supernatant of TCL-Na1 cells by preparative isoelectric focusing, gel filtration on AcA-34 and gel filtration on 3,000SWG in the presence of 0.1% Triton-X.   The activity to induce proliferation of BCL$_1$ cells or DXS-stimulated B cells was

Table II
Augmentation of IgM secretion in human
B blast cells by BCGF-II

Factors	IgM-PFC
Medium	65 ± 12
BCGF-I + BCDF	300 ± 26
BCGF-I + BCDF + BCGF-II	1,272 ± 114

detected in the fraction with a PI of 5 to 6 and with a molecular weight of more than 60K. The activity to induce IgM secretion in BCL_1 cells or DXS-stimulated B cells was also observed exactly in the same fraction and both activities to induce proliferation and IgM secretion were not separated by any chromatographycal procedures. The result strongly suggests that BCGF-II has the activity to induce both proliferation and Igs-secretion in B cells. Therefore, BCGF-II may belong to the same category of the factors, such as BRMF by Melchers et al. (22), BGDF by Pike et al. (23) and T15 TRF by Takatsu et al. (24), which show both growth and differentiation activities.

Partially purified BCGF-II (BGDF) induced proliferation of normal human B cells with low density, which had been activated in vivo. Conventional T cell factors, which included both BCGF-I and BCDF, induced IgM secretion in in vivo activated human B blast cells or in SAC-stimulated human B cells. The addition of BCGF-II to conventional T cell factors (BCGF-I + BCDF) augmented IgM secretion in activated human B cells, indicating that at least three B cell stimulatory factors, BCGF-I, BCGF-II (or BGDF) and BCDF are required for the maximum induction of Ig-secretion in B cells (Table II).

IL-2 and γ-IFN as B cell stimulatory factors:

As has been described, the involvement of B cell specific growth and differentiation factors in the activation of B cells to Igs-secreting cells has been clearly demonstrated. However, the role of IL-2 or γ-IFN in the activation of B cells, i.e., whether IL-2 or γ-IFN has any direct effect on proliferation or differentiation of B cells or not, has not yet been solved. In order to prove or disprove the direct effect of IL-2 on B cells, IL-2 preparation should not include any other lymphokine activities and B cell preparation should not include any T cells which might be activated to secrete B cell stimulatory factors in the presence of IL-2. Cloning of cDNA for IL-2 by Taniguchi et al. (25) has made it possible to obtain theoretically pure IL-2 as a transcription product of a cloned cDNA.

The study with recombinant IL-2 and highly purified human B cells showed that IL-2 is able to induce proliferation of SAC- or anti-μ-activated B cells. In this study, 20 to 30% of activated B cells expressed Tac antigen and anti-Tac antibody completely inhibited IL-2-induced proliferation of activated B cells. IL-2 induced proliferation of SAC-stimulated B cells, but no Igs-secretion. The addition of γ-IFN with IL-2 induced Igs-secretion in activated B cells and the amount of Igs was comparable to that induced with conventional T cell factors. The possibility that IL-2 activated contaminated T cells to secrete B cell stimulatory factors is very unlikely, since no Leu 1- or Leu 4-positive cells were detected in a highly purified B blast population. However, above mentioned possibility can not be completely excluded. In order to prove the direct effect of IL-2 on B cells, theoretically pure B cell population should be employed. Thus, we established hybridomas between human activated B cells and a mouse B lymphoma, M12.4.5, which was kindly provided by Dr. R. Asofsky (NIH), and IL-2 responsive clones were selected. A hybrid clone, SGB3, was responsive to IL-2 and IL-2 induced IgG secretion in SGB3 cells in a dose-dependent manner. As shown in Fig.4, 10 units/ml IL-2 (3×10^8 units/mg IL-2) could induce IgG secretion but more than 1,000 units/ml of IL-2 was required for the maximum IgG secretion. SGB3 cells expressed Tac antigen and anti-Tac antibody inhibited IL-2-induced IgG secretion in SGB3 cells. Purified BCDF also induced IgG secretion in SGB3 cells, but BCDF-induced IgG secretion was not affected by anti-Tac antibody. All of these results clearly showed that IL-2 could directly act on B cells and could induce even Igs secretion in B cells at a certain activation stage.

Conclusion:
It was shown that three distinct kinds of B cell stimulatory factors, i.e. i) B cell specific growth

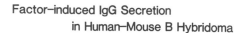

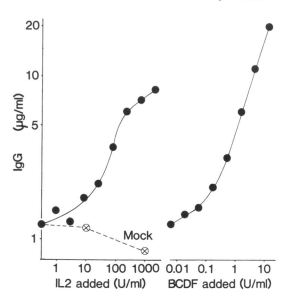

Fig.4.   Induction of IgG in a human B hybrid clone with
recombinant IL-2.

factor (BCGF-I or BSF-p1), ii) B cell specific growth and
differentiation factor (BCGF-II or BGDF) and iii) B cell
specific differentiation factor (BCDF), are required for
the maximum activation of human B cells into Igs-
secreting cells. HTLV-transformed T cell lines secreting
a relatively large amount of BCGF-II or BCDF have been
established.   By employing a HTLV-transformed T cell
line, TCL-Na1, BCDF has been highly purified to an
apparent homogeneity. BCDF is responsible for the final
maturation of activated B cells and induces a high-rate
transcription of mRNA for secretory type heavy chains.

By employing a monoclonal B hybrid clone and recombinant IL-2, a direct effect of IL-2 on B cells to induce Ig-secretion was demonstrated.   IL-2 was shown to act directly on activated B cells as one of growth factors as well as differentiation factors.

Isolation and chemical characterization of B cell stimulatory factors and their receptors on target cells will provide an essential information for the elucidation of molecular mechanism of B cell activation.

Reference

1) Sugiyama, H., Akira, S., Kikutani, H., Kishimoto, S., Yamamura, Y. and Kishimoto, T.   Nature 303, 812 (1983).

2) Hieter, P.A., Korsmeyer, S.J., Waldmann, T. and Leder, P. Nature 290, 368 (1981).

3) Dutton, R.W., Falkoff, R., Hirst, J.A., Hoffman, M., Kappler, J.W., Kettman, J.R., Lesley, J.R. and Vann, P. Prog.Immunol. 1, 355 (1971).

4) Schimpl, A. and Wecker, E.   Nature New Biology. 237, 15 (1972).

5) Kishimoto, T. and Ishizaka, K. J.Immunol. 111, 1194. (1973).

6) Rubin, A.S. and Coombs, A.H. J.Immunol. 108, 1597 (1972).

7) Amerding, D. and Katz, D.H. J.Exp.Med. 140, 19 (1974).

8) Kishimoto, T. and Ishizaka, K. J.Immunol. 144, 585 (1975)

9) Kishimoto, T., Miyake, T., Nishizawa, Y., Watanabe, T. and Yamamura, Y. J.Immunol. 155, 1179 (1975).

10) Parker, D.C., Fothergill, J.J. and Wadsworth, D.C. J.Immunol. 123, 931 (1979).

11) Yoshizaki, K., Nakagawa, T., Kaieda, T., Muraguchi, A., Yamamura, Y. and Kishimoto, T. J.Immunol. 128, 1296 (1982).

12) Okada, M., Sakaguchi, N., Yoshimura, N., Hara, H., Shimizu, K., Yoshida, N., Yoshizaki, K., Kishimoto, S., Yamamura, Y. and Kishimoto, T. J.Exp.Med. 157, 583 (1983).

13) Butler, J.L., Muraguchi, A., Clifford, H. and Fauci, A.S. J.Exp.Med. 157, 60 (1983).

14) Butler, J.L., Falkoff, R.J.M. and Fauci, A.S. Proc.Natl.Acad.Sci.,USA 81, 2475 (1984).

15) Muraguchi, A., Kishimoto, T., Miki, Y., Kuritani,
     T., Kaieda, T., Yoshizaki, K. and Yamamura, Y.
     J.Immunol. 127, 412 (1981).
16) Miki, Y., Kishi, H., Muraguchi, A., Kishimoto, S.,
     Yamamura, Y. and Kishimoto, T. J.Immunol. 128,
     675 (1983).
17) Kishi, H., Miki, Y., Kikutani, H., Yamamura, Y.
     and Kishimoto, T. J.Immunol. 131, 1961 (1983).
18) Kishimoto, T., Miki, Y., Kishi, H., Muraguchi, A.,
     Kishimoto, S. and Yamamura, Y. J.Immunol. 129,
     1367 (1982).
19) Kaieda, T., Okada, M., Yoshimura, N., Kishimoto,
     S., Yamamura, Y. and Kishimto, T. J.Immunol. 129,
     46 (1982).
20) Yoshizaki, K., Nakagawa, T., Fukunaga, K., Kaieda,
     T., Maruyama, S., Kishimoto, S., Yamamura, Y. and
     Kishimoto, T. J.Immunol. 130, 1241 (1983).
21) Swain, S.L., Howard, M., Kappler, J., Marrack, P.,
     Watson, J., Booth, R., Wetzel, G.D. and Dutton,
     R.W. J.Exp.Med. 158, 822 (1983).
22) Melchers, F., Adnersson, J., Lernhardt, W. and
     Schreier, M.H. Eur.J.Immunol. 10, 679 (1980).
23) Pike, B.L., Vaux, D.L., Clark-Lewis, I., Schrader,
     J.W. and Nossal, G.J.V.   proc.Natl.Acad.Sci.,USA
     79, 6350 (1982).
24) Takatsu, K., Tanaka, K., Tominaga, A., Kumahara, Y.
     and Hamaoka, T. J.Immunol. 125, 2646 (1980).
25) Taniguchi, T., Matsui, H., Fujita, T., Takaoka, C.,
     Kashima, N., Yoshimoto, R. and Hamuro, J. Nature
     302, 305 (1983).

THE HUMAN B CELL CYCLE: ACTIVATION, PROLIFERATION, AND DIFFERENTIATION

Julian L. Ambrus, Jr., and Anthony S. Fauci

Laboratory of Immunoregulation, National Institute of Allergy and Infectious Diseases, National Institutes of Health, Bethesda, Maryland 20205

INTRODUCTION

The full expression of a competent immune response, either cell mediated or humoral, requires the precise cooperation of a number of cell types which communicate either by cell-to-cell contact or by soluble immunoregulatory factors. With regard to the humoral immune response, B lymphocytes play the central role as they progress through the cell cycle from the resting to the fully differentiated state whereby they evolve into immunoglobulin (Ig)-secreting cells. Dutton et al.[1] first suggested that soluble helper factors, presumably produced by T lymphocytes, could activate B cells to become Ig-secreting cells. Several laboratories have subsequently been involved in delineating the events which occur between activation of B cells and their production of Ig. Kishimoto et al.[2] demonstrated in the rabbit model that the crosslinkage of surface Ig by anti-Ig combined with T cell-derived helper factors could induce B cells to produce Ig. This was confirmed in the murine system by Parker et al.[3] and led to the development of a similar model in the human system by Yoshizaki et al.[4] and by our own laboratory[5] to further study B cell function. This model basically maintains that resting B cells can be activated by antigen or other surface Ig crosslinking agents to express receptors for growth factors. In the presence of growth factors, B cells enter S phase and express receptors for

differentiation factors. In the presence of differentiation
factors, these cells produce and secrete Ig.

Human B cell activation in most antigen nonspecific in
vitro studies is initiated by two surface Ig crosslinking
agents, F(ab')$_2$ fragments of goat antihuman μ chain
(anti-μ)[6] and Staphylococcus aureus Cowan strain I (SAC)[7].
Resting cells (G$_0$ phase) exposed to one of these agents
sequentially express a number of activation markers,
including 4F2 and 5E9 (the transferrin receptor)[8,9,10].
Both of these markers are expressed before S phase. B cells
express the 4F2 marker early in G$_1$ phase and are already
responsive to B cell growth factors (BCGF). In contrast, B
cells express the 5E9 marker in late G$_1$ phase and are
responsive to different BCGF (see below).

B CELL GROWTH FACTORS

Early studies of B cell growth utilized crude
supernatants from mixed lymphocyte cultures as a source of
BCGF[11]. Because these supernatants inevitably contained a
wide variety of factors, it was unclear whether BCGF and T
cell growth factor, now called interleukin-2 (IL-2), were in
fact distinct lymphokines. Although IL-2 and BCGF were
found to be biochemically similar[12], their existence as two
distinct factors has been supported by several lines of
evidence: (1) IL-2-dependent T cell lines can absorb out
IL-2 activity but not BCGF activity from crude mixed
lymphocyte culture supernatants[12-14], (2) T-T hybridomas
have been established which produce BCGF in the absence of
IL-2[15,16], and (3) several studies have demonstrated that
highly purified IL-2 or recombinant IL-2 cannot induce B
cell proliferation in the conventional BCGF
assay[13,14,17,18]. Subsequently, several laboratories have
demonstrated that there are at least two different BCGF.
Swain et al.[19] reported a 50-70 kd BCGF from the Dennert
line which maintains the growth of the BCL$_1$ tumor line in
vitro, and an 18 kd BCGF which enhances the proliferation of
anti-μ-stimulated normal B cells. Yoshizaki et al.[14]
reported the production of a 50 kd BCGF by a human helper T
cell clone and a 17 kd BCGF by phytohemagglutinin
(PHA)-stimulated peripheral T cells which could act
synergistically on normal anti-Ig-stimulated B cells. We
have reported an 18 kd BCGF produced by a human T-T

hybridoma[15] and a 60 kd BCGF produced by a human T cell
line[20] (Table 1); these factors can act synergistically on
normal, small anti-μ-stimulated human B cells. Our T cell
line-derived factor acts perferentially, but not
exclusively, on large in vivo activated B cells and may,
therefore, be specific either for a particular stage in the
B cell cycle and/or a particular subset of B cells.

B CELL DIFFERENTIATION FACTORS

Differentiation of proliferating B cells has long been
felt to be dependent upon antigen nonspecific B cell
differentiation factors (BCDF), also known as T
cell-replacing factors[1,21-23]. Human T-T hybridomas have
been used by Okada et al.[16] and by our laboratory[24] to
produce BCDF. These factors are distinct from BCGF as
evidenced by the fact that the BCDF-responsive cell line
CESS can absorb BCDF but not BCGF activity from the
hybridoma supernatant. In contrast, anti-μ-activated B

TABLE 1
HUMAN BCGF*

	3B3 or $2B_{11}$ (BCGF 1)	Namalva or T-ALL (factor) (BCGF II)
Source	T-T hybridoma	B or T cell lymphoma line
Molecular weight	~ 20,000	60,000
Isoelectric point	6.3-6.6	6.7-7.8
Activtity on anti-μ stimulated small B cells	++++	++
Activity on unstimulated large B cells	+	++++

*Taken from ref. 24.

cells absorb BCGF but not BCDF activity from hybridoma
supernatant[24] (Table 2). In vivo activated B cells obtained
from normal volunteers immunized with keyhole limpet
hemocyanin or tetanus toxoid can be triggered in vitro to
produce specific antibody by BCDF alone[25]. This suggests
that the clonally expanded antigen-specific B cells express
receptors for the antigen-nonspecific, major
histocompatibility complex-nonrestricted factor BCDF.
Isotype-specific BCDF have been described for IgE in the rat
system[26], IgG in the mouse system[27], and IgA in both the
mouse[28] and human[29] systems. Recently, Hirano et al.[30] have
shown that two distinct, sequentially acting BCDF exist in
the supernatant of PHA-stimulated mononuclear tonsillar
cells. Both of these factors must act on SAC-activated B
cells to produce maximal amounts of IgG.

OTHER B CELL-INDUCING FACTORS

        The role of other well-characterized lymphokines in the
activation, proliferation, and differentiation of B cells
has been of interest to several laboratories. IL-1 has been
shown to effect the proliferation of both murine[31] and

TABLE 2
ABSORPTION OF BCGF AND BCDF ACTIVITIES
FROM THE SUPERNATANT OF THE HUMAN T-T HYBRIDOMA 7D$_5$*

Control activity	Cells used for absorption			
	None	Anti-µ stimulated B cells	PHA stimulated T cells	CESS
% BCGF	100	14	98	96
% BCDF	100	85	102	2

human[32] B cells. However, IL-2 does not directly induce the
proliferation of resting human B cells, and although IL-2
can synergize somewhat with anti-μ in the induction of
proliferation of human B cells, it does not enhance the
proliferation of B cells which are proliferating maximally
in response to BCGF[32]. IL-1 can enhance the production of
Ig induced by BCDF in both murine[33] and human[34] systems but
is probably not a requirement for B cell differentiation to
occur. In contrast, Lipsky et al.[35] found in the human
system that antibody to IL-1 could block Ig production by
pokeweed mitogen (PWM)-driven peripheral blood mononuclear
cells. However, this discrepancy may reflect certain
peculiarities of the PWM-driven system which is a T cell and
monocyte-dependent system.

THE ROLE OF IL-2 IN THE B CELL CYCLE

The ability of IL-2 to directly affect B cells has been
a source of considerable controversy. Swain et al.[36] and
Marrack et al.[37] suggested that IL-2 may play a role in B
cell responses, while Kishimoto et al.[38] found no effect of
purified or recombinant IL-2 on B cell lines. However,
Korsmeyer et al.[39] recently demonstrated IL-2 receptors on
hairy cell leukemia B cells. Muraguchi et al. (manuscript
submitted) in our laboratory have found that
anti-μ-activated B cells express receptors for IL-2. These
receptors are similar to the IL-2 receptors on T cells as
demonstrated by immunoprecipitation although they occur in
fewer numbers and with lower binding affinities than the
receptors on PHA-stimulated T cell blasts. Highly purified
human B cells have been prepared by Lê thi Bich-Thuy in our
laboratory and were found to respond to high doses of
recombinant IL-2 with enhanced proliferation. These cells
remain 95% surface Ig positive after 6 days in culture.
Furthermore, the addition of up to 2.5% T cells to these
purified B cells did not affect their proliferation in
response to IL-2 (Lê thi Bich-Thuy et al., manuscript
submitted). In addition, Muraguchi et al.[18] have
demonstrated direct stimulation by IL-2 of the human T cell
leukemia/lymphoma virus (HTLV)-I transformed B cell line
HS-1. However, it is unclear at present whether this line
is merely the expansion of a small subpopulation of B cells
which can respond to IL-2 normally or is an aberrantly
behaving, virally infected B cell population.

B CELL-DERIVED BCGF

Besides T cell- and monocyte-derived lymphokines,
several laboratories have recently been studying B
cell-derived lymphokines. Clark-Lewis et al.[40] noted the
production of IL-1, T cell replacing factor, colony
stimulation factor, and P cell stimulation factor by the
murine B cell line WEHI-231.1. Yoshizaki et al.[41]
demonstrated the production of BCDF by a subclone of the
Epstein-Barr virus (EBV)-transformed cell line CESS. During
our studies on the human B cell cycle, several observations
suggested to us that B cells themselves might be capable of
elaborating factors which support the growth and/or
differentiation of B cells: (1) the ability of B cell
lymphomas/leukemias to induce diffuse immunologic
abnormalities, (2) the density dependence of several B cell
lines[42,43], and (3) the ability of SAC-activated B cells to
respond to BCDF in the absence of exogenous BCGF[44]. We thus
screened a panel of B cell lines to determine if in fact
certain of these lines secreted BCGF. We found that certain
EBV-positive and EBV-negative B cell lines could be induced
to produce BCGF in the presence of PHA (Ambrus and Fauci,
manuscript submitted). The BCGF produced by these lines has
a molecular weight of 60 kd and isoelectric points of 6.7
and 7.8. This B cell-derived BCGF enhances the
proliferation of large in vivo activated B cells more than
that of small anti-μ-stimulated B cells (i.e., activated in
vitro). Furthermore, this BCGF manifests synergy with the
20 kd BCGF produced by the T-T hybridoma $2B_{11}$[15] in enhancing
the proliferation of small anti-μ-stimulated B cells. Thus,
B cells clearly can produce factors to regulate some of
their own functions.

FACTORS WHICH DIRECTLY ACTIVATE B CELLS

Factors which directly activate B cells in an antigen
nonspecific manner and are produced by peripheral blood
mononuclear cells are being studied both in the murine and
human systems. Sidman et al. (45) and Howard et al. (46)
described a factor, BMF, found in the supernatant of
antigen-stimulated helper T cell lines or the supernatant of
EL-4 which can activate resting B cells and cause them to
produce Ig in the absence of proliferation. We (Bowen
et al., manuscript in preparation) have been studying an

~ 10 kd factor produced by a T4+ lymphoma line which can
activate resting B cells and induce them to a state of
responsiveness to BCGF (this line also produces a 60 kd
BCGF). However, this factor does not cause terminal
differentiation of B cells as noted in the mouse models.

CONCLUSIONS

The study of lymphokines has expanded our knowledge of
the various aspects of B cell activation, proliferation, and
differentation. Many cell types are involved with the
production of these lymphokines including B cells.
Purification of these lymphokines in large quantities will
eventually allow not only exact comparisons of these various
lymphokines but also dissection of the various aspects of B
cell function at the molecular biologic level.

REFERENCES

1. Dutton, R. W. et al. Prog. Immunol. 1, 335-369 (1971).
2. Kishomoto, T. et al. J. Immunol. 115, 1179-1184 (1975).
3. Parker, D. C., Fothergill, J. J., Wadsworth, D. C.
   J. Immunol. 123, 931-941 (1979).
4. Yoshizaki, Y. et al. J. Immunol. 128, 1296-1391 (1982).
5. Muraguchi, A., Butler, J. L., Kehrl, J. H., & Fauci,
   A. S. J. exp. Med. 157, 530-546 (1983).
6. Sieckmann, D. G. Immunol. Rev. 52, 181-210 (1980).
7. Romagnani, S. et al. J. Immunol. 127, 1307-1313 (1981).
8. Haynes, B. F. et al. J. Immunol. 126, 1409-1414 (1981).
9. Haynes, B. F. et al. J. Immunol. 127, 347-351 (1981).
10. Kehrl, J. H., Muraguchi, A., Butler, J. L., Falkoff,
    R. J. M. & Fauci, A. S. Immunol. Rev. 78, 75-96
    (1984).
11. Muraguchi, A. & Fauci, A. S. J. Immunol. 129, 1104-1108
    (1982).
12. Muraguchi, A., Kasahara, T., Oppenheim, J. J. & Fauci,
    A. S. J. Immunol. 129, 2486-2489 (1982).
13. Maizel, A. et al. Proc. natn. Acad. Sci. U.S.A. 79,
    5998-6002 (1982).
14. Yoshizaki, K. et al. J. Immunol. 130, 1241-1246 (1983).
15. Butler, J. L., Muraguchi, A., Lane, H. C. & Fauci,
    A. S. J. exp. Med. 157, 60-68 (1983).

16. Okada, M. et al. Proc. natn. Acad. Sci. U.S.A. 78, 7717-7721 (1981).
17. Farrar, J. J. et al. Immunol. Rev. 63, 129-166 (1982).
18. Muraguchi, A., Kehrl, J. H., Longo, D. L., Volkman, D. J. & Fauci, A. S. Fed. Proc. 43, 1676 (1984).
19. Swain, S. L. et al. J. exp. Med. 158, 822-835 (1983).
20. Ambrus, J. L., Jr., & Fauci, A. S. J. clin. Invest. (in the press).
21. Dutton, R. W. Transplant. Rev. 23, 66-77 (1975).
22. Shimpl, A. & Wecker, E. Nature 237, 15-17 (1972).
23. Shimpl, A. & Wecker, E. Transplant. Rev. 23, 176-180 (1972).
24. Butler, J. L., Falkoff, R. J. M. & Fauci, A. S. Proc. natn. Acad. Sci. U.S.A. 81, 2475-2478 (1984).
25. Peters, M. & Fauci, A. S. J. Immunol. 130, 178-180 (1983).
26. Kishimoto, T. & Ishizaka, K. J. Immunol. 114, 1177-1184 (1975).
27. Isakson, P., Pure, E., Vitetta, E. S., Krammer, P. H. J. exp. Med. 155, 734-748 (1982).
28. Kiyana, H. et al. J. exp. Med. 156, 1115-1130 (1982).
29. Mayer, L., Fu, S. M. & Kunkel J. exp. Med. 156, 1860-1865 (1982).
30. Hirano, T., Teranishi, T., Lin, B., Onoue, K. J. Immunol. 133, 798-802 (1984).
31. Howard, M. et al. J. exp. Med. 157, 1529-1543 (1983).
32. Falkoff, R. J. M. et al. J. Immunol. 131, 801-805 (1983).
33. Liebson, H. J., Marrack, P., Kappler, J. J. Immunol. 129, 1398-1402 (1982).
34. Falkoff, R. J. M., Butler, J. L., Dinarello, C. A. & Fauci, A. S. J. Immunol. 133, 692-696 (1984).
35. Lipsky, P. E., Thompson, P. A., Roschwasser, L. J. & Dinarello, C. A. J. Immunol. 130, 2708-2714 (1983).
36. Swain, S., Dennert, G., Warmer, J. F., Dutton, R. W. Proc. natn. Acad. Sci. U.S.A. 78, 2517-2521 (1981).
37. Marrack, P. et al. Immunol. Rev. 63, 33-49 (1982).
38. Kishimoto, T. et al. Immunol. Rev. 78, 97-118 (1984).
39. Korsmeyer, S. J. et al. Proc. natn. Acad. Sci. U.S.A. 80, 4522-4526 (1983).
40. Clark-Lewis, I., Schrader, J. W., Wu, Y., Harris, A. S. Cell. Immunol. 69, 196-200 (1982).
41. Yoshizaki, K. et al. J. Immunol. 132, 2948-2954 (1984).

42. Blazar, B. A., Sutton, L. M., Strome, M. Cancer Res.
     43, 4562-4568 (1983).
43. Gordon, J. et al. J. exp. Med. 159, 1554-1559 (1984).
44. Falkoff, R. J. M., Zhu, L. P. & Fauci, A. S.
     J. Immunol. 129, 97-102 (1982).
45. Sidman, C., Paige, C. J., Schreier, M. H. J. Immunol.
     132, 209-222 (1984).

POSSIBLE AUTOREGULATORY ROLES OF INTERLEUKIN 1 FOR NORMAL

HUMAN EPITHELIAL CELLS, MONOCYTES AND B LYMPHOCYTES

J. J. Oppenheim[1], K. Matsushima, K. Onozaki
A. Procopio, and G. Scala[2]
[1]Laboratory of Molecular Immunoregulation,
NCI, NIH, Frederick, MD and [2]Institute of
Biological Chemistry, 2nd University Medical
School, Napoli, Italy

Of all the hormones and growth factors that have been tested only interleukin 1 and 2 (IL 1 and 2) have been documented to be costimulants of thymocyte proliferation. Consequently the operational definition of IL 1 is that of a comitogenic factor for thymocytes that, in contrast with IL 2, does not support the growth of IL 2 dependent lymphocyte cell lines. Another difference between these two cytokines is that IL 2 is produced only by T lymphocytes and some large granular lymphocytes (LGL) (1), whereas IL 1 is produced by many types of cells including monocyte/macrophages, LGL, keratinocytes, mesangial cells of the kidney, astrocytes, some EBV transformed B cell lines fibroblasts, melanoma cell lines, endothelial cells, and glioma cell lines (as reviewed in 2). Although some of the IL 1 activities derived from non-macrophage cell sources have been partially purified, their precise relationship to macrophage-derived IL 1 will be clarified only when their amino acid sequences become known.

Many pathophysiological roles have been proposed for IL 1 in immunity, inflammation and even wound healing. On the basis of its amplifying effects on the growth and differentiation of T and B lymphocytes, IL 1 certainly may serve as an important amplifier of immunity (3). The stimulating effects of IL 1 on the growth and functions of fibroblasts, endothelial cells, the hypothalamic fever center, neutrophils, hepatocytes, LGL, synovial cells,

muscle cells, mesangial cells, osteoclasts and chondrocytes certainly suggest that IL 1 functions as an important promulgator of inflammatory reactions (as reviewed
in 4). The diversity of target cells of IL 1, the capacity of IL 1 to function as an intercellular messenger and
the presence of IL 1 activity in urine (5) all provide a
basis for the suggestion that IL 1 acts as a regulatory
hormone.

     A review of the list of cell types that produce and
respond to IL 1 identifies a number of cell types that
are capable of both functions (e.g. fibroblasts, endothelial cells, LGL, mesangial cells). This suggests that
IL 1-like factors may also have autoregulatory roles. In
this paper we will show that human B lymphocytes which
have been reported to respond to IL 1 (6), also can be
stimulated to produce an IL 1-like factor. Furthermore,
murine epithelial cells and human monocytes as well as
producing IL 1 (2,4) also react to IL 1; epithelial cells
by producing collagen and monocytes by killing tumor cells.

IL 1 Stimulation of Murine Epithelial Cells

     Collagen type IV, a major constituent of basement
membrane (7) is commonly found at sites of potential IL 1
producing cells in the placenta, kidney, cornea, endothelium of blood vessels, gingival epithelium and skin (8).
We therefore, hypothesized that IL 1 may also induce
collagen type IV production by epithelial cells at these
sites. Primary cultures of normal murine mammary epithelial cells were stimulated by IL 1 derived from silica
stimulated human peripheral blood monocyte (PBM) cultures.
Crude culture supernatants of silica stimulated PBM failed
to augment epithelial cell production of collagen type IV.
However, IL 1 partially purified by ammonium sulfate precipitation followed by Sephacryl S200 gel chromatography
and isoelectrofocusing did possess considerable epithelial
cell stimulating activity suggesting the elimination of
coexistant and unidentified inhibitors by these procedures.
In addition, more purified IL 1 also was capable of
stimulating collagen type IV production by the epithelial
cells. The thymocyte comitogenic and epithelial cell
stimulating activities that were present in supernatants
of cultured PBM consistently cochromatographed after se-

quential purification by isoelectrofocusing, anion exchange
(AX300) on high performance liquid chromatography (HPLC)
followed by a final gel filtration using TSK 3000.

Table 1:   Effect of HPLC (TSK 3000) Purified Human IL 1 on
           Type IV Collagen Production by Normal Murine
           Epithelial Cells

Doses of IL 1	Collagen	(% of Control)
None	631*	–
0.35 units/ml	1,677	266**
0.070 "	1,320	209**
0.014 "	1,703	270**
0.007 "	965	153
0.0035 "	996	163

*cpm of ^{3}H lysine incorporated by collagenase susceptible
 fraction of TCA precipitable protein.

**Greater than two-fold increases over control were
  significant (p <0.05).

This purification scheme yielded only two bands on SDS-
PAGE by silver staining in the region of IL 1. Although
not completely pure, such preparations of IL 1 were presumably free of fetal calf serum derived EGF which also
has the capacity to promote epithelial cell production of
collagen type IV.   Furthermore, of all the fibroblast
growth factor (e.g. IL 1, PDGF, FGF, EGF and MSA) only
IL 1 also acted as a comitogen for thymocytes, and as a
stimulant for epithelial cells (9).

    The assay for epithelial cell collagen production was
100 times more sensitive to IL 1 than the thymocyte comitogenic assay.   In contrast, the in vivo fever inducing and
acute phase protein-inducing capacities of IL 1 are about
10-100 times less sensitive than the thymocyte assay (10).
The dramatic enhancement of epithelial cell function by
relatively minute levels of IL 1 may contribute not only to
inflamation induced thickening of basement membrane, but
may also play a role in repair processes as well as in the
maintainance of normal basement membrane production.   Since

keratinocytes, mucosal and corneal epithelial cells can all
produce IL 1-like activities, it is plausible that IL 1 may
function as an autocrine signal for epithelial tissues.

IL 1 stimulation of Human Monocytes

It has been observed that partially purified IL 1 is
a chemoattractant for human monocytes (11) and that monocytes can produce PGE_2 in response to IL 1 (12). Since
monocytes produce IL 1 constitutively (13) low levels of
IL 1 activity may always be available in monocyte/macro-
phage-rich tissues. IL 1 may therefore be able to act as
an autocrine signal for monocytes. We therefore examined
the possibility that IL 1 may promulgate human monocyte
tumoricidal functions.

For this purpose preparations of $\geq$ 97% peripheral
blood human monocytes (PBM) were obtained by sequential
Ficoll-Hypaque and Percoll gradient centrifugation and
selection of cells adherent to flat microtiter wells.
Such monocytes were incubated for 24 hrs w/wo stimulants
and supplemented with ^{125}IUdR labelled human melanoma
(A375) target cells for another 24 hrs. The nonadherent
tumor cells were then washed off and the extent of tumor
cell lysis by monocytes was assessed 48 hrs later by
measuring the residual ^{125}IUdR remaining adherent to
the wells as follows:

$$\% \text{ cytotoxicity} = \left(1.0 - \frac{\text{cpm in target cells + test PBM}}{\text{cpm in target cells + control PBM}}\right) \times 100$$

The ^{125}IUdR released into the supernatant was shown to
be associated either with non-viable cells and debris or
in a soluble form (14).

It was observed that partially purified human IL 1,
prepared as previously described (15), markedly increased
monocyte mediated killing of A375 melanoma cells in this
long term in vitro cytotoxicity assay. Concentrations as
low as 2 units IL 1/ml were effective. The effect on
monocytes achieved by our preparations of IL 1 could not
be attributed to contaminating endotoxin since it was
blocked by polymyxin B (20 ug/ml). The IL 1 preparation
was also free of endotoxin by the limulus lysate assay,

and did not exhibit any antiviral activity. Consequently,
neither interferon nor endotoxin were responsible for
these results. Treatment of the adherent PBM with monoclonal antibody (3G8) and rabbit complement to eliminate
LGL with natural killer activity also did not reduce the
observed effect of IL 1 on cytotoxicity. The thymocyte
comitogenic activity of IL 1 coeluted exactly with monocyte cytocidal activity from the final TSK 3000 gel HPLC,
supporting the hypothesis that IL 1 is responsible for
promulgating monocyte tumoricidal activities.

The mechanism of IL 1 enhancement of monocyte cytotoxicity was investigated. Our studies showed that indomethacin could block IL 1 induced monocyte cytotoxicity,
whereas addition of exogenous PGE_2 and PGE_1 but not $PGF_2\alpha$
could promote monocyte cytotoxicity. Since PGE_1 and
PGE_2 but not $PGF_2\alpha$, stimulate adenyl cyclase, this data
suggested that the intracellular messenger, cAMP, might
participate in IL 1 induction of monocyte cytotoxicity.
This hypothesis was supported by the observations that
theophylline, which reduces degradation of cAMP, and
dibutyryl cAMP both promoted monocyte cytotoxicity.
Control studies indicated that dibutyryl cAMP, PGE_2,
theophylline and indomethacin had no direct lytic effects
on tumor cells. Thus, the augmenting effect of IL 1, on
monocyte tumoricidal activity appears to be sequentially
mediated by PGE and cAMP.

It is perplexing that IL 1 which acts as a second
augmenting signal in promoting the reactions of lymphocytes, appears to be able by itself to activate monocytes
to be tumoricidal. However, since the IL 1 preparation
was not completely pure we cannot rule out a role for a
contaminant. It is also possible that a fetal calf or
human serum component served as cofactors for IL 1 during
the in vitro incubation. It is more likely, since fresh
PB monocytes have been shown to be spontaneously cytotoxic
(16) that monocytes are induced by a prior in vivo signal
to become tumoricidal. Thus, IL 1 may function as a
second signal that retains the cytocidal functions of
cultured monocytes at their prior in vivo level. This
hypothesis is supported by data showing that the effect
of IL 1 is maximal when it is added at the onset of incubation and decreases progressively to background levels
if it is added after the second day of preincubation.

Table 2:   Effect of Increasing Duration of Preincubation
           in Medium on Capacity of IL 1 or Lymphokines to
           Promote Monocyte Cytotoxicity

Duration of Preincubation in Days	Medium	24 hr Incubation in IL 1 (8 u/ml)	Lymphokines[**] (1:5 dil.)
0	35[*]	73	65
1	29	47	50
2	15	24	29
3	7	10	28
4	9	15	28

[*]% of ^{125}IUdR released by A375 human melanoma cells after
72 hrs of incubation with preincubated monocytes.
Melanoma cells incubated for 72 hrs with fresh human PBM
released 63% of their ^{125}IUdR due to spontaneous monocyte
cytoxicity. Changes in cytotoxicity of $\geq$ 10% are significant (p <0.05).

[**]Lymphokines consisted of supernatants of concanavalin A
(5 ug/ml) stimulated human mononuclear cells.

In contrast, "aged" monocytes that were preincubated in
medium for up to four days still could be induced to
become moderately cytotoxic for melanoma cells by activating agents such as endotoxin or an unfractionated
lymphokine containing supernatant. Control supernatants
as well as IL 1 were inactive. Since in vitro
"aged" monocytes apparently cannot be stimulated to become
cytocidal by IL 1, IL 1 presumably functions predominantly as a second signal that maintains preexisting cytotoxic
activity of monocytes.

     The identity of the prior in vivo "first" signals that
induce monocyte cytotoxicity remains unclear. Since low
levels of gamma interferon (IFN γ) are probably continually
produced in vivo (17) and since IFN γ exhibits macrophage
activating factor (MAF) activity for human monocytes in
short term cytocidal assays (18), IFN γ is a plausible
candidate. However, IFN γ by itself is not active in
stimulating monocytes to be tumoricidal in the longer
term ^{125}IUdR release assay, unless low doses of endotoxin

are also present (19). However, we could not demonstrate
any interaction between IL 1 and IFN γ in our assay for
monocyte cytotoxicity (unpub. data). Thus, IL 1 apparently promulgates monocyte cytotoxicity independent of
IFN γ and the proposed in vivo "MAF" which induces the
monocytes to be cytotoxic remains to be identified.

IL 1 Production by Human B Lymphocytes

There is considerable evidence that IL 1 can augment
both proliferation antibody production by B lymphocytes
(20). IL 1-like factors have also been reported to be
produced by some but not all EBV transformed human B
cell lines (21). In order to ascertain whether IL 1 can
act as a potential autoregulatory signal for B lymphocytes,
we have therefore investigated whether normal human B
lymphocytes produce an IL 1-like factor with thymocyte
comitogenic activity.

A major hurdle to surmount for such a study is to
obtain purified normal B lymphocytes that are rigorously depleted of other IL 1 producing cells such as macrophages and LGL. Human peripheral blood B lymphocytes
were purified by gradient centrifugation on Ficoll-Hypaque
followed by depletion of T lymphocytes by two rounds of
E-rosetting with AET treated SRBC (22,23). The non-
rosetted cells were isolated from Ficoll-Hypaque and
fractionated further by a three step discontinuous gradient of Percoll. This yielded an upper low density fraction which was enriched in monocytes (>90%), a second
fraction consisting of a mixture of <5% monocytes, 5-20%
LGL and ~70% B lymphoblasts (B_L) and a third high density
cell layer containing small resting B (B_S) lymphocytes
(97 $\pm$ 2% SIg$^+$) as determined by a fluorescense activated
cell sorter (FACS). The B_L and B_S fractions were further
treated with a cocktail of monoclonal antibodies (anti-
tac, OKT11 and T101) and rabbit complement to eliminate
any residual contaminating cells. This procedure yielded
cell fractions consisting of $\geq$ 90% B_L and 99% pure B_S
cells respectively. The B_S fraction was devoid of any
monocytes by morphological criteria.

These B cell subpopulations were then incubated with
a variety of stimulants. The culture supernatants of
endotoxin and anti μ stimulated B_L and B_S lymphocytes

both were observed to contain considerable thymocyte
comitogenic activity.

Table 3:   IL 1-like Factor Production by Normal Human
           Peripheral Blood B Lymphocytes

	Medium Alone	LPS 1 ug/ml	anti- μ	
			25 ug/ml	100 ug/ml
B_L *	<1.0 U/ml **	52.2	6.5	33.6
B_S *	<1.0	15.6	10.0	15.6

*1 x 10^6/ml large B lymphocytes (B_L) or small B lymphocytes
(B_S) were cultured in RPMI 1640 and 5% FCS for 48 hr and
the supernatant IL 1-like activity was measured by a
thymocyte comitogenic assay.

**An IL 1 unit equals the reciprocal value of the dilution
at which 50% of the maximal response of thymocytes to a
standard human monocyte-derived IL 1 was obtained.

The apparent molecular weight of B_L and B_S derived thymocyte comitogenic activities were in the 20,000 and 25,000
dalton range respectively by HPLC gel filtration (TSK 3000).
The B cell supernatants did not support the growth of an
IL 2 dependent CTLL-2 cell line. We cannot be certain
that the anti μ antibodies used in this study actually
stimulated B cells to produce the factor since they were
contaminated by $\leq$ 100 ng/ml endotoxin. Nevertheless,
these observations suggest that normal human B lymphocytes can produce such a factor.

     In conclusion IL 1 appears more and more to have the
properties of a classical hormone. Il 1 is a peptide
which functions as an intercellular messenger and acts
on many target cells. Since systemic administration of
IL 1 results in fever and elevation of serum acute
phase proteins and IL 1 has also been recovered from
inflammatory sites, IL 1 appears to be able to act in
vivo over long as well as short distances. In contrast
with hormones, which are generally produced by discreet
glands, many different tissues appear to produce IL 1.
Although it remains to be established whether the same

cell that produces IL 1 can also react to it, it appears that several additional cell types including epithelial, B lymphocyte and monocytic can both produce and react to this cytokine.

References:

1. Scala, G., Allavena, P., Djeu, J.Y., Kasahara, T., Ortaldo, J. R., Herberman, R. B. & Oppenheim, J. J. Nature 309, 56-59 (1984).

2. Oppenheim, J. J., Scala, G., Kuang, Y. K., Matsushima, K., Sztein, M. B. & Steeg, P. S. Prog. in Immunol. 5, 285-294 (1983).

3. Smith, K. A., Lachman, L. B., Oppenheim, J. J. & Favata, M. F. J. Exp. Med. 151, 1551-1556 (1980).

4. Oppenheim, J. J. & Gery, I. in T Lymphocytes Today (ed Inglis, J. R.) 89-95 (Elsevier, Amsterdam, 1983).

5. Kimball, E. S., Pickeral, S. F., Oppenheim, J. J. & Rossio, J. L. J. Immunol. 133, 256-260 (1984).

6. Falkoff, R.J.M., Butler, J. L., Diharello, C. A. & Fauci, A. S. J. Immunol. 133, 692-696 (1984).

7. Timpl, R., Glanville, R. W., Wick, G. & Martin, G. R. Immunology 38, 109-112 (1979).

8. Laurie, G. W., Leblond, C. P. & Martin, G. R. J. Cell. Biol. 95, 340-346 (1982).

9. Matsushima, K., Bano, M., Kidwell, W. & Oppenheim, J. J. J. Immunol., in press.

10. Dinarello, C. A. Rev. Infectious Dis. 6, 51-95 (1984).

11. Luger, T. A., Charon, J. A. & Oppenheim, J. J. J. Immunol. 81, 187-190 (1983).

12. Dinarello,, C. A., Marnoy, S. A. & Rosenwasser, L. J. in Interleukins, Lymphokines and Cytokines (eds Oppenheim, J. J. & Cohen, S.) 769-772 (Academic Press, New York, 1983).

13. Treves, A. J., Barak, V., Tal, T. & Fuks, Z. Eur. J.
     Immunol. 13, 647-651 (1983).

14. Kleinerman, E. S., Schroitt, A.J., Fogler, W. E. &
     Fidler, I. J. J. Clin. Invest. 72, 304-315 (1983).

15. Oppenheim, J. J., Onozaki, K. & Matsushima, K. in
     Fourth Conference on Mononuclear Phagocytes (ed
     Van Furth, R.) in press.

16. Fischer, D. G., Hubbard, W. J. & Koren, H. S. Cell.
     Immunol. 58, 426-435 (1981).

17. Palacios, R., Martinez-Maza, O. & DeLey, M. Eur. J.
     Immunol. 13, 221-225 (1983).

18. Le, J., Prensky, W., Yip, Y. K., Chang, Z., Hoffman,
     T., Stevenson, H. C., Balaes, I., Sadlik, J. R. &
     Vilcek, J. J. Immuno. 131, 2821-2826 (1983).

19. Kleinerman, E. S., Zicht, R., Sarin, P. S., Gallo,
     R. C., Fidler, I. J. Cancer Res., in press.

20. Howard, M. & Paul, W. E., Annu. Rev. Immunol. 1,
     307-333 (1983).

21. Scala, G., Kuang, Y. D., Hall, E., Muchmore, A. V. &
     Oppenheim, J. J. J. Exp. Med. 159, 1637-1652 (1984).

22. Procopio, A.D., Scala, G., Herberman, R. B.,
     Oppenheim, J. J. & Ortaldo, J. R. Fed. Proc. 43,
     1607 (1984).

23. Madsen, M. & Johnsen, H. C. J. Immunol. Meth. 27,
     61-74 (1979).

Acknowledgement:

     We are grateful for the constructive criticisms of
the manuscript to Drs. Scott Durum, Luigi Varesio and
Harriet Gershon and for the last minute secreterial
assistance of Ms. Bobbie Unger.

CLONING OF AN IgE IMMUNOREGULATORY FACTOR

BY EXPRESSION IN MAMMALIAN CELLS

C. Martens, T. Huff[1], P. Jardieu[1], K. Ishizaka[1], K. Moore

DNAX Research Institute of Molecular and Cellular Biology, 1450 Page Mill Road, Palo Alto, CA 94304

[1]Johns Hopkins University, Good Samaritan Hospital, 5601 Loch Raven Blvd., Baltimore, MD 21239

INTRODUCTION

   T lymphocytes and their products regulate synthesis of immunoglobulin by B lymphocytes at several levels. T-cells may help or suppress immune responses in an antigen-specific or non-specific way, or may regulate idiotype or isotype-specific responses. Several researchers have described isotype specific regulation of the synthesis of IgE, IgA, and IgG in rodents as well as humans. Certain characteristics appear to be common to such regulation: the T cells which regulate the synthesis of a heavy-chain isotype by B-cells bear Fc receptors specific for that isotype and these Fc receptor-bearing lymphocytes secrete factors which are active in regulating immunoglobulin synthesis by B-cells. In general, the soluble factors bind specifically to the Fc region of the immunoglobulin isotype which they regulate, and appear to be related structurally to the lymphocyte Fc receptor. We refer to this family of isotype-specific regulatory factors as "immunoglobulin-binding factors", or Ig-BF.

The IgE-specific immunoregulatory factors have been
well characterized in rats by Ishizaka and colleagues (1).
Two factors produced by mesenteric lymph node cells from
parasite infected rats have been described. Both have
affinity for the Fc region of IgE, but they have different
effects on in vitro IgE responses: the IgE-potentiating
factor selectively enhances the IgE response, while IgE-
suppressive factor inhibits the IgE response. These two
factors appear to share some structural characteristics,
including affinity for IgE, molecular size (approx. 13,000
daltons), and some antigenic determinants, but they differ
in glycosylation as reflected by different lectin affinity
profiles. In fact, the two factors may share the same
precursor molecules, as the nature of the factor obtained
from rat T lymphocytes may be altered simply by changing
culture conditions of the producing cells. For example,
mesenteric lymph node cells cultured with 10 µg/ml ConA
produce IgE-potentiating factor; addition of tunicamycin or
glucocorticoids to these cultures leads to production of
IgE-suppressive factor. Thus, a single T lymphocyte can
produce either the potentiator or the suppressor factor,
and the two factors may be very similar or possibly
identical polypeptide chains which differ in glycosylation
and perhaps in other post-translational modifications.

Recently, Huff et al. (2) have described a rat-mouse T
hybridoma line, 23B6, which produces at least three
IgE-binding factors when cultured in the presence of 3 to
10 µg of IgE per ml of medium. One factor has a molecular
weight of about 13,000 daltons, and is active in
suppressing an in vitro IgE response. A second factor of
about 26,000 daltons does not have potentiating or
suppressing activity, though it binds to IgE. In recent
studies (Jardieu and Ishizaka, unpublished results) a
60,000 dalton IgE-binding factor has also been found to be
secreted by this hybridoma cell line. The possible
precursor/product relationship of these three factors has
not been studied. We chose to study the molecular biology
of the IgE-binding factors produced by the 23B6 hybridoma
by constructing cDNA libraries from RNA isolated from the
hybridoma cells and isolating from those libraries clones
which encode the IgE-binding factors. The data presented

here describe the identification of these clones and some
biochemical characterization of the factors produced from
cDNA templates in mammalian cells, and demonstrate that the
genes which encode an IgE binding factor are a subset of an
endogenous retrovirus-like gene family.

IDENTIFICATION OF IgE-BF cDNA CLONES

To isolate and identify clones which encode IgE-binding
factors, we constructed cDNA libraries using RNA from the
IgE-BF-producing hybridoma cell line 23B6 as template. The
first cDNA library was made in the phage vector λgt10.
Initially, we selected clones from this library using a
"subtraction" probe, that is, a radioactively labeled
first-strand cDNA copy of 23B6 RNA which was hybridized in
liquid phase with an excess of RNA from the fusion partner
cell line, BW5147 (3). Sequences common to 23B6 and BW5147
formed RNA-DNA duplexes, while sequences which were unique
to or more prevalent in the hybridoma remained single-
stranded. These single stranded molecules were
fractionated on hydroxylapatite to isolate the "hybridoma-
enriched" labeled cDNA probe. About 300 λgt10 clones were
isolated from the 23B6 cDNA library, and these phage clones
were recloned as EcoRI fragments into the plasmid vector
pUC8 for ease of handling. These clones were screened by
hybrid selection of 23B6 RNA followed by translation of the
selected RNA in Xenopus oocytes. The oocyte supernatants
were tested for the presence of IgE-binding factor by the
inhibition of IgE-specific rosettes formed between mouse
spleen cells bearing Fc receptors and IgE-coated ox red
blood cells. Several clones were identified which were
active in hybrid selecting RNA which directed synthesis of
IgE-BF in oocytes. The IgE specificity of the oocyte
supernatants was confirmed by demonstrating that rosette-
inhibiting activity could be bound to, and eluted from,
IgE-Sepharose but not IgG-Sepharose.

These results were very encouraging, but hybrid
selection can be misleading if unrelated messages share
some regions of near-homology or if an unrelated, abundant
message physically traps small amounts of active message on

the filter. To confirm that our cDNA clones were active in
encoding the IgE-BF, we constructed a second cDNA library
from 23B6 RNA, this time using the mammalian expression
vector system, pcD. This vector, developed by H. Okayama
(4), allows efficient cloning of full-length cDNA molecules
within SV40 control sequences, and the cloned sequences may
be expressed in cells which constitutively synthesize SV40
T antigen, such as the monkey kidney cell line COS7. This
second cDNA library was screened with pUC8 clone A18, the
largest of the cDNA fragments identified as sharing
homology with IgE-BF genes by hybrid selection and oocyte
injection. About 70 clones were isolated which were
homologous to A18, and these were tested by transfecting
DNA from each clone into COS7 cells for transient
expression, followed by assay of the supernatant fluids for
the presence of IgE-BF. Of the 70 clones tested in this
way, eight were shown to direct synthesis of IgE-Bf in COS7
cells. Again, the IgE-binding activity found in the
supernatants was absorbed specifically to an IgE-Sepharose
column but not to an IgG-Sepharose column.

Four of the IgE-BF produced by cDNA clones by transient
expression in COS7 cells were characterized further. IgE-
binding factors purified from IgE-Sepharose columns were
included in cultures of antigen-primed rat mesenteric lymph
node cells to test for suppression or potentiation of IgE
responses. Table I shows the results: expression of
clones 8.3 and 9.5 in COS7 cells results in IgE-BF which
potentiate the IgE response, increasing the number of
IgE-containing plasma cells about four-fold relative to the
control cultures without added factor. This potentiation
is comparable to that seen when IgE-binding factors from
mesenteric lymph node cells of a parasite infected rat are
included in the culture. The IgE-binding factors produced
by expression of clones 4.2 and 10.2 had little effect on
the in vitro IgE response. None of the factors tested were
active in suppressing the IgE response, and none had any
detectable effect on the IgG2 response. Thus, although the
hybridoma from which the cDNA library was made produces
IgE-suppressive factor and no detectable potentiator
factor, two of these clones, when expressed in a foreign
host cell, potentiate the IgE response.

TABLE I

EFFECT OF IgE-BINDING FACTORS FROM COS7 CELLS ON IN VITRO
IgE   RESPONSES

IgE-BF from	IgE-containing cells (x10^6)	IgG2-containing cells (x10^6)
none	22	120
Nb*-infected rat	84	122
8.3	86	120
9.5	82	115
10.2	36	118
4.2	40	128

*Nb = Nippostrongylus brasiliensis

There are two possible explanations for this result. First, the 23B6 hybridoma may transcribe the genes for potentiator factors, but translation, processing, or secretion of the products may be inhibited. A second explanation is that the IgE-potentiator and IgE-suppressor factors may in fact be encoded by the same message, but differ in features of their post-translational processing depending upon conditions within the host cell. In fact, as described above, several studies have suggested that the two factors are very closely related. Our results support the view that the biological activity of IgE-binding factors is governed by the nature or extent of glycosylation of the same protein precursor, in that factors with potentiator activity have been cloned from a cell line which produces suppressor factor(s). It is likely that the polypeptides translated from these cDNA clones are processed differently in the rat-mouse T cell hybridoma and in the monkey kidney cells, resulting in different biological activities.

BIOCHEMISTRY OF CLONED IgE-BF

We have analyzed the biochemical properties of IgE-

binding factors produced by transient expression of two of
the cDNA clones, 8.3 (a potentiator factor), and 10.2 (a
biologically inactive IgE binding factor) in COS7 cells.
First, molecular sizes of the transient expression
products of these two cDNA clones were determined by gel
filtration, with IgE binding activity monitored by assaying
inhibition of IgE-specific spleen cell rosettes. The
IgE-BF produced by expression of clone 10.2 eluted at
approximately 70,000 daltons. The IgE-BF encoded by 8.3
eluted in two peaks, of about 70,000 and 11,000 daltons;
both of the two factors were active in potentiating an in
vitro IgE response. All three of these IgE-BF bind to
lentil lectin, as do IgE-potentiating factors from other
sources (e.g., rat mesenteric lymph node cells). These
factors are similar in size to some of the IgE binding
species produced by 23B6 (see above); the small size
difference in the small IgE-binding factor (11,000 daltons
from COS7 expressing clone 8.3; 13,000 daltons in 23B6) may
be attributable to differences in glycosylation.

The complete nucleotide sequence of the IgE-potentiator
factor clone 8.3 was determined. The cDNA appears to
encode a polypeptide of 556 amino acids (63,000 daltons),
including two potential sites for N-linked glycosylation
and several possible sites for proteolytic cleavage at
tandem basic amino acid residues. The 11,000 dalton IgE-BF
observed in the 8.3-transfected COS7 cell supernatant is
probably generated by such post-translational cleavage of
the 70,000 dalton factor; clearly the larger molecule is a
precursor of the smaller factor, as the COS7 cells were
transfected with a single cDNA clone.

MOLECULAR CHARACTERIZATION OF CLONES

Restriction map analysis of the eight pcD clones which
encoded IgE-BF in COS7 cells showed that these clones
ranged in size from about 3400 bp to nearly 7000 bp. The
eight clones shared many restriction sites, especially at
the 3' ends, but differed in details of their restriction
maps. Cross-hybridization experiments using restriction
fragments of clone 8.3 as probes showed that the eight

clones shared sequence homology at the 5' and 3' end, with
the longer clones apparently having additional coding
information in the middle.

RNA blot analysis using restriction fragments of clone
8.3 as probes showed that the 23B6 hybridoma transcribes
large amounts of mRNAs which are homologous to the IgE-BF
clone. The sizes of these transcripts ranged from about
3400 bases to about 7000 bases, in good agreement with the
sizes of cDNA clones we isolated. RNA from 23B6 cells
which had not been induced with IgE and were not making
detectable IgE-BF contained essentially the same population
of homologous transcripts. The rat IgE-producing myeloma,
IR162, and rat basophilic leukemia cell line RBL-2H3 did
not contain homologous transcripts. Southern blot analysis
of genomic DNA from rats using fragments of clone 8.3 as
probe showed a fairly simple pattern, with from two to five
bands hybridizing, depending on the restriction enzyme
used. Analysis of mouse genomic DNA and DNA from the 23B6
hybridoma gave a more complex pattern: the sequences
appeared to be highly reiterated, even with short
restriction fragment probes.

HOMOLOGY TO INTRACISTERNAL A PARTICLE GENES

The amino acid sequence predicted by the nucleotide
sequence of clone 8.3 was compared by Dr. Russell Doolittle
to published amino acid sequences in his computer database.
The unexpected result was that the N-terminal 437 amino
acids shared no apparent homology with any published
sequence, but there was a short region (amino acids 438 -
488) of exceptionally high homology to the polymerase gene
products of several retroviruses. This homology,
schematically shown in Figure 1, is found in a region
which is highly conserved among polymerases of retroviruses
of avian, rodent, and primate species. The homology is
found in a part of the polymerase which is cleaved from the
polymerase β subunit to become p32, an endonuclease which
may be important in integration of the retrovirus into the
host genome. We investigated this homology further by
testing for hybridization of fragments of clone 8.3 with

cloned genes from several retroviruses. Strong
hybridization was found only with clones of intracisternal
A particles (IAP); the 8.3 sequences appeared to be
homologous to genes in the pol and env regions of the IAP
clones.

FIGURE 1

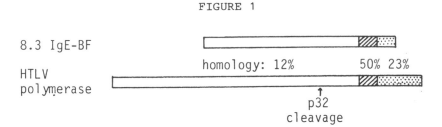

The restriction maps of the 8 pcD clones which encoded
IgE-BF in COS7 cells are very similar to published maps of
intracisternal A particle genes (5). Some of the 8 clones
appear to contain a full genome-size insert (about 7 kb);
others, including the potentiator factors 8.3 and 9.5, are
shorter and appear to have lost genetic material from the
middle of the IAP genome. Southern blot analysis of mouse
genomic DNA, and blot analysis of RNAs derived from many
tumor cells, using cloned IAP genes as probes give results
very similar to those we obtained using IgE-BF clone 8.3.
Thus we conclude that the IgE-BF cDNA clones we have
identified are a subset of the gene family of
intracisternal A particles.

Intracisternal A particles are noninfectious,
morphologically distinctive virus-like particles found in
the cisternae of the endoplasmic reticulum of
preimplantation embryos and some tumor cells (6). The
genes comprise a family of about 1000 copies in the genome
of Mus musculus, but are much less prevalent in other
rodent species, and rare in other species which have been
investigated. The structure of the endogenous IAP genomes
is similar to those of infectious retroviruses, in that
long terminal repeat sequences are located on the 5' and 3'
ends, and there are several genes encoding structural

proteins. Transcripts of IAP genes are widely found in murine tumor cell lines, including all plasmacytomas, and several groups have cloned genomic IAP genes to study their structure. However, no physiologically relevant function has previously been ascribed to any member of this gene family.

Although IgE-BF are members of the IAP gene family, apparently only a small subset of these highly reiterated genes encode IgE-BF. Of 70 clones which shared nucleic acid homology in the pcD library, only 8 were shown to encode IgE-BF. Further, cells which do not express detectable IgE-BF or Fc receptors do contain IAP transcripts (e.g., mouse L cells, NIH-3T3 cells, and uninduced 23B6 hybridoma cells).

In view of the striking homology between IAP genes and IgE-BF genes, it is tempting to suggest that the mechanism by which Ig-BF may regulate expression of immunoglobulin genes may be related to functions of IAPs. IAP genes appear to be mobile elements which can move around in the genome of the host; integration of IAP genes into or near other genes can activate (as in the c-mos gene of plasmacytoma XRPC24 [7]) or decrease (as in two mutant hybridomas which are defective in Ig synthesis [8]) expression of those genes. Homology between IgE-BF genes and infectious retroviruses is in a portion of the polymerase gene which functions as an endonuclease and may be important in integration of viral DNA into the host genome; a similar function may be important in regulation of heavy- or light-chain transcription by B cells.

SUMMARY

We have isolated genes from a cDNA library which encode T lymphocyte factors which bind to the Fc region of IgE and which regulate the IgE response of B lymphocytes. The translation products of two of these genes expressed in a foreign host cell, monkey COS7, are similar in molecular weight to a subset of the IgE binding factors produced by the T hybridoma cell, 23B6, which was the RNA source for the cDNA library. The expressed factors, however, differ

from the hybridoma-produced IgE-BF in lectin-affinity
characteristics and in their immunoregulatory nature: the
factors produced upon transfection of clones 8.3 and 9.5
bind to lentil lectin and potentiate the IgE response,
while factors isolated from the hybridoma do not have
affinity for lentil lectin and suppress the IgE response.
The differences between the cloned, expressed factors and
the hybridoma-produced factors appear to be in the nature
or extent of glycosylation of the molecules. The genes
which encode the IgE-BF appear to be a subset of the
intracisternal A particle genes, a highly reiterated gene
family in mice. Features of these retrovirus-like genes
may be important in the mechanism of action of the Ige
regulatory factors.

REFERENCES

1. Ishizaka, K. Lymphokines 8, 41-80 (1983).

2. Huff, T.F., Uede, T., & Ishizaka, K. J. Immunol. 129,
    509-514 (1982).

3. Davis, M.M., et al. Proc. Nat. Acad. Sci. USA 81,
    2194-2198 (1984).

4. Okayama, H., & Berg, P. Mol. Cell. Biol. 3, 280-289
    (1983)

5. Kuff, E.L., Smith, L.A., & Lueders, K.K. Mol. Cell.
    Biol. 1, 216-227 (1981).

6. Wivel, N.A., & Smith, G.H. Int. J. Cancer 7, 167-175
    (1971).

7. Canaani, E., et al. Proc. Nat. Acad. Sci. USA 80,
    7118-7122 (1983).

8. Hawley, R.G., et al. Proc. Nat. Acad. Sci. USA 79,
    7425-7429 (1982).

Normal and abnormal B cell regulation

Summary of workshop A2 by David W. Scott and Klaus
Eichmann, The University of Rochester Cancer Center,
Immunology Unit, Rochester, N.Y.,U.S.A. and Max-Planck-
Institut fur Immunbiologie, D-7800, Freiburg, FRG.

In its first part the workshop was concerned with the
role of T cells in controlling the expression of idio-
typically defined B cell responses. Several systems
were discussed. Firstly, experiments were presented
which address the role of suppressor T cells in
controlling the expression of the NP^b idiotype in strain
B6 mice. After neonatal injection of anti-NP^b monoclonal anti-idiotypic antibody, the expression of this
idiotype is prevented for prolonged periods. In cell
transfer experiments it could be shown that the
suppressed population contains T cells by which
idiotype-specific suppression can be transferred. It
was concluded that suppressive T cells play a role in
the negative control of idiotype expression. In a
second system, the question of a role for idiotype-
specific helper T cells was addressed in the arsonate
system. In adoptive transfer experiments using carrier-
primed T cells and in attempts to deplete idiotype-
specific cells on idiotype-coated plates, no evidence
could be obtained that idiotype-specific helper cells
play a role for the expression of the arsonate idiotype.
A discussion followed in which a number of other systems
were mentioned in which idiotype-specific help and
suppression has been demonstrated in the past.
Moreover, the discussion extended to isotype-specific
help and suppression. Taken together, it was agreed
that experimental examples exist that argue both for and
against the control of idiotype expression by T cells
with apparent idiotypic specificity.

Further discussion during the first half of the workshop
included a study on the maturation of the anti-
phosphorylcholine response in mice. It was shown that
primary and secondary responses to this antigen were
dominated by different immunoglobulin classes, idiotypes
and fine specificity behaviour. The study suggested
that not all antibodies that appear late after

immunization are the products of somatic mutations of clones that appear early in immunization. This phenomenon needed further evaluation. Moreover, experiments on idiotypes of human antibodies to group A streptococcal carbohydrate were discussed. A variety of idiotypes, defined by monoclonal anti-idiotypic antibodies showed various degrees of cross-reactivity between different antibody clonotypes of the same and of several individuals. Interestingly, although most idiotopes showed more or less pronounced cross-reactivity between different antibody populations, no shared idiotopes were observed between IgG and IgM antibodies. It was discussed whether this was indicative of different distribution patterns of B cells in human individuals or, perhaps, a lack of IgM-IgG switching among human B cells. Furthermore, an example of idiotype sharing between T cells and antibodies was reported for rabbits. Rabbits injected with antigen produce T cells which can be restimulated in vitro with the anti-idiotypic antibody in the presence of IL-2. These T cells also show positive fluorescence when stained with fluoresceinated anti-idiotypic antibody. The significane of this study was that it showed idiotype sharing between T cells and antibodies in species other than mice and that, in contrast to the studies on mice, positive immunofluorescence could be shown for T cells stained with anti-idiotypic antibody.

Normal and abnormal regulation of growth and differentiation in neoplastic B cells was discussed in the second half of the workshop in several model systems. Murine and human B lymphomas have been described which respond to extrinsic agents such as anti-u and T cell factors or non-specific agents like PMA and butyrate. Interestingly, both murine and human B lymphomas were shown to produce BCGF activity either constitutively or after stimulation. Whether this factor activity is present in normal B cells upon activation is not known. In some cases, differentiation to antibody secretion or increased IgM synthesis was demonstrated in response to lymphokines, mitogens or other agents. Such agents may affect the tumorigenicity and metastatic ability of certain tumors by causing their differentiation.

In addition, murine hybrids have been prepared from
myeloma fusions; these hybridomas have the morphology of
Mott cells with Russell bodies. Such cells were shown
to produce u-chains, and have defective secretory
ability. As another model of defective immune
regulation, experiments were described in which CLL
small lymphocytes may degrade intracellular u-chains but
can be induced to secretion (at which point catabolism
ceases). Other CLL behave like activated B cells and
secrete IgM spontaneously. Markers for B lymphomas and
myelomas relating to associated kappa chains or kappa:
lambda ratios were described in certain human diseases.

Overall, this workshop highlighted a number of model
systems to evaluate the regulation of V_H expression in
normal animals and in disease, as well as the growth and
differentiation of neoplastic (abnormal) B cells.

PROBING THE T-CELL REPERTOIRE

A. Moretta[1] and C.J.M. Melief[2]

[1]Ludwig Institute for Cancer Research, Lausanne
Branch, 1066 Epalinges, Switzerland
[2]Central Laboratory of the Netherlands Red
Cross Blood Transfusion Service, Amsterdam,
Netherlands

The T-cell repertoire is built on the following elements 1) available germ-lines genes, allowing diversity of antigen receptors on T cells, 2) available class I and class II MLC restriction elements, 3) the need for tolerance of self structures and 4) other genetically determined immune mechanisms tuning the T-cell repertoire, 5) diversification due to environmental priming. Many of these points were discussed at the workshop dealing with "Probing of T-cell repertoire", notably MHC control or immune response (Ir) gene control of class II MHC restricted T-cell responses (T helper cells, T_H) and class I MHC restricted T-cell responses (cytotoxic T lymphocytes, CTL). The T-cell repertoire can be most fruitfully studied by comparing T-cell responses a) in bulk cultures, b) in short term limiting dilution, c) with long term antigen-specific T-cell clones. Short term limiting dilution assays offer the advantage of allowing analysis of precursor frequency of T_H or CTL and in addition allow limited fine specificity studies of individual T-cell clones. Long term antigen-specific T-cell clones on the other hand, cannot be considered representative of the overall repertoire, but offer the possibility to study specificity,lymphokine production immunoregulation and in vivo activity of well defined cell lines, of which relatively large members can be grown.

It was illustrated at the workshop that class I H-2 molecules regulate CTL responses (and thus influence the

135

expressed repertoire) in much the same way in which class
II H-2 molecules, the products of classical Ir genes, regulate T-helper cell responses. In the T-helper cell response
to hapten-carrier conjugates not only class II H-2 molecules were found to influence the response but also chromosome 12-linked gene(s) different from IgH. Competition was
seen between carrier and hapten-specific T cells for class
II molecules on antigen presenting cells. Limited amino
acid (AA) substitutes in class I or class II molecules can
have profound effects on the expressed T-cell repertoire
as demonstrated with T-cell responses in class I or class
II H-2 mutants bearing 1-3 AA substitutions in the mutant
molecule, probably on the basis of gene conversion. An
example is the CTL response against Sendai virus of a
series of H-2 K^b mutants. These mutants are intermediate
responders, low responders or non-responders in bulk culture. The intensity of bulk culture responses is reflected
in precursor CTL frequencies in limiting dilution cultures,
low and non-responders showing low and immeasurable precursor frequencies, respectively. No evidence for suppressor
cells was found. The biologic importance of this type of
immunoregulation was demonstrated by the finding that the
bm1 H-2 K^b mutant CTL non responder was at least 100-fold
more sensitive to the lethal effect of virulent Sendai
virus than the strain of origin B6, a CTL responder. While
these studies indicate various levels of loss of H-2 K^b
retriction sites for Sendai virus in the K^b mutants, the
T-cell repertoires of the same K^b mutants in limiting dilution analysis of the CTL response against TNP showed 13-43%
mutant-unique CTL clones and all mutants generated good
H-2 K restricted CTL responses. Thus novel restriction elements
for antigen-specific CTL responses occur in H-2 mutants if
looked for in the appropriate system. An interesting study
concerned the role of Class II antigens in the recognition
of Mls determinants by T cells. It was shown that anti-Ia
antibodies inhibited the response to Mls determinants and
that this was not due to direct or indirect blocking of
lymphokine production. Thus recognition of Mls appears to
require concomitant recognition of class II antigens. Whether this constitutes actual H-2 restriction remains to be
explored. H-2 genes are also implicated in the anti-Mls
response, because AKR spleen cells are strong stimulators
of an anti-Mls proliferative response, whereas cells from
the H-2 congenic strain AKR-H-2^b are not. Several reports

dealt with the in vitro and in vivo properties of long term
T-cell clones. Class II restricted murine clones were reported that provided help for both B lymphocytes and cytotoxic precursor cells, delivered by signals distinct from
interleukin-2 and interferon- . It was also reported that
only very few cells of a T-helper clone actually have to
localize after intravenous injection to the site of immune
response (CTL activation) in order to deliver help. It is
not clear whether the help was delivered locally by very
few cells or systemically (e.g. by lymphokine release).
In general, the field of in vivo activity of T-cell clones
needs to be further developed and many problems such as the
homing of T-cell clones in vivo have to be resolved. A
major area of interest is also the ontogeny of the development of the T-cell repertoire in relation to the role of
the thymus. Evidence is accumulating that the thymus exerts
a major influence on the T-helper repertoire but not on the
CTL repertoire. Advanced culture techniques, including CTL
precursor development in the bone marrow and thymus organ
culture, coupled to molecular genetic (T-cell receptor) and
functional studies will allow further incisive probing of
the T-cell repertoire.

The second part of the workshop dealt with studies on
the human T cell functional repertoire. In the human, as
well as in the mouse, these studies have been greatly facilitated by the use of cloned T cells and by the analysis of
the frequencies of different functional precursors. In fact,
it is now evident that the simple analysis of T cell subset
functions in bulk culture is insufficient and may even be
misleading. For example, studies of cell subpopulations
suggested the existence of correlations between given surface phenotypes and cell function, up to the point that T
cell functional capabilities are often extrapolated on the
basis of the expression of surface antigens such as T4 or
T8. However, a more careful analysis at the clonal level
has shown a striking heterogeneity in cell functions within
T lymphocytes expressing the same phenotype and considered
to be functionally homogeneous on the basis of studies carried out at the population level. First, CTL clones were
discribed which instead of the expected T8+ phenotype,
expressed the T4 surface antigen; more recently, several
T8+ cytolytic clones were shown to be capable of autonomous
proliferation and to produce lymphokines such as IL-2 in
response to antigens or mitogens.

As clearly demonstrated at the workshop, even studies based on the use of combinations of surface markers were proven to be unsatisfactory. For example, clones having the same T4+, Leu8+ phenotype displayed different functional activities. Thus, while one of such clones provided help for B cells (in the presence of T cells or T cel factors), the other suppressed B cell Ig production under the same culture conditions.

It should be stressed, however, that the classical clonal approach does not allow the procurement of precise information on the actual representation of functional T cells within a T cell subset identified by the expression or surface markers. To this purpose, limiting dilution analysis of the frequency of functional precursors appears, at the present time, the most reliable assay for studying the actual functional composition of a given T cell population. By applying this analysis it has been previously shown that the precursors of cytolytic cells (CTL-P) represent about 1/3 of the human peripheral blood T cells, in addition, virtually all T8+ cells have this functional potential, whereas CTL-P are relatively infrequent among T4+ cells (1/15 to 1/40). At the workshop, data have been presented on the analysis of the frequency of T cells producing IL-2 and/or BCGF. It was shown that about 60% of the peripheral T cells consists of precursors of IL-2 producing cells; perhaps more importantly, a large fraction ($\sim$ 20%) of T8+ (cytolytic) cells have this functional potential, thus confirming preliminary data obtained by the analysis of CTL clones and showing that CTL able to release IL-2 are relatively frequent among human T lymphocytes. Another important application of T cell clones that has been discussed at the workshop is the analysis, at the clonal level, of the functional modifications induced by HTLV-1 infection. One T cell clone released γ-IFN, BCGF, BCDF and IL-2 only following an appropriate stimulus; however, after infection, this clone constitutively produced γ-IFN, BCGF and BCDF whereas no detectable IL-2 release occurred even in response to mitogens such as ConA or PHA. Such a functional variation was associated with a sharp decrease in the number of T3 molecules expressed at the cell surface of the infected cells.
A similar effect on the T cell receptor-related T3 molecule has been reported by another group in influenza virus-specific helper clones. One such clone, in the presence

of HLA-DR matched cells, was able to respond to a synthetic
peptide corresponding to the 24 amino acid C terminal
portion of the haemagglutinin HA1 molecule. It was shown
that preincubation of the cloned T cells with an excess
peptide induced a loss of the proliferative capacity of
the cells together with "modulation" of the T3 structure;
other T cell antigens such as T4, T1, T11 and 3A1 were not
affected.

Thus while the limiting dilution analysis is the most
precise system to study the functional composition of T cell
populations, the clonal approach certainly represents the
most important tool for studying the functional involvement
of molecules expressed by human T cells, as well as for
analyzing functional and biochemical correlations of such
molecules with antigen and/or MHC recognition structures.

ROLE OF THYMUS T CELL DIFFERENTIATION:

J.J.T. OWEN* AND R. SCOLLAY **

*DEPT. OF ANATOMY, UNIVERSITY OF BIRMINGHAM, U.K.

**WALTER & ELIZA HALL INSTITUTE, MELBOURNE, AUSTRALIA.

The first part of the Workshop was addressed to a number of questions concerning the role of the thymus in the generation of the T cell repertoire. In particular, the way in which the thymic environment might influence tolerance and MHC restriction of emerging T cell populations was discussed and evaluated. A first question - to what extent does contact of differentiating thymic T cells with MHC antigens expressed on thymic stromal cells determine restriction? - was taken up by Golding and Singer (NIH, U.S.A.). They indicated that whereas Ia-restricted T helper cells are restricted by the thymic Ia haplotype, class I restricted cytotoxic T cells are not necessarily restricted by the thymic haplotype. They argued that this discrepancy is due to an inherent difference between the ontogeny of T helper and T cytotoxic precursors. In the discussion that followed a number of points emerged - (i) it is still unclear whether class II MHC antigens on thymic epithelial cells or on thymic dendritic (interdigitating) cells might direct restriction of T helper cells (ii) difficulties in resolving the roles of different thymic stromal types in restriction are due to uncertainties concerning the regenerative capacity of dendritic cell populations following thymic transplantation or irradiation. Thus, in instances where thymic epithelial cells have been implicated, the restriction patterns seen might be due to persisting dendritic cells and their precursors.

141

Do MHC antigens expressed on thymic epithelial cells render differentiating thymic T cells tolerant to them? This was a question taken up by Ready, Jenkinson, Kingston and Owen (Birmingham, U.K.). They described experiments in which deoxyguanosine was used to eliminate lymphoid and dendritic cells from embryonic thymus organ cultures. Epithelial thymuses were then colonized by lymphoid and dendritic cell precursors of a different MHC haplotype to themselves. It was reported that epithelial cells do not induce tolerance in the lymphoid cells which are, however, tolerant to the haplotype of the dendritic cells. It was concluded that dendritic cells might be the dominant element in tolerance induction. Robinson (Newcastle, U.K.) reported that thymic rudiments depleted of lymphoid cells by culture at suboptimal temperatures do induce tolerance to their own MHC antigens when they are colonized by host lymphoid stem cells after grafting to nude mice. He argued that this result suggests that thymic epithelial cells can induce tolerance but in the discussion that followed it was not clear whether thymic rudiments treated in this way are totally devoid of dendritic cells which might play a crucial part. Teh and Ho, (Vancouver,Canada) were able to detect in fetal thymus and organ cultures of fetal thymus suppressor activity against alloresponsiveness. Cells derived from these sources are especially potent in suppressing cytotoxic T lymphocyte responses but without specificity i.e. not limited to antigens syngeneic to the thymus. Hence the possible involvement of these cells in establishing tolerance to self is unclear.

Finally, the discussion turned to the question of whether inflowing stem cells undergo clonal development within the thymus. A number of reports in the literature have suggested that this is the case. Jenkinson,Kingston and Owen (Birmingham,U.K.) described experiments in which single stem cells, micromanipulated from early embryonic thymuses, were added to alymphoid, deoxyguanosine-treated thymic lobes in "hanging-drops" in vitro. In some cases, a single stem cell was shown to produce a fully lymphoid thymic lobe and to generate cell populations of helper and cytotoxic phenotype. In was concluded that lymphoid stem cells migrating into thymus have considerable proliferative potential.

The second part of the Workshop was concerned with factors which are effective in the thymus and the target cells for these factors. Thymic lymphocytes fall into at least five well defined subpopulations and which of these includes the cells which can respond to various factors, hormones or stimuli has been controversial. The five types are best defined with the lineage markers Ly 2 and L3T4 in the mouse or T4 and T8 in the human. Two of these five are the mature medullary cell types expressing one or other of the markers but not both. The other three are the early cortical blasts expressing neither antigen (5% of the thymus), the typical cortical blasts expressing both antigens (15% of the thymus), and the small dense cells expressing both antigens (65% of the thymus). The two medullary populations are peanut agglutinin (PNA) negative, while the cortical populations are PNA$^+$. Data from Scollay, Andrews and Shortman (Melbourne) who used Con A stimulated limit dilution cultures optimised for clonal growth of mature T cells, suggested that murine PNA$^+$ cells (i.e. cortical cells) could not be "pushed" into mature cell growth and response patterns by IL-2 or by a range of well known thymic hormones. This was true whether the hormones were added before or during the cultures. They concluded that all mitogen responsive cells were of medullary phenotype. Lopez-Botet and Moretta (Lausanne) using a similar mitogen driven high cloning efficiency system in humans also found most responsive cells to be medullary phenotype (T3$^+$, T6$^-$). They found some functional cells among the T6$^+$ population, but the possibility of contamination by T6$^-$ cells could not be absolutely ruled out. They also found that a large proportion of thymic CTL-p were T4$^+$, rather different from the mainly T8$^+$ CTL-p found in blood. Thus both these studies suggested that cortical cells were unable to proliferate extensively in response to mitogens and that addition of growth factors and hormones to the cultures did not change this. However, several posters addressed the question of short-term, limited proliferation by various cell populations, particulary in the guinea pig. Sandberg and Soder (Stockholm) showed how guinea pig thymus could be fractionated by density and rosette forming ability into populations corresponding to medullary cells, cortical blasts and small cortical cells, although the exact comparison with the mouse and human systems was difficult in the absence of markers for the guinea pig functional

lineages, Kolare and Sandberg(Stockholm) showed using PNA
and tritiated thymidine both <u>in vivo</u> and <u>in vitro</u>, that
the large PNA$^+$ cortical cells gave rise to small PNA$^+$
cortical-type cells, but also to PNA$^-$, medullary type
cells.   However, in the absence of markers it could not
be determined whether the blasts which gave rise to the
PNA$^-$ cells were typical cortical blasts (double positive
for lineage markers) or perhaps the immature cortical
blasts (double negative for the functional markers). Thus
the question whether the typical cortical cells could be
induced to mature remained unanswered. However, the
guinea pig experiments demonstrated a new factor,
designated thymocyte growth factor (Ernstrom, Soder and
Jungstedt, Stockholm), which at nanomolar concentrations
pushed cortical blasts through one (and one only) cycle
of cell division.   The factor purified from calf or
guinea pig thymus is a peptide of about Mr. 1600 which
appears to be distinct from other known factors and
hormones. A similar factor from human thymus was described
by the same group. Thus, despite the interesting data
presented, the question whether typical cortical cells can
be induced to mature under appropriate conditions remained
unanswered.

Papiernik and El Rouby (Paris) described a phagocytic
cell of the thymic reticulum which is dependent on CSF-1
for its growth. These cells secrete IL-1 and
prostaglandins form rosettes with a particular minority of
cortical cells(5%), but appear to stimulate only medullary
cells.   They suggested that the thymic lymphocytes
trigger IL-1 production by these cells, initiating a factor
cascade.   However, the exact role of these cells (or any
others for that matter!) in the maturation of thymocytes
remains unclear.

REGULATION OF NK ACTIVITY

Chairpersons: Dr. John Ortaldo, Biological
Response Modifiers Program, National Cancer
Institute, Frederick, MD 21701; Dr. Graham
Flannery, Department of Genetics and Human
Variation, LaTrobe University, Bundoora,
Victoria 3083, Australia.

Twenty-two abstracts were submitted to the "Regulation
of NK Activity" Workshop. These varied widely in the
topics of discussion and particularly in their approaches
to regulation of natural cytotoxicity. Fifteen of the 22
proferred papers were presented as oral communications,
while all were displayed as posters. The abstracts were
divided broadly into in vitro and in vivo regulation. A
major theme of in vitro activity was that of IL-2 regulation of natural killer cells (papers presented by Drs.
Ortaldo, Djeu, Kabelitz, and Shaw). A second area of in
vitro regulation centered on discussion of the role of the
transferrin receptor and inhibition by transferrin of
natural killer activity (papers presented by Drs. Kay,
MacDougall, and Borysiewicz). The remainder of the workshop centered around various aspects of in vivo regulation
or ontogeny. Ontogeny was discussed by Drs. Hurme and
Flannery. Modulation by BRMs or other substances was
presented by Drs. Wiltrout and Masihi and tumor modulation
of NK activity was discussed by Dr. Ljunggren. The association of large granular lymphocytes with various diseases
was discussed by Dr. Reid with two abstracts on lymphoproliferative disease and the role of the parent virus in
lymphoproliferative diseases of large granular lymphocytes.
Finally, Dr. Clancy discussed the role of natural killer
cells in his graft-vs.-host disease model.

145

I. Regulation of Activity In Vitro

It was the consensus of all the presentations regarding natural killer cells and IL-2 regulation that IL-2, both natural and recombinant, was a potent regulator of NK cytolysis. Some differences were stated regarding the kinetics of activation with various preparations of IL-2, but7no comparison was made with the various preparations, and each investigator was using a different preparation. Clearly, recombinant homogeneous IL-2 from several sources should be tested in parallel to address this issue of possible differences in the kinetics of activation. It was generally agreed that natural killer cell activity is enhanced in the absence of a detectable level of Tac expression. All the presentations indicated that antibodies to Tac produced little or no inhibition of the activation, using either PBL or purified LGL, and indicate the lack of involvement of the Tac receptor in the immunoregulatory effect. In addition, it was generally agreed that the IL-2 activation of natural killer cells resulted in significant levels of interferon gamma being produced from these lymphocyte preparations. However, experiments presented here raised some questions as to whether interferon gamma might be the mediator of NK boosting by IL-2, since a number of monoclonal antibodies directed against gamma interferon failed to inhibit boosting by IL-2 and only anti-IL-2 antibodies consistently inhibited this IL-2-mediated event. Experiments presented by several investigators indicated that interferon gamma was a very poor augmenter of natural killer activity and that the levels of interferon gamma produced during IL-2 stimulation did not result in significant augmentation to the level of that of IL-2. Very high doses (10,000 units or more) of interferon gamma never achieved the level of activation induced by IL-2 and the consensus opinion was that interferon gamma was not a potent regulator of natural killer activity as was IL-2.

There was some discussion regarding whether or not natural killer activity is enhanced through a non-Tac receptor or a low affinity Tac receptor. Some disagreement occurred regarding the ability of anti-Tac antibody to block IL-2-mediated proliferation of natural killer cells in a normal mitogen-driven, PHA-stimulated response. It was generally agreed, however, that considerably more investigation is necessary using a radiolabeled IL-2 in an attempt to clarify this question regarding the mechanism of IL-2 activation.

Results discussing possible synergy between beta interferon and IL-2 were reported by Dr. Shaw. A discussion followed which indicated the general consensus by the investigators that the modulation and synergy was not seen in combinations of IL-2 with beta interferon, alpha interferon, or gamma interferon. In addition, a question by Dr. Kirchner addressing whether gamma interferon could synergize in NK cell activation with other interferons, either alpha or beta, was aired. None of the investigators had convincing evidence that this occurred, and in fact only additive effects were seen when these types of experiments were performed. Therefore, the synergy that is seen in some of the antiviral systems with gamma + alpha interferons appears not to be evident in the augmentation of NK cell-mediated cytolytic activity.

The next series of presentations concerned the role of transferrin receptor as the target for natural killer activity and transferrin itself as an inhibitor of natural killing. Dr. Kay presented some interesting data regarding variability among concerned transferrin lots and indicated that some lots were totally noninhibitory within physiological ranges. Further investigation of this issue seemed to indicate that the active substance within the transferrin reponsible for the inhibition was hemopexin, a protein whose role in regulation of NK activity is not presently known. Experiments with hemopexin demonstrated that dose-dependent inhibition of NK function could be seen with highly purified hemopexin. Discussion by other presenters within the session demonstrated correlations between the expression of transferrin receptor on NK-susceptible target cells and their NK susceptibility. It was felt, however, that although such indirect evidence is certainly interesting, it did not directly indicate a role for the transferrin receptor. In fact, no information was presented concerning the involvement of the transferrin receptor in binding between NK targets and highly purified NK populations. The consensus from the discussion was that one should very carefully examine transferrin and other agents showing similar correlations, to be sure that such molecules are involved in either binding or lysis by natural

killer cells. Either spatial arrangement or parallel regulation of receptors like transferrin and other structures
on the cell surface certainly are possible and these events
could lead to erroneous conclusions. The feeling of the
participants at the meeting was that no convincing direct
evidence exists that the transferrin receptor plays a role
in the binding of natural killer cells to their targets.
However, further investigations are necessary to determine
whether transferrin is important, either in mediating or
stabilizing recognition of NK-susceptible targets.

II. Regulation of Activity In Vivo

   A number of papers addressed the issues of the in vivo
relevance of NK cells, especially with respect to agents
which modulate NK activity in various organs, NK activity
relative to various tumors, as well as NK cells in various
disease states, and their role in lymphoproliferative
diseases.

   Several papers described approaches for examination
of ontogeny and development of natural killer cells, and
included investigation of rat spleen and liver at various
days of development, before and after birth. A presentation by Dr. Flannery indicated that levels of NK activity
in liver decrease quite dramatically during the second and
third trimester of gestation and become considerably lower
after birth and remain low in normal situations beyond 5
to 7 weeks. The converse, however, is seen in the spleen,
with no activity detectable until birth, and a slow rise
until 5 to 6 weeks, at which time maximal activity is seen.
These results indicate that early fetal development and
differentiation of natural killer cells occurs in the liver.

   In an adoptive transfer model (paper by Dr. Hurme),
use was made of an F_1 antiparent chimera system to examine
the passive transfer of bone marrow (depleted of Thy-1-
positive cells) into x-irradiated recipient mice. This
model system demonstrated rapid repopulation of donor type
(F_1) NK activity in the spleen and blood of the recipient
mice (days 7-12). Such approaches will allow a better
understanding of hemopoietic sites which exhibit NK activity
during gestation and identification of the phenotypic
markers present on the bone marrow progenitors of natural
killer cells. The repopulation properties of such

progenitors could then be examined in a similar way. In
addition studies are planned to examine the repopulation
of myelomonocytic cells and thymus in order to determine
the donor phenotype, for validation of the chimeric state.

Several abstracts dealt with the issue of modulation
of natural killer cell activity in various organs using
Biological Response Modifiers such as C. parvum, MVE, BCG,
and trehalose dimycolate. A number of investigators felt
examinations of the peripheral organs, such as the spleen
or the blood, may not adequately reflect activity which
may be present in other organs such as the lung or the
liver, where distant metastases often will reside. A very
good example of this, pointed out by Dr. Wiltrout, was that
MVE-2 treatment dramatically increases the level of activity
in the liver and lungs, at a time when it is not seen in
the peripheral circulation or in the spleen. These latter
organs, however, are sites examined in many metastatic
tumor models. A point emerged relative to clinical studies
in that peripheral circulating NK activity may not
adequately reflect the level which has been achieved at the
tumor site or within various organs such as the lung and
liver, and therefore inconclusive or misleading results may
be obtained because of the limitation of assessing only
peripheral natural killer function.

Finally, several instances relating large granular
lymphocytes to various types of lymphoproliferative disease
were reported by Drs. Reid and Clancy in a herpes virus-
associated lymphoproliferative disease and in an acute GVH
reaction, respectively. Discussion prompted by these
papers stressed the fact that we must begin now to broaden
the ranges of our investigations regarding natural killer
cells and their functions in and relationships to diseases
other than cancer. The association of large granular
lymphocytes in a number of T-gamma lymphocytoses has
indicated that these cells develop a pseudoleukemic state
(in the Fischer 344 rat), where a lethal lymphoproliferative
disease results and indicates that LGL indeed may play a
significant role in pathogenesis of some lymphoproliferative
diseases. However, it was also emphasized that in T-gamma
lymphocytosis patients no treatment is generally required,
and in fact treatments are generally detrimental to the
long-term survival of such patients. These patients
present a high percentage of large granular lymphocytes in

their peripheral circulation. Without any treatment and
with routine monitoring, these patients survive quite well
with the chronic lymphocytosis. It certainly seems that a
great deal more investigation and awareness must be given
to large granular lymphocytes since they do possess a
potent cytotoxic potential and more recently have demonstrated a very active and varied capacity to secrete
different cytokines. The examination of LGL and their
role in a variety of nonmalignant diseases reinforces the
view that their in vivo relevance may not be confined to a
surveillance role against malignancy and in fact may support
the alternate hypothesis that natural killer cells regulate
normal hemopoietic development and differentiation, as
their primary in vivo function.

RECEPTORS INVOLVED IN T CELL ACTIVATION

Dominique J. CHARRON[+] and Michaël J. CRUMPTON[o]

[+]Lab. Immunogénétique CHU Pitié-Salpétrière
91, bd de l'Hôpital, PARIS

[o]Imperial Cancer Research Fund. Lincoln's.
Inn Fields LONDON

T lymphocytes are able to respond specifically to a diverse set of foreign determinants. Among the molecules which are critical in regulating the immune system is the elusive T cell receptor for antigens. After years of speculation, the molecular nature of the T cell receptor has at last begun to emerge. Thus, biochemical studies of T cell clones and T cell hybrids have identified the clonotypic structure which determines antigen specificity as a 90 Kd heterodimeric disulfide-linked molecule comprising two chains of 40-45 Kd (α chain) and 42-44 Kd (β chain). cDNA clones encoding the β subunit of the T cell antigen receptor have been isolated in mouse and man and are the subject of intensive investigation. The workshop was devoted to the molecular nature of the β chain of the T cell receptor and some of the biological consequences of T cell activation.

Restriction maps and sequence analyses have indicated that the genomic organisation of the β chains of the T cell receptor is very similar to that of the immunoglobulin genes with variable (V), constant (C) and joining (J) segments as well as the presence of a diversity (D) segment. As reported and discussed by N. GASCOIGNE and M. COLLINS the functional β gene is formed by VDJ rearrangement followed by splicing of the VDJ segment to the constant region. The origin of the structural diversity emerged as a central question and the role played by the J region in particular was discussed in detail. Four different poten-

tial mechanisms could account for the diversity provided
by the J region genes. First the large number of J genes.
Thus, two J clusters have been identified that could encode for as many as 11 functional J elements. The variability of each gene, the variable length of the coding
sequences, and finally the indeterminate position of rearrangement with the use or not of D, potentially provide
further bases for extensive variability. Similar mechanisms
operate in the rearrangement of these genes when compared
with those of the immunoglobulin genes. Not only are the
J 5' flanking sequences remarkedly similar to the 5' flanking sequences of the immunoglobulin J regions, but also
the 11/12.12.12/13 rule, first described in the immunoglobulin system, is preserved in the formation of the T cell
receptor variable region, with the additional possibility
of direct VH-JH joining (by-passing D), although this has
yet to be confirmed experimentally. The important question
of the number of V genes cannot yet be answered, although
all present indications are that it is smaller than for
immunoglobulin. In this case, the less diverse set of V
regions could be easily compensated for by the greater polymorphism of the J system. Although each J region is different, the two C regions are closely similar differing by
4 amino acids only in the carboxy-terminus. In contrast,
the 3' untranslated regions are highly divergent indicating
that duplication of the C gene may have occurred at the
time of speciation.

The cell types in which the differentiation stage at
which T cell receptor genes rearrangement occurs were also
considered. This topic was only briefly discussed in the
workshop, since it had been extensively reported by
S. HEDRICKS and E. REINHERZ in the first symposium that
most T cell types including thymic cells, peripheral blood
resting T cells, T cell leukemias and hybridomas undergo
somatic rearrangement. This is also the case for T cells
with specific immune functions such as helper, CTL's and
possibly, although not definitely, suppressor cells. It is
important to appreciate that notable quantitative differences were observed at the transcript level. Moreover, all
the present data stem from the examination of the β chain
only and thus should not be regarded as definitive. Not
only has the α chain to be taken into account, but various
post-translational modifications may be necessary to express
a fully active T cell receptor at the cell surface. When
the predicted protein structure was deduced from the nucleotide sequence, R. MAGE noted that the presence of an

extra CYS residue raises the possibility of an additional
disulphide bridge in the T cell receptor β chain of mouse,
man and rabbit. Obviously, free-SH groups, alternative
intra- or inter-chain S-S bonds may affect the conformation and the level of surface expression of the β chains
in an identical way with that proposed for the rabbit K1
gene.

The biological consequences and the functional diversity of MHC-restricted antigen specific T cell recognition
may be more complex than hitherto suspected. In addition
to the established partners of the T cell antigen receptor
such as the T3 and MHC antigens, novel molecules were depicted. As well, unexpected reactivities were suggested
for other known structures. A.W. BOYLSTON reported on a
monoclonal antibody which mimicked all the properties of
antibodies against the T3 antigen but which appeared to
recognise a different molecular species, namely one of
about 60 Kd molecular weight. The biological significance
of this molecule will have to await the description of new
data. A monoclonal antibody against T3 was reported by
H. SPITS to induce non-specific cytolytic activity in CTL
clones and to convert proliferative T cells to CTL's. One
explanation for the non-specific killing is the presence
of Fc receptors on the cells. This explanation could be
easily evaluated by using F(ab')2 fragments. Whilst the
previous work may have unveiled a lytic machinery in a
non-lytic cell, P. BEVERLEY presented clear evidence that
an antigen specific T cell clone reponds to stimulation
by a monoclonal antibody against T3 by increasing its Ca^{++}
intracellular concentration. Although the use of the Ca^{2+}
sensitive fluorescent dye, Quin-2, to measure intracellular Ca^{2+} concentration presents some uncertainties this
approach has clearly yielded interesting data. An important
point is whether the same response is induced by interaction of the antigen with the receptor. The nature of the
biochemical events following Ca^{++} mobilisation are also of
great physiological interest.

Numerous differences in the spectra of polypeptides
expressed by different T cell clones were documented by
F. TRIEBEL et al. This structural heterogeneity was further
emphasised by S. HEDRICKS who reported that comparisons of
the spectra of mRNA's from different T cell clones by the
substraction method, revealed as many as 40 genes which
were both T cell specific and which coded for proteins
synthesised on membrane bound polysomes. These data argue
in support of the view that a variety of T cell specific

genes and proteins exist for which no serological probe
or function have yet been designated. Such molecules are
of course attractive candidates for mediating important
biological activities.

Several experiments were presented that served to
illustrate the complexity of the molecular network regulating T cell function. WASSMER et al. reported that a
monoclonal antibody against L3T4 inhibited the activation
of a T cell hybridoma. Since the absence of class II antigens on the target cell ruled out the possibility of an
interaction between the L3T4 and class II antigens, it was
suggested that the L3T4 molecule may interact directly
with the T cell receptor. A parallel approach was presented by LODBERG who indicated that the Ly1 molecule may
function as a receptor for the lymphokine IL1. This suggestion was based on the observation that a monoclonal
antibody recognising a second epitope on the L3T4 molecule
was able to enhance the response to IL1 in the thymocyte
co-stimulator assay and augment the response of thymocytes,
properties which are known to belong to IL1 perse. Although
the above experiments were competently executed, a definitive conclusion cannot be drawn from studies in which monoclonal antibodies were used to block functional traits.
Thus, it is possible that the binding of antibody to an
irrelevant site may induce changes in another molecule or
site which will in turn affect the function. Similarly,
fail_ure of a particular antibody to inhibit may reflect
low antibody affinity rather than failure of the antigen
to mediate the particular function. The provocative claim
that the β chain is shared by the MaC-1 molecule and the T
cell receptor needs further study at the molecular level.

Knowledge of the structural organisation of the T
cell antigen receptor has accumulated at an impressive
rate over the past two years and this was well reflected
in the workshop. Several important questions, however, remain to be answered. For example, do CTL's, suppressor and
helper T cells use the same pool of genes and undergo similar somatic rearrangements ; do they carry the same or
distinct C regions and what is the role of the C region
in mediating the effector function ; do the various V and
D gene segments overlap or are they distinct ; how and to
what extent does the presence of two polymorphic chains
contribute to the structural and functional diversity of
the T cell receptors.

In spite of the notable strides which have been made
in respect of delineating molecules on the lymphocyte

surface, little progress has been made in describing their putative interaction with the cytoskeleton or the nature of the intracellular signals which activate the effector cells.

One of the disappointments of the workshop was the absence of data at the molecular level addressing the question of the nature of the association of the T cell receptor with class I or class II molecules. The predictable weakness of the association may well be of relevance physiologically as well as a contributory cause to the lack of information.

Finally, because the T cell receptor associates with other molecules especially the T3 antigen to form a macromolecular complex, a topological approach is likely to be required to fully understand the structural and functional diversity of the system.

SECTION III

LYMPHOCYTE TRANSFORMATION

TRANSFORMATION OF CELLS BY EPSTEIN-BARR VIRUS:

AN HYPOTHESIS

Beverly E. Griffin

Department of Virology,

Royal Postgraduate Medical School,
Hammersmith Hospital, London, W12.

INTRODUCTION

Epstein-Barr virus (EBV) has been found in association
with three different diseases of B-cell origin and one
originating from epithelial cells. With regard to the
former, the virus has been shown to be the causative agent
of infectious mononucleosis, and to be present in most
monoclonal Burkitt's lymphomas. In addition, viral
association with increasing numbers of lymphoproliferative
disorders, in response to immunosuppressive agents, is
being recognised. EBV is also found in epithelial cells
derived from poorly differentiated carcinomas of the naso-
pharynx (NPC). One of the most striking and unexplained
aspect of both Burkitt's lymphomas and NPC is the uneven
distribution of the disease among ethnic groups. The role
of EBV in the B-cell diseases has been frequently speculated
to be related to its ability to induce unlimited proliferation in infected cells.[1] A similar role in the
epithelium disorder may exist, but this has been more
difficult to study in vitro, largely because no epithelial
cell has yet been identified that has receptors for EBV.
This has led to the suggestion and experiments to show
that the entry of the virus into this cell type might be a
consequence of fusion with an infected B-cell.[2]

Several lines of evidence from both epidemiological
and laboratory studies implicate EBV in induction of
immortalisation, or continuous growth proliferation, of

159

cells. For example, a detailed study by Nilsson et al.[3]
of established B-lymphoblastoid lines (derived from
healthy human donors infected in vitro by EBV) showed them
to be incapable of growing in soft agar and non-tumourigenic
in nude mice as long as the cells remained diploid.
Subsequent chromosomal alterations, however, which resulted from passaging of cells in culture were apparently
accompanied by genotypic alterations in that the cells
frequently became tumourigenic. Most lines established
directly from Burkitt's lymphomas were found to be
aneuploid and tumourigenic in nude mice. The possibility
that the event involved in going from a "passively
immortalised" to a malignant cell may involve the relocat-
ion of the myc "oncogene" in these cells is currently
being given very serious consideration.[4]

EXPERIMENTAL APPROACH TO STUDIES ON IMMORTALISATION
USING SPECIFIC SUB-GENOMIC FRAGMENTS OF EBV DNA
     Our studies over the past few years have been direct-
ed toward localising a function, or functions, within the
EBV genome that may be responsible for cellular immort-
isation of epithelium, or B-cells.   To initiate such
experiments, we first made a recombinant DNA library (in a
cosmid vector) that encompassed the entire viral genome
within six cloned fragments, as illustrated in Fig. 1.
Transfection experiments were than carried out to introduce
each of the specific DNA fragments into an essentially
mixed primary culture of fibroblast and epithelial cells
from African green monkey kidneys (AGMK) in the presence
of calcium phosphate. This so-called "calcium method" in
our hands has in the past always proved reliable and
reproducible, conveniently allowing a large enough sample
of cells to be investigated for a minor event to be
observed. However, the method has been found to be
generally too toxic for B-lymphocytes. Our experiments to
date have therefore all been carried out on epithelial cell
populations on the assumption that any uncovered pathway
to immortalisation might be (but need not be) also
similar in B-lymphocytes. By this approach we were able
to produce continuously proliferating cultures from AGMK
cells transfected with either of the two overlapping fragments of EBV DNA designated p13 and p31 in Fig.1. All
other experiments were negative. Individual established
cell lines were found to be entirely epithelial, to grow
continuously in vitro even in low serum, and to contain

"footprints" of EBV DNA which remained in cells carried
for more than a year in culture. On the other hand, they
showed only a limited ability to grow in soft agar and did
not produce tumours in nude mice.[5] The remarkable aspect
was that epithelial cells were produced that could overgrow fibroblasts in the population. As a model, AGMK
cells proved useful but have numerous disadvantages in
that, in general, they are prone to spontaneous transformation, may carry their own EBV-related herpes viruses, and
have a diploid number of 60 which complicates chromosomal
analysis.

Having established that, in the presence of a specific
sub-genomic fragment of EBV, immortalised cells could be
produced, we elected to repeat the experiment in a more
advantageous cell. We chose kidneys from the "common
marmoset" (Callithrix jacchus) as having none of the
disadvantages elaborated for AGMK cells. (They have a
diploid chromosomal number of 46[6]). In addition, primary
source material could be obtained and animals are available
for subsequent in vivo studies. Primary marmoset kidney
cells were thus transfected with individual members of the
cloned EBV library, and in this case, combinations of
cloned fragments were also used. The results obtained
were as follows:[7]

1. When the fragment designated p31 was transfected onto
the cell population, immortalised epithelial cells were
again obtained. These could be shown to be poorly
differentiated, and capable of unlimited proliferation in
culture. They produced very dense cell monolayers, and
could also grow in low serum. As observed in the case of
the respective cultures from AGMK cells, they had only
limited capacity to divide in soft agar and to date have
not produced tumours in nude mice. "Footprints" of viral
DNA could be detected in cells, even after more than 200
doubling times. Again, the consequence of transfection
with a specific fragment of EBV DNA was found to be the
production of an apparently immortalised subpopulation of
epithelial cells, that could overgrow fibroblasts but were
not in the normal sense of the word "transformed".

2. Transfection experiments with the fragment designated
p13, or with any of the other fragments, were negative.

3.   An experiment involving co-transfection of fragments p31 and p5 onto the marmoset kidney cells gave rise to an unexpected result.   Cells that could grow continuously in culture, but more slowly than observed in the case where transfection was carried out with p31 alone, were obtained. Although these could be shown by immunofluorescent staining with anti-keratin antibodies to be entirely epithelial, morphologically different cell types were evident in the population.   Moreover, upon reaching confluence these cells produce hemi-cysts or "domes", characteristic of high-polarised, active ion-transporting cells.   Dome formation could be enhanced by agents such as dimethylsulfoxide or sodium butyrate, chemicals which stimulate cells to differentiate, or abolished by ouabain which interferes with ion-transport.   The cells appeared more highly differentiated than those immortalised by p31 alone, having, for example, well-defined desmosomes.

Studies similar to the above have now been carried out with human breast milk cells obtained from lactating females,[7] and with cells derived from foetal kidneys.   In both cases growth stimulation was observed in cells transfected with DNA from the p31 clone.   The results with foetal kidneys are particularly encouraging in that cells are still actively growing after nearly four months in culture (unpublished data).

A MODEL FOR TRANSFORMATION OF CELLS BY EBV DNA
Based in the experimental results described above a "working hypothesis" is proposed to explain how EBV might be involved in cellular transformation, at least of epithelial cells.   The assumptions are:

1.   EBV per se lacks the ability to transform a cell "fully", as measured in vitro by the soft agar assay or in vivo by tumour formation.

2.   The virus contains (at least) two functions relevant to transformation, however.

A. An immortalising function (as encoded within p31).
B. A function associated with differentiation (as encoded within p5).

3.   Expression of A. plus B. does not lead to cellular immortalisation.

4.   Expression of A. in the absence of B. leads to production of an immortalised "susceptible" cell that can undergo further alterations to produce a fully-transformed or malignant cell.

Conclusions: Transformation is a step-wise, or continuum, consequence of infection of an immature cell by a sub-population of EB virions that immortalise and block cellular maturation, and a non-virally coded event (such as a genetic accident that leads to a chromosomal translocation, or a mutation of a cellular gene) that may lead to altered genetic expression in these cells, and in some cases to malignancy.

Some aspects of this hypothesis are capable of being tested in the laboratory. In particularly, it should be possible to answer the question of whether sub-populations of the virus exist, and whether the immortalised cells can be stimulated by chemical mutagens or carcinogens, tumour promoters, or "oncogens" to produce fully-transformed and tumourigenic cells. It will be of great interest to determine whether any of the data derived from studies on epithelial cells will be pertinent to B-lymphocytes.

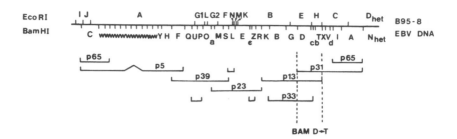

Figure 1. A cosmid library of EBV DNA. EB virion DNA
from B95-8 cells was partially digested with BamHI,
fragments about 40 Kb in size ligated to the BamHI cleaved
cosmid pHC79 DNA (from which the 5'-phosphates had been
removed), and the resulting hybrid DNAs cloned according
to the procedure of Hohn and Collins[8]. Individual
recombinant DNAs were isolated and analysed as previously
described[5]. Those that yielded results consistent with the
known physical maps of EBV DNA (as shown) were selected to
make up a library of largely overlapping fragments which
consisted of six clones designated p65, p5, p39, p23, p13
and p31, as indicated. (p33 was selected originally as
part of the library because "miniprep" analysis showed it
to contain the BamHI R fragment, necessary to provide an
overlap of p23 and p13. Further characterisation failed
to confirm this). The overlapping region between p13 and
p31, both of which produced immortalised cells when
transfected onto AGMK cultures, are indicated. Successful
immortalisation of primary marmoset kidney cells was only
achieved with p31. Recombinant clone p5 contains a
number of regions thought to be of considerable interest
with regard to the biology of EBV, in that they are expressed in latently infected B-lymphocytes.[9]

REFERENCES

1. zur Hausen, H. In, Molecular Biology of Tumor Viruses,
    2nd ed. (ed. J. Tooze) 747-795. Cold Spring Harbor
    (1980).

2. Li, Y. et al. Sicentia Sinica (Series B) 27,
    284-293 (1984).

3. Nilsson, K., Giovanella, B. C., Stehlin, J. S. and
    Klein, G. Int. J. Cancer 19, 337-344 (1977).

4. Dallas-Favera, R., Bregeni, M., Erikson, J.,
    Patterson, D., Gallo, R. C. and Croce, C. M. Proc.
    Natl. Acad. Sci. USA 79, 7824-7827 (1982).

5. Griffin, B. E. and Karran, L. Nature 309, 78-82
    (1984).

6. Wohnus, J. F. and Benirschke, K. Cytogenetics 5,
    94-105 (1966).

7. Griffin, B. E., Karran, L., King, D. and Chang, S. E.
    Soc. Gen. Microbiol., Cambridge Univ. Press, in press.

8. Hohn, B. and Collins, J. Gene 11,291-298 (1980).

9. Miller, G. In, Progress in Medical Virology,
    30 (ed. J. L. Melnick) 107-128. Karger, Basel (1984).

HUMAN T-CELL LYMPHOTROPIC RETROVIRUSES (HTLV) ASSOCIATED

WITH T-CELL MALIGNANCY AND IMMUNODEFICIENCY: IN VITRO

STUDIES

Mikulas Popovic and Robert C. Gallo

Laboratory of Tumor Cell Biology, National

Cancer Institute, Bethesda, Maryland

The first human retrovirus, human T-cell leukemia/
lymphoma virus type I (HTLV-I) was discovered in the
cultured leukemic cells of a patient with mature T-cell
malignancy[1,2]. Using the new methodology for culturing
of mature T-cells[3] and the experience with the first HTLV
isolates, hundreds of HTLV isolates were obtained in our
and other laboratories within a relatively short period of
time[4,5]. Propagation of these isolates in the appropriate
host cell type provided a system for large scale production
and, thus, enabled their extensive characterization[1,4,6].
Based on specific features, at present time, this rapidly
expanding family of human retroviruses can be subdivided
into three subgroups called HTLV-I, HTLV-II and HTLV-III[7].
This family of HTLV is naturally occuring retroviruses.
In the past, this group of relatively commonly occuring
retroviruses in nature were extensively studied in animals
and they are called chronic leukemia viruses[5,7]. They are
replicative competent and the cause of naturally occuring
leukemia in chickens, mice, cats, cows, and gibbon apes.
They contain the complete set of genes for replication: the
gag gene coding for internal structural proteins, the pol
gene coding for the reverse transcriptase, and env gene coding for the viral envelope. These viruses do not contain
cellular onc genes, however, in vivo produce a malignancy
after long latency, and in general they do not transform
cells in vitro. The mechanism of tumor induction by these

167

retroviruses involving a specific integration event is a
subject of great current interest[8].

Initially, HTLV-I and HTLV-II were classified as a
chronic leukemia virus, however, detailed sequence analysis
of the cloned provirus showed that, in addition to all
three genes for replication, they contain a sequence of
about 1.6 Kb at the 3' end of the viral genome originally
termed pX[9]. Recent sequence analysis of HTLV-III, a
retrovirus which is a primary cause of the acquired immunodeficiency syndrome (AIDS) suggests a similar genomic structure[10]. Therefore, this group of retroviruses, which also
include bovine leukemia virus (BLV) and primate T-cell
leukemia virus (PTLV), represent a new category of retroviruses[11]. All of the viruses display the phenomenon of
trans-acting transcriptional regulation (TAT) which is defined as a greatly increased rate of transcription directed
by the viral large terminal repeats (LTR) in infected as
compared to uninfected cells. The high rate of transcription is induced by viral infection and acts in trans[12].
Trans-activation is strain (subgroup) specific, since one
type of virus does not, in general, activate transcription
directed by the LTR of another type of virus[11,12]. Moreover, like chronic leukemia viruses, they produce monoclonal tumors after a long latency period, and do not contain a cellular derived onc gene. However, HTLV-I and
HTLV-II do transform (immortalize) fresh primary human T-
cells in vitro apparently due to their lor (large open
reading frame) genes (pX) coding for 42 Kd and 36 Kd proteins, respectively, which could be involved in the first
stages of HTLV induced neoplasia[11].

Here we summarize the properties of each subgroup of
HTLV and briefly describe their role to cause malignancy
and immunodeficiency emphasizing the latest results from
in vitro studies.

COMMON FEATURES OF THE HTLV FAMILY OF RETROVIRUSES

Despite distinctive differences between HTLV-I, HTLV-
II and HTLV-III, there are several common properties among
all three subgroups of these retroviruses[5,7] (see Table 1)
which are: (1) T-cell tropism, particularly with the T4
(OKT4/Leu3a) phenotype; (2) a major core protein of about

Table 1.   Common Characteristics of HTLV-I, HTLV-II
and HTLV-III

Property	Subgroup of HTLV		
	I	II	III
Particular cell tropism	T4	T4	T4
Major core	p24	p24	p24
RT size	~100K	~100K	~100K
Common envelope epitope	+	+	+
Nucleic acid homology to I (stringent)		±	-
Genome contains a lor gene (pX)	+	+	+
Trans-acting transcriptional regulation	+	+	+
Produces giant multinucleated cells	+	+	+
African origin	Likely	?	Likely
Homology to other retro-viruses	0	0	0

24 Kd; (3) a 100 Kd reverse transcriptase (RT), favoring
Mg^{++} for its catalytic activity; (4) they share some common
cross-reactive determinants; (5) sequence homology can be
demonstrated in certain regions of their genomes; (6) as
mentioned above, they have a coding capacity for an additional gene besides gag, pol, and env at the 3' end of the
viral genome coding for a novel protein called lor gene
(pX) product; (7) and their high rate of transcription is
induced by virus infection and acts in trans which is determined by LTR of a particular subgroup of HTLV; (8) the capability to exert a cytopathic effect on some of the infected
cells and to induce multinucleated giant cells, and (9)
the probable origin is Africa.

HTLV-I

The first two HTLV-I isolates were obtained from two
black patients respectively, in the United States with what
were diagnosed as an unusually aggressive variant of cutaneous T-cell lymphoma/leukemia (Sezary syndrome and mycosis
fungoides)[1,2]. The virus isolate showed a type-C morphology, the size of virus particles varied from 900 to 1400
Å and, although rarely, budding from the cell membranes

was observed[1]. HTLV-I is distinct from other animal retroviruses by nucleic acid hybridization, by protein serology,
and is exogeneous to man[5]. The virus is transmitted hori-
zontally[5].

Since the first isolations of HTLV-I, many additional
isolates have been obtained in this laboratory from patients and their close clinically healthy relatives from
the U.S.[4,5], the Caribbean[4,5], Japan[4], Africa[13] and
Israel[4]. Several isolates were obtained independently by
investigators in Japan[14,15], the U.S.[16], Holland[17] and
England[18]. These isolates have mainly been obtained from
T cells of patients with adult T-cell leukemia (ATL)[4,15].
Comparative studies of various isolates, namely immunological cross-reactivities of the viral proteins, sequence
homology by molecular hybridization, cleavage sites of
several restriction endonucleases, and more recently by
nucleotide sequence analyses clearly indicate that these
isolates belong to a group of very closely related viruses
of the same HTLV-I subgroup[5,7]. Extensive seroepidemiological survey showed that in addition to sporadic cases
found in the southeastern U.S., two geographic regions
were noted in which disease was endemic and clinically
resembled those from which the first two HTLV-I isolates
originated[5]. These two regions were the Caribbean[19] and
southwestern Japan[14].

HTLV-II

In collaboration with UCLA investigators we isolated
a new retrovirus from a patient with a T-cell variant of
hairy cell leukemia. This retrovirus is related to, but
substantially different from HTLV-I and is called HTLV-II[20].
Recently, a second isolate of HTLV-II was obtained in our
laboratory from an intravenous drug user with AIDS[21]. At
the present time, HTLV-II has not been linked epidemiologi-
cally to any diseases. Other variants having minor differences from HTLV-I in their genome were also recognized[13].

HTLV-III

Retroviruses classified as HTLV-I or HTLV-II have
occasionally been isolated from tissues obtained from AIDS

and pre-AIDS (persistent lymphadenopathy syndrome)[22]. In
contrast to these observations, retroviruses belonging to a
distinct new subgroup of HTLV, termed HTLV-III, have been
isolated at a very high frequency from AIDS and pre-AIDS
patients and individuals at high risk for AIDS[6,23]. HTLV-
III has been isolated in approximately 50% of patients
with AIDS and 80% of pre-AIDS syndrome. HTLV-III was not
found in 125 samples of normal heterosexual donors[23].
This incidence of virus isolation from the AIDS samples is
clearly an underestimate of the true frequency since many
more patients have been exposed to the virus as indicated
by high percentage seropositive cases for antibody to
viral proteins[24].

For the first time, HTLV-III was detected in this laboratory in November 1982, but because of difficulty in
growing the infected T-cells adequate characterization was
not feasable. Eventually, permissive subclones of an
established leukemic T-cell line were obtained which could
be infected by HTLV-III and yielded large amounts of virus[6].
This development facilitated the preparation of immunological and nucleic acid reagents for detailed characterization of the virus, enabled extensive seroepidemiological
survey and comparison of isolates obtained from patients
with AIDS, thus, allowing us to demonstrate that HTLV-III
is the etiological agent of AIDS[24,25]. This was clearly
documented in patients with AIDS who received blood transfusion from donors positive for HTLV-III[26]. In addition,
this development opened the way to large-scale blood bank
assays for serum antibodies to the virus.

The first isolate, called lymphadenopathy associated
virus (LAV), was originally reported by F. Barre-Sinoussi
et al.[17] Comparison of HTLV-III and LAV-1 showed that
both viruses are closely related and belong to the same
HTLV subgroup[28].

BIOLOGICAL EFFECTS OF HTLV

Infection and Immortalization of Fresh Human T Lymphocytes by HTLV-I and HTLV-II

Following identification of HTLV-I positive leukemic T-cells after in vitro cultivation, these cells were lethally irradiated or treated with mitomycin-C, and co-cultivated with normal T-cells to transmit the virus to these recipient cells and to study their biological proper-ties. The most sensitive target cells for these studies were T-cells from cord blood (CB) of newborns and adult bone marrow[4,29,30]. Infected, replicating cells were observed within 3 to 6 weeks after exposure to HTLV-I and these cells eventually grew to populate the culture. A susceptibility and immortalization by HTLV-I of three different T-cell subsets separated from CB of newborns and peripheral blood (PB) of adults (data not shown) were assayed. T-cells were separated according to cell surface markers which expressed only T4 (OKT4+), T8 (OKT8+) or were negative for both (OKT4- and OKT8-) antigens. As shown in Table 2, all three T-cell populations from CB predefined by cell surface markers were susceptible to HTLV-I infection. After infection, they exhibited the capacity for indefinite growth in vitro. Percentage of HTLV-I positive T-cells determined by immunofluorescence assay (IFA) was in the range of 42 to 59% for the viral core protein HTLV-Ip19. Similarly, four different T-cell fraction separated according to the size of cells by Percoll gradient were susceptible to HTLV-I infection (data not shown). However, attempts to infect and immorta-lize large granular lymphocytes (LGL) by co-cultivation with HTLV-I, gave consistently negative results. Thus, these data indicate that different subsets of T cells separated for cell surface markers or by size can be in-fected and immortalized by HTLV-I with exception of LGL cells.

Properties of HTLV-I and HTLV-II Transformed T-Cells

Previous extensive in vitro studies clearly estab-lished that HTLV-I infected T cells exhibited several characteristic features which distinguish them from uninfected T-cells and show similarities to T-cell lines originated from patients with HTLV-I positive T-cell

Table 2. Infection of T-Cell Subsets with HTLV-I$_{TK}$

Cells	Cell Surface Markers			IFA for HTLV-Ip19
	OKT3	OKT4	OKT8	
	(Percent Positive Cells)			
C145	68	95	0.5	0
C145/TK*	72	92	0	59
C145	81	0	85	0
C145/TK*	85	0	78	42
C201	91	1	0	0
C201/TK*	94	1	0	56
LGL**	60	0	50	0
LGL/TK	ND	ND	ND	<1

Cord blood T cells (C145 and C201) were separated by
sepharose column using OKT4, OKT8, and OKT3 moabs.
Large granular lymphocytes (LGL) were separated by
Percoll gradient. Cells were infected with HTLV-I$_{TK}$
by cocultivation and showed a permanent growth (e.g.,
C145/TK*, etc.) with the exception of LGL. **Cytotoxicity to K562 cells of LGL was 1000 lytic units per
10^6 effectors at 15% specific lysis. ND, not done.

malignancies[29,31]. Here we briefly describe the main characteristics of in vitro transformed T-cells by HTLV-I and
HTLV-II. Like primary neoplastic T-cells, the HTLV-I and
-II transformed T cells in vitro exhibit indefinite growth
potential, show a decreased requirement for exogeneous
TCGF and eventually become completely independent of the
growth factor[29,30]. They have generally helper/inducer
(OKT4+/Leu3a+) phenotype and become a constitutive producer
of various lymphokines[32]. However, constitutive TCGF production at least in the case of in vitro transformed T-
cells was rarely observed. HTLV-infected T-cell populations
display growth, morphological (presence of multinucleated
giant cells) and cell surface alterations[29]. The most
consistent findings in HTLV-I and -II transformed CB T-
cells were high density of TCGF (detected by anti-Tac) and
transferrin receptors, and expression of HLA class-II
antigens (HLA-Dr)[29]. The only difference between HTLV-I
and HTLV-II infected T-cells was in expression of additional HLA antigen[33]. Unlike HTLV-II infected T-cells,
HTLV-I positive T-cells consistently expressed an additional antigenic determinant(s) in HLA-A or HLA-B loci

detected by alloantisera and a monoclonal antibody (4D12)
reacting with a polymorphic HLA class-I antigen[33,34].

Alteration of T-Cell Functions by Infection with HTLV-I and HTLV-II

Although both HTLV-I and HTLV-II infect and immortalize
different subsets of T-cells, precise comparison of HTLV-
transformed T-cells with its uninfected conterparts is not
feasable due to enormous heterogeneity of T-cells obtained
from CB, PB or bone marrow. Moreover, HTLV-I or HTLV-II
transformed T-cells represent an oligo- or monoclonal T-
cell population as determined by restriction pattern of
flanking sequences of integrated HTLV provirus into genome
of infected T-cells. These results indicate that transformed T-cells represent a highly selected cell population[5,7]
while normal "conterpart" of mitogen activated T-cells grown
in presence of TCGF is a very heterogeneous cell population.
To overcome these obstacles, HTLV infection of functionally
predefined T-cell populations originated from a single-cell
was studied[34-36]. Two different classes of human T-cell
clones, with specific helper and cytotoxic functions were
infected with different isolates of HTLV-I and -II. Morphological, growth and cell surface changes were essentially
the same as those described in HTLV-I or -II transformed T-
cells from CB (see above). However, virus-induced functional
alterations of HTLV-infected T-cells exhibited a very broad
spectrum of changes. These results are summarized in Table
3. Before HTLV infection the T-cell clones with helper
function proliferate and provide "help" to B-cells only in
presence of both a specific solubile antigen [keyhole limpet
hemocyanin (KLH)] and histocompatible antigen presenting
cells (APC). HTLV-I infected helper cells responded with
increased proliferation and indiscriminant stimulation of
polyclonal immunoglobulin production by B-cells, regardless
of the histocompatibility of APC or the presence of the soluble antigen[34]. On the other hand, tetanus-toxoid specific
helper T cells infected with HTLV-I lost requirement for
presence of APC and responded with increased proliferation
to the antigen[35]. Similarly, a broad spectrum of functional
changes in cytotoxic T-cells was found after HTLV-I and
HTLV-II infection[34-36].

A T-cell line derived from a HTLV-I infected ATL
patient with a prolonged survival possessed specific

Table 3. Alterations of Specific Functions of Helper and Cytotoxic T-Cell Clones Infected with HTLV-I or HTLV-II

T-Cell Clones	Functional Characteristics		
	Proliferative Response	Ig Production by B-Cells	Cytotoxic Activity
Before the Virus Infection			
Helper T-Cells specific to:			
KLH	High (only in the presence of both KLH and compatible APC)	High	
Tetanus-toxoid	High (only in the presence of both the antigen and compatible APC)		
Cytotoxic T-Cells specific to:			
HTLV-Infected T cells with class I (HLA-A1) antigen	High		High
Cells with class II (DR2 or DR7) antigen			High
After the Virus Infection			
Helper T-Cells specific to:			
KLH	High (independent of KLH and histocompatibility of APC)	High	
Tetanus-toxoid	High (independent of APC)	NT	
Cytotoxic T-Cells specific to:			
HTLV-I infected T-cells with class I (HLA-A1) antigen	Low or Absent*		Low or Absent
Cells with Class II (DR2 or DR 7) antigen			Low or Absent

NT, not tested; KLH, keyhole limpet hemocyanin; APC, antigen presenting cells. *K7 cytotoxic clone positive for HTLV-I responded by cell death[36].

cytotoxic activity to neoplastic T-cells expressing HTLV-I,
provided that the target tumor cells expressed at least
one HLA antigen (HLA-A1) in common with effector cells[36].
However, a clone (K7) derived from the parental cell line
and carried one copy of HTLV-I provirus per cell appeared
to have lost its normal immune functions. When exposed to
tumor cells expressing HTLV-I antigens, this clonal population ceased to proliferate and eventually died[36]. Furthermore, two clones of cytotoxic T-cells generated in
vitro with specificity to class II antigens, DR-2 and DR-7,
respectively resulted in a diminution or loss of the cytotoxic function after HTLV-I or HTLV-II infection[34]. Thus,
in addition to morphological, growth and cell surface alterations, HTLV infection of functionally predefined helper
or cytotoxic T cell populations originated from a single
cell leads to alteration or complete loss of specific
functions.

Biological Properties of HTLV-III

In contrast to HTLV-I or HTLV-II, transmission of HTLV-
III to fresh human lymphocytes was highly effective with
cell-free virus preparations[7]. Like HTLV-I and HTLV-II
the primary targets of HTLV-III are T-cells with helper
phenotype (OKT4/Leu3a+)[37]. The usual consequence of HTLV-
III infection was a burst of virus production, usually
within 1 to 3 weeks following infection[6,22]. During this
period of time a pronounced cytopathic effect on the infected cells was also observed[6,37]. As shown in Fig. 1,
one effect is the formation of multinucleated giant cells
which can be readily recognized in freshly infected T-cell
cultures as large cells which rapidly died out during cultivation. As mentioned above, certain established human
leukemic T-cell lines can be productively infected by
HTLV-III[6,38]. Detailed studies of HTLV-III infection of
leukemic T-cell lines showed that the virus can productively infect first of all those cells which express T4
antigen[38]. After infection, HTLV-III producing T-cell
lines failed to express T4 antigen detected by moabs
(OKT4, OKT4a and Leu3a). Further detailed analyses of
requirement of T4 antigen expression for HTLV-III infection
showed that at least part of the T4 molecule composes a
receptor for HTLV-III[39-41]. This was established by four
different assays utilizing moabs directed against T4 antigenic determinants which blocked HTLV-III and VSV pseudotype

(vesicular stomatitis virus bearing HTLV-III envelope)
infection, binding of the virus particles to the cell surface and syncytia induction in T4+ cells. The capability
of the virus to utilize a differentiation antigen (T4)
suggests that "early" infection (adsorption, penetration
and uncoating) may occur in nonactivated T-cells, which
can considerably facilitate the virus transmission in vivo
due to the availability of the receptors. To examine this
possibility, we attempted to infect non-activated T-lympho-
cytes from peripheral blood. After exposure to the virus,
the lymphocytes had been cultured for one hour, 2 and 4
days and then at each time point, stimulated by phytohemagglutinin (PHA). The virus expression was followed by
both IF and RT assays. To determine HTLV-III inactivation
in vitro, HSB_2 cells which are resistant to the virus and
do not express T4 antigen were exposed to the same viral
inoculum. The virus rescue from these cells was performed
by cocultivation procedure with PHA activated lymphocytes.
As shown in Fig. 2 the virus infection took place even
when nonactivated T lymphocytes had been cultured for 4
days after exposure to the virus. Both assays, percentage
of positive cells for HTLV-III core protein p24 and RT
activity, showed full expression of the virus. In contrast,
the virus could not be recovered from HSB_2 cells already
after 2 days of exposure. Similarly, the viral inoculum

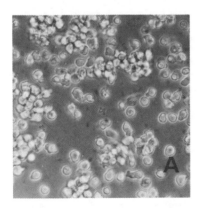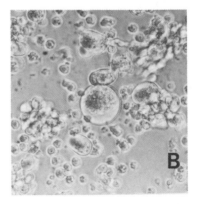

FIG 1. Growth pattern and morphology of H9 cells before (A)
and after (B) HTLV-III$_{RF}$ infection. Note the polymorphism
and presence of large cells in the infected cultures (X210).

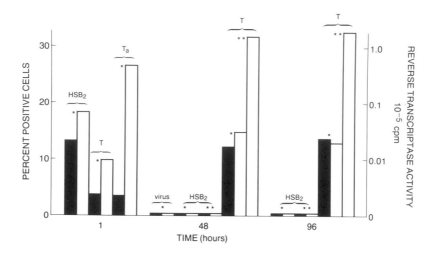

FIG. 2. HTLV-III infection of non-activated human T-cells
from peripheral blood. Percentage of infected cells
expressing HTLV-IIIp24 (■) and reverse transcriptase (RT)
activity (⊓) in culture fluids were assayed 3rd[*] day, and
RT activity only on 7th[**] day as previously described. The
following controls were done: (1) the same virus inoculum
were kept for 48 hours at 37°C and then used for infection
of activated T lymphocytes. HTLV-III$_B$ expression was
scored by IF and RT assays at 3rd[*] day. (2) Lethally irradiated HSB$_2$ cells were exposed to the same virus inoculum
and after one, 48 and 96 hours of cultivation, HTLV-III$_B$
from these cells was rescued by cocultivation procedure
using activated T lymphocytes and the virus expression was
tested 3rd and 7th day after cocultivation. The susceptibility of these T-cells (Ta) was tested by one hour exposure
to the virus.

kept for 2 days at 37°C was not biologically active. Thus,
these results indicate that the virus can utilize the
receptors on non-activated lymphocytes and full expression
of the virus takes place after blastogenic transformation.
It is conceivable that spreading of the virus infection
in vivo can under substantially more complex conditions go
through similar sequences as demonstrated in vitro which

involve "early" infection, T-cell activation, virus release, eventually T-cell death and again reinfection of non-activated T4 antigen positive T cells.

REFERENCES

1. Poiesz, B. J., et al. Proc. Natl. Acad. Sci. U.S.A. 77, 7415-7519 (1980).
2. Poiesz, B. J., Ruscetti, F. W., Reitz, M. S., Kalyanaraman, V. S. & Gallo, R. C. Nature 294, 268-271 (1981).
3. Morgan, D. A., Ruscetti, F. W. & Gallo, R. C. Science 193, 1007-1008 (1976).
4. Popovic, M., et al. Science 219, 856-859 (1983).
5. Gallo, R. C., in Cancer Surveys (eds. Franks, L. M., Wyke, L. M. & Weiss, R. A.) 113-159 (Oxford University Press, Oxford, 1984).
6. Popovic, M., Sarngadharan, M. G., Read, E. & Gallo, R. C. Science 224, 497-500 (1984).
7. Wong-Staal, F. & Gallo, R. C. Blood (in the press).
8. Hayward, W. S., Neel, B. G. & Astrin, S. M. Nature 290, 475-480 (1981).
9. Seiki, M., Hattori, S., Hirayama, Y. & Yoshida, M. Proc. Natl. Acad. Sci. U.S.A. 80, 3618-3622 (1983).
10. Ratner, L., et al. Nature (in the press).
11. Haseltine, W. A., et al. (submitted).
12. Sodroski, J. G., Rosen, C. A. & Haseltine, W. A. Science 225, 381-385 (1984).
13. Hahn, B. H., Shaw, G. M., Popovic, M., LoMonico, A. & Gallo, R. C. Int. J. Cancer 34, 316-618 (1984).
14. Hinuma, Y., et al. Proc. Natl. Acad. Sci. U.S.A. 78, 6476-6480 (1981).
15. Yoshida, M., Miyoshi, I. & Hinuma, Y. Proc. Natl. Acad. Sci. U.S.A. 79, 2031-2035 (1982).
16. Haynes, B. F., et al. Proc. Natl. Acad. Sci. U.S.A. 80, 2054-2058 (1983).
17. Vyth-Drees, F. A. & de Vries, J. E. Lancet ii, 993 (1983).
18. Greaves, M. F., et al. Int. J. Cancer 33, 795-806 (1984).
19. Blattner, W. A., et al. Int. J. Cancer 30, 257-264 (1982).
20. Kalyanaraman, V. S., et al. Science 218, 571-573 (1982).

21. Popovic, M., et al. (submitted).
22. Gallo, R. C., et al. Science 220, 865-867 (1983).
23. Gallo, R. C., et al. Science 224, 500-503 (1984).
24. Sarngadharan, M. G., Popovic, M., Bruch, L., Schupbach,
        J. & Gallo, R. C. Science 224, 506-508 (1984).
25. Schupbach, J., et al. Science 224, 607-610 (1984).
26. Feorino, P. M., et al. Science 225, 69-72 (1984).
27. Barre-Sinoussi, F., et al. Science 220, 868-871 (1983).
28. Wong-Staal, F., et al. (submitted).
29. Popovic, M., Lange-Wantzin, G., Sarin, P., Mann, D. &
        Gallo, R. C. Proc. Natl. Acad. Sci. U.S.A. 80,
        5402-5406 (1983).
30. Markham, P. D., Salahuddin, S. Z., Macchi, B.,
        Robert-Guroff, M. & Gallo, R. C. Int. J. Cancer
        33, 13-17 (1984).
31. Popovic, M., Wong-Staal, F., Sarin, P. S. & Gallo,
        R. C., in Advances in Viral Oncology (ed. Klein, G.)
        45-70 (Raven Press, New York, 1984).
32. Salahuddin, S. Z., et al. Science 223, 703-706 (1984).
33. Mann, D. L., et al. Nature 305, 58-60 (1983).
34. Popovic, M., et al. Science 226, 459-462 (1984).
35. Mitsuya, H., et al. Science 225, 1484-1486 (1984).
36. Mitsuya, H., et al. Science 223, 1293-1296 (1984).
37. Klatzmann, D., et al. Science 225, 59-63 (1984).
38. Popovic, M., Read-Connole, E. & Gallo, R. C. Lancet
        ii, 1472-1473 (1984).
39. Dalgleish, A., et al. Nature 312, 763-767 (1984).
40. Klatzmann, D., et al. Nature 312, 767-768 (1984).
41. Popovic, M., Read-Connole, E., Neuland, C. & Mann, D.
        (submitted).

Stage Specific Transforming Genes in Lymphoid Neoplasms

M.A. Lane,[1,2] H.A.F. Stephens;[1,2]
M.B. Tobin[1] and Kevin Doherty[1]
[1] Laboratory of Molecular Immunobiology
Dana Farber Cancer Institute
and
[2] Department of Pathology
Harvard Medical School

The NIH 3T3 transfection assay has now been employed successfully for over five years in the identification of activated transforming genes of neoplasms from multiple species. The first genes to be identified utilizing this assay were members of the ras gene family, including ras^H and ras^K which had been retrovirally transduced by Harvey and Kirsten Sarcoma Viruses, and ras^N, first identified in a human neuroblastoma cell line, SK-N-SH, a ras family member which had not been transduced by a retrovirus. To date, ras genes have been found to be activated in 10-20% of all neoplasms tested. As ras genes are transcribed in virtually all cells at most stages of differentiation, it is not surprising that these genes fall "at risk" to neoplastic transformation at some low level in tumors representative of every lineage and stage of differentiation (Reviewed in 1).

In contrast to the ras genes, activated at a low level in neoplasms of multiple different lineages, stage specific genes have been identified whose activation is uniquely confined to cells of a particular lineage, at a particular stage of differentiation. Several years ago we reported the identification of five different stage-specific transforming genes activated within neoplasms of T- and B-lymphoid cells (2). To date, we have examined over two hundred leukemias, lymphomas and myeloma/plasmacytomas and have not found stage specific transforming genes activated in inappropriate stages of lineages.

Within the B-lymphoid lineage, three different genes

181

are consistently activated. The gene activated in pre B
neoplasms which express cytoplasmic heavy chains but no
surface immunoglobulin has been identified in 24 human
or mouse neoplasms of this phenotype. Expression of this
gene is inactivated by digestion with the enzymes BAM Hl
and Xho I. The intermediate B gene Blym-l, is found to
be activated in B- cell tumors which express surface Ig,
but have not undergone morphologic transition to plasma-
cytes, and has been found activated in forty different
neoplasms from chicken (3), mice and humans (2). This
group includes Burkitts lymphomas, Hairy B- cell leukemias,
chronic lymphatic leukemias and diffuse histiocytic
lymphomas covering a range of disease states between slowly
progressive and acute. This gene can be differentiated
from the pre B gene by its susceptibility to inactivation
by digestion with the enzyme BAM Hl, but not XhoI.

     Within plasmacytomas and myelomas of mouse or human
origin which are active secretors of immunoglobulins and
have undergone characteristic end stage morphologic differentiation, a third gene is activated and has been
identified in 17 different plasmacytomas or myelomas, both
in mice and humans. The mature B gene is inactivated only
by the enzyme Sac I.

     Within T lineage neoplasms, two predominant stage
specific genes have been identified. The Tlym-I gene has
been found to be activated in 18 mouse or human early to
mid thymic entry neoplasms and differs by restriction
analysis from the gene activated in 8 mature stage T
lymphoid tumors. A third gene has been identified to be
activated in a single human tumor possessing mixed phenotypic markers and which shares no homology with either of
the two previously identified genes. One other human T
cell tumor appears to have three linked activated genes,
one of which is Tlym-I, while the other two represent genes
which have not previously been encountered activated in
either T- or B- lymphoma neoplasms.

     Of these stage specific genes from the T- and B-
lineages, none shares homology with retrovirally transduced
oncogenes including ras and myc family members. The Blym-l
gene is one member of a family containing 6-8 family members, and it is likely that these members include the Pre
B and mature B genes. Tlym-I, because of its shared
homology with MHCI genes may represent a family of as many
as 36 members but shares no homology with the B lineage
genes.

     Two of these genes have been successfully cloned.

Human Blym-1, isolated from a Burkitts lymphoma recombinant library, using Chicken Blym as a probe, encodes a
small protein of 8 kd which shares homology with transferrin molecules (4). The bulk of the protein encoded by
chicken Blym appears to be expressed in the nucleus; however, at this point, rapid cycling between the nucleus,
cytoplasm and cell surface cannot be excluded. The mechanism of activation of human Blym is currently being
examined by comparison of nucleotide sequences obtained
from normal and neoplastic cells (4).

Mouse Tlym-I isolated from the S49 TLymphoma, appears
to encode a secreted protein of 43-44kd. This gene both
at the protein level and by southern blot hybridization
appears to share some homology with genes from the MHCI
region (5). As restriction site analysis has ruled out
identity to genes encoding conventional H2 molecules, it
is likely that Tlym-I is either a gene encoded within the
TL-QA region (6) or may represent a novel gene from this
region activated as a result of a gene conversion event.
Sequence analysis and further hybridization to genes within
the MHCI cluster should serve to precisely define the
nature of this gene.

It is one of our goals to define the role of proteins
encoded by transforming genes both in normal and neoplastic
cells. As transferrins have been reported to behave under
certain circumstances as lymphoid cell mitogens, it is
attractive to speculate that Blym-1 may act in this manner,
as an aberrant growth stimulus which alters the ability of
B-cells to terminally differentiate and end their life
cycle. Tlym-I, which encodes a secreted MHCI like protein
may, we speculate, form an aberrant association with the
T-cell receptor which recognizes viral antigen and an
MHCI product to produce an abnormal growth stimulus in situ
in the thymus. Thus far we have determined that while
Tlym-I does not substitute for IL2, it does have the ability to stimulate growth of splenic cells in a short term
assay, and is activated in T-cell clones which have become
antigen and feeder layer independent.

Sequencing of the Tlym-I gene is in progress and
approximately 2.2kb has now been completed. Preliminary
computer assisted analysis has indicated that this gene
shares no complete homology to any genes currently
included in the mouse sequence data base. Short sequences
of 30-40 nucleotides have been identified which share as
much as 70% homology with genes within the MHCI region and
with members of immunoglobulin gene family. These findings

are consistent with this gene's being a member of the
super gene family. Two truncated Kappa R repeats have
additionally been identified which are located before the
first open reading frame. Conserved in these repeats are
the regions which share homology with SV40 enhancer sequences. Kappa R repeats have previously been detected
associated with functional immunoglobulin genes, globin
genes, one H-2 gene and preceeding several intracisternal
A partical genes.

The authors wish to thank S. Hunt, G.M. Cooper and
J. Strominger for useful discussions, and J. Strominger
for assistance with the computer analysis. This work was
supported by CA 33108. M.A.L. is a Leukemia Society Scholar.
H.A.F.S. is a fellow of the Cancer Research Institute.

References

1. Cooper, G.M. and Lane, M.A. (1984) Biochem. Biophys.
    Acta, Elsevier (in Press).

2. Lane, M.A., Sainten, A. and Cooper, G.M. (1982) Cell
    28: 873.

3. Goubin, G., Goldman, D.S., Luce, J., Nieman, P.E. and
    Cooper, G.M. (1983) Nature 302:114.

4. Diamond, A., Cooper, G.M., Ritz, J. and Lane, M.A.
    (1983) Nature 305:112.

5. Lane, M.A., Sainten, A., Doherty, K.M. and Cooper, G.M.
    (1984). P.N.A.S.

6. Lane, M.A., Stephens, H.A.F., Doherty, K. and Tobin,
    M. (1984) Modern Trends in Human Leukemia VI, Springer-
    Verlag (in Press).

MOLECULAR CLONING AND EXPRESSION OF cDNAS ENCODING

THE HUMAN INTERLEUKIN-2 RECEPTOR

Warren J. Leonard. Joel M. Depper,
Gerald R. Crabtree, Stuart Rudikoff.
Janet Pumphrey, Richard J. Robb*,
Martin Krönke, Penny B. Svetlik.
Nancy J. Peffer, Thomas A. Waldmann,
and Warner C. Greene

National Cancer Institute, Bethesda,
    MD 20205
*E.I. du Pont de Nemours & Co.,
Glenolden, PA 19036

ABSTRACT

We have identified cDNAs encoding the human interleu-
kin-2 (IL-2) receptor from a cDNA library constructed from
HUT-102B2 cell mRNA. and have expressed them in eukaryotic
cells. Based on the deduced amino acid sequence from the
DNA sequence, the IL-2 receptor is initially synthesized as
a preprotein of 272 amino acids and then processed to a
mature form of 251 amino acids. The protein has a very
short positively charged cytoplasmic region at the carboxy
end of the molecule that contains potential phosphorylation
sites. The protein has two potential N-linked carbohydrate
addition sites and multiple potential O-linked carbohydrate
addition sites. Although the IL-2 receptor appears to be
encoded by a single structural gene, there are two distinct
mRNAs that encode the protein that differ in the polyadenylation signal used. Further, there is evidence that
alternate mRNA splicing may also occur.

INTRODUCTION

Activation of resting T lymphocytes results in the de
novo synthesis and secretion by some T cells of IL-2, also
known as T-cell growth factor.[1] The same or other T cells,
when activated, express IL-2 receptors. The cells with
receptors, in the presence of IL-2, proliferate and result
in the evolution of T cells capable of mediating helper
and cytotoxic functions.[2-4] Both IL-2 and IL-2 receptor
expression are inducible events whose regulation is critical to the evolution of an immune response. Human IL-2 has
been purified[5], molecularly cloned[6], and identified as
being encoded by a single gene[7,8] on chromosome 4. IL-2
receptors have been characterized as glycoproteins that are
both sulfated and phosphorylated with apparent M_r's of
approximately 55,000 on normal activated T cells.[9-13]
Receptors are also present on human T-cell leukemia/
lymphoma virus-I (HTLV-I) infected T cells.[12-14] These
cells have uniformly large numbers of IL-2 receptors.[14] We
now describe the purification of the IL-2 receptor protein,
and identification, expression, sequencing of IL-2 receptor
cDNAs, and utilization of the cDNAs to explore receptor expression. A more detailed discussion of these data is
provided in reference 15.

PURIFICATION AND SEQUENCE OF THE IL-2 RECEPTOR

As shown in Figure 1, we purified the IL-2 receptor on
HTLV-I infected HUT-102B2 cells to apparent homogeneity
using an anti-Tac[16,9] immunoaffinity column. The purified
protein was able to block IL-2 induced proliferation and
thus represented a protein capable of binding IL-2. The
protein was sequenced by gas phase microsequencing.
Certain positions were confirmed by sequencing receptor
biosynthetically radiolabeled with select amino acids. The
sequence obtained is as follows:

H_2N-glu-leu-cys-asp-asp-asp-pro-pro-glu-ile-pro-his-ala-thr
-phe-lys-ala-met-ala-tyr-lys-glu-gly-thr-met-leu-asn-cys-glu

MOLECULAR CLONING OF THE HUMAN IL-2 RECEPTOR

An oligonucleotide probe of length 17 and 64-fold
degeneracy was prepared based on amino acids 3 through 8

AFFINITY PURIFIED TCGF RECEPTOR
FROM HUT-102B2 CELLS

$M_r \times 10^{-3}$

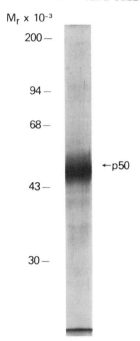

Figure 1· Purification of the human IL-2 receptor.
4×10^9 HUT-102B2 cells were solubilized on ice in 10 mM
tris pH 7.4 containing 0.15 M NaCl, 100 ug/ml phenylmethyl-
sulfonylfluoride and 0.5% NP-40. Nuclei and other debris
were pelleted by centrifugation, and the supernatant was
passed first over a control column and then over an anti-Tac
sepharose column. The column was washed extensively at
varying salt concentrations, and the bound protein then
eluted with 2.5% acetic acid in water. This material was
concentrated and an aliquot electrophoresed on an 8.75%
SDS gel. Reproduced from reference 15 with permission of
Nature.

(generously provided by Drs. R.M. Balagaje and J.P. Burnett,
Lilly Research Laboratories), underlined above, and this
pool of 17mers was used to screen a cDNA library prepared
from HUT-102B2 mRNA in the bacteriophage lambda gt10 (see
ref. 15 for details regarding the cDNA library).

SELECTIVE HYBRIDIZATION
WITH IL-2 RECEPTOR cDNAs

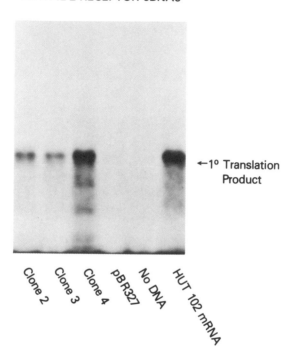

←1° Translation
Product

Clone 2 Clone 3 Clone 4 pBR327 No DNA HUT 102 mRNA

Figure 2: Selective hybridization of IL-2 receptor mRNA.
DNA from clones 2, 3, or 4 and from control pBR327 were
bound to nitrocellulose (see ref. 15 for details) and
hybridized to HUT-102B2 mRNA. The filters were washed,
the specifically associated mRNA eluted in water, translated
in a wheat germ cell free translation system and immunoprecipitated with anti-IL-2 receptor heteroantiserum, and
electrophoresed on an 8.75% SDS gel. Shown are results
using clone 2, 3, 4, pBR327, nitrocellulose to which no
DNA was bound, and on the right, the primary translation
product of HUT-102B2 mRNA. Reproduced from reference 15
with permission of Nature.

        Candidate cDNA clones were identified from the cDNA
library by hybridizing with the ^{32}P-end-labeled 17mer. In
order to confirm that these cDNAs were clearly associated
with the IL-2 receptor, the inserts from three clones were

subcloned into pBR322 and then selective hybridization experiments were performed, as shown in Figure 2. On the right, the primary translation product for IL-2 receptor mRNA is indicated. As can be seen, candidate clones 2, 3, and 4 were all capable of selectively hybridizing IL-2 receptor mRNA, but pBR327 and nitrocellulose without DNA could not.

We next proceeded to sequence clones 2, 3, and 4, which contained inserts of approximately 900, 2300, and 1600 base pairs, respectively. Shown in Figure 3 is the restriction map of the sequence for clones 3 and 4. The two clones differ in two principal ways. First, clone 3 is longer and extends further 3' than clone 4. Second, clone 3 contains a segment 216 base pairs long that is not present in clone 4. Examination of the sequence in detail revealed that this region is bounded by the repeated sequence TTCCAGGT, and therefore has typical donor and acceptor mRNA splice signals. Thus, it was possible either that the larger cDNA had retained an intron, or that the shorter cDNA had lost part of an exon. The clone 4 cDNA encoded a protein 72 amino acids shorter which shared both amino and carboxy termini with clone 3. It was therefore critical to determine which cDNA-- the spliced or the nonspliced form-- would encode a functional IL-2 receptor.

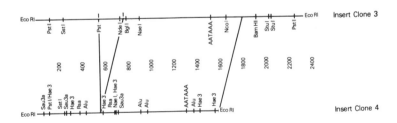

Figure 3: Restriction maps of clones 3 and 4. The lines extending from clone 4 to clone 3 demark the regions absent in clone 4. Reproduced from reference 15 with permission of Nature.

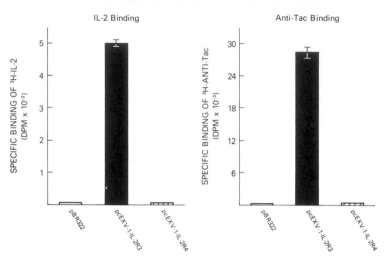

EXPRESSION OF IL-2 RECEPTOR cDNAs IN COS-1 CELLS

Figure 4: The unspliced cDNA encodes a functional IL-2
receptor. COS-1 cells were transfected by calcium phosphate
precipitation with 5 ug of either pBR322 or the expression
vector pcEXV-1 containing the insert from either cDNA
clone 3 or 4. The cells were grown overnight, the media
changed, and the cells cultured for another 48 hours. Cells
were then washed, incubated at 4°C for 90 minutes in RPMI
1640 containing 3% fetal bovine serum and either 45,000
dpm of ^{3}H-IL-2 or 194,000 dpm of ^{3}H-anti-Tac, with or
without excess unlabeled IL-2 or anti-Tac, respectively.
Cells were washed, dissolved in 0.1 M NaOH, and associated
radioactivity determined. Specific IL-2 and anti-Tac
binding are indicated.

     We made use of the expression vector pcEXV-1, prepared
and generously provided to us by Drs. J. Miller and R.
Germain, NIH, for this purpose. This vector contains the
enhancer and early promoter regions of SV40. The inserts
from cDNAs 3 and 4 were subcloned into pcEXV-1 in the
correct orientations, and then COS-1 cells were transfected
by calcium phosphate precipitations. As shown in Figure 4,
COS-1 cells transfected with the clone 3 construct resulted
in expression of IL-2 receptors. In contrast, cells transfected with the clone 4 construct were incapable of binding

either IL-2 or anti-Tac. Thus, the functional IL-2 receptor
is encoded by the unspliced cDNA. Indeed, COS-1 cells
transfected with the clone 3 cDNA express on their surface
an IL-2 receptor identical in apparent M_r to that seen on
HUT-102B2 cells. Using either anti-Tac or an anti-IL-2
receptor heteroantiserum, we have not been able to precipitate any protein from COS-1 cells transfected with the
clone 4 construct, although we identify clone 4 associated
mRNA in these cells. Thus, we do not know with certainty
whether the existence of clone 4 represents an alternate
form of processing of IL-2 receptor mRNA which encodes a
protein of some other function, or whether it might
represent a cloning artifact, although this latter possibility is perhaps minimized by the presence of perfect
donor and acceptor mRNA splice signals.

ONE GENE, BUT DIFFERENT mRNA SIZE CLASSES

We next used an IL-2 receptor cDNA to hybridize to a
Southern blot of genomic DNA digested with EcoRI. As
shown in Figure 5, a relatively simple pattern of hybridization is identified, consistent with the existence of a
single gene. In contrast, as shown in Figure 6, mRNA of
two different sizes, approximately 1500 and 3500 bases
long, are identified. In data detailed elsewhere[15], we
demonstrate that these two classes of mRNA almost certainly
differ because of the utilization of different polyadenylation signals. Within each size class, we propose that
there may be two forms of mRNA-- one containing and one not
containing the 216 base segment that can be spliced. Thus,
we propose that there are a total of four or possibly even
six different forms of mRNA (six because in addition to two
AATAAA polyadenylation signals, there is also an ATTAAA,
which may sometimes function as a polyadenylation signal).
IL-2 receptor mRNA, as expected, is found in induced but
not in uninduced peripheral blood T cells. It is also
found in all HTLV-I infected T cells and B cells that we
have studied to date. So far, there is complete concor-
dance between the expression of Tac antigen and the
presence of IL-2 receptor mRNA.

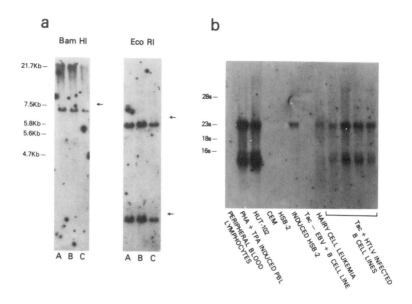

Figure 5:   Panel a-- DNA from placenta (A) or tonsils
(B and C) were digested with BamHI and EcoRI, electrophoresed, transferred to nitrocellulose, and hybridized
with an IL-2 receptor cDNA probe. When full length cDNAs
have been used in subsequent digests, 2 BamHI fragments
(25 and 7.5 kb) and 5 EcoRI fragments (10 kb, 6 kb, 2.4
kb, and two smaller fragments) are identified.
Panel b-- Northern blot of 10 ug mRNA from the indicated
cell types, hybridized to IL-2 receptor cDNA. Reproduced
from reference 15 with permission of Nature.

ANALYSIS OF THE IL-2 RECEPTOR PROTEIN

        The complete amino acid sequence of the IL-2 receptor
was deduced from the nucleic acid sequence[15] (see Figure 6).
The receptor is initially synthesized as a preprotein of 272
amino acids and then processed to a mature receptor of 251
amino acids. There are a total of 13 cysteine residues. We
know that at least one and perhaps multiple disulfide bonds
form, as the mature protein migrates faster on SDS gels
electrophoresed under nonreducing conditions as opposed to

DEDUCED AMINO ACID SEQUENCE OF THE HUMAN IL-2 RECEPTOR

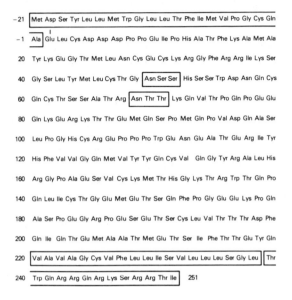

Figure 6: Deduced amino acid sequence of the human IL-2
receptor. Boxed are the signal peptide (amino acids -21
to -1), two potential N-linked glycosylation sites
(asn-ser-ser and asn-thr-thr), the hydrophobic transmembrane region (beginning val-ala-val-ala), and the
intracytoplasmic domain (beginning thr-trp-gln).

reducing conditions. There are two potential N-linked
carbohydrate addition sites, both of which must be utilized
based on our earlier studies of the protein wherein we
demonstrate that there are two N-linked precursors with
apparent M_r's of 35,000 and 37,000.[10,13] The receptor also
contains multiple potential O-linked carbohydrate addition
sites.

    Near the C-terminus, there is a long hydrophobic region
that almost certainly represents an alpha helical transmembrane crossing. There are only 13 amino acids carboxy
to this region, forming a very short cytoplasmic domain.
This domain contains six positively charged amino acids and
therefore presumably serves as a cytoplasmic anchoring

region. This regions also contains two potential phosphorylation sites (one serine and one threonine). We have previously shown that IL-2 receptors are phosphoproteins and therefore hypothesize that at least one of these is phosphorylated. The intracytoplasmic region is so short that it is difficult to imagine that it contains an enzymatic function. It is therefore puzzling to hypothesize the mechanism of signal transduction for the IL-2/IL-2 receptor system. Perhaps the receptor serves only to bind IL-2 and IL-2 itself provides the actual initial intracellular signal. Alternatively, it is possible that a receptor complex exists. Above, we have only considered the binding protein for IL-2. We have previously hypothesized[9] that two other proteins that we routinely coimmunoprecipitate with anti-Tac (apparent M_r's 113,000 and 180,000) might be subunits in a receptor complex.

We hope the availability of cDNAs corresponding to the IL-2 receptor will help to elucidate the unanswered questions regarding IL-2 receptor regulation and the mechanisms of signal transduction. Further, we hope to clarify the nature of the relationship between HTLV-I infection and IL-2 receptor expression.

REFERENCES

1. Morgan, D.A., Ruscetti, F.W. & Gallo, R.C. Science 193, 1007-1008 (1976).
2. Watson, J. J. exp. Med. 150, 1510-1519 (1979).
3. Coutinho, A., Larsson, E-L, Gronvik, K-O, & Andersson, J. Eur. J. Immun. 9, 587-592 (1979).
4. Gillis, S., Baker, P.E., Ruscetti, F.W. & Smith, K.A. J. exp. Med. 148, 1093-1098 (1978).
5. Robb, R.J., Kutny, R.M. & Chowdhry, V. Proc. natn. Acad. Sci. U.S.A. 80, 5990-5994 (1983)
6. Taniguchi, T., Matsui, H., Fujita, T., Takeoka, C., Kashima, N., Yoshimoto, R. & Hamura, J. Nature 302, 305-309 (1983).
7. Fujita, T., Takeoa, C., Matsui, H. & Taniguchi, T. Proc. natn. Acad. Sci. U.S.A. 81, 1634-1638 (1983).
8. Holbrook N.J., Smith, K.A., Fornace, A.J., Jr., Comeau, C.M., Wiskocil, R.L., and Crabtree, G.R. Proc. natn. Acad. Sci. U.S.A. 81, 1634-1638 (1984).

9. Leonard, W.J., Depper, J.M., Uchiyama, T., Smith, K.A., Waldmann, T.A. & Greene, W.C. Nature 300, 267-269 (1982).

10. Leonard, W.J., Depper, J.M., Robb, R.J., Waldmann, T.A., & Greene, W.C. Proc. natn. Acad. Sci. 80, 6957-6961 (1983).

11. Wano, Y., Uchiyama, T., Fukui, K., Maeda, M., Uchino, H., and Yodoi, J. J. Immun. 132, 3005-3010 (1984).

12. Leonard, W.J., Depper, J.M., Waldmann, T.A. & Greene, W.C., in Receptors and Recognition, Series B, Vol 17, (ed., Greaves, M.), pp 45-66 (1984).

13. Leonard, W.J., Depper, J.M., Krönke, M., Robb, R.J., Waldmann, T.A. & Greene, W.C. J. Biol. Chem. (in the press).

14. Depper, J.M., Leonard, W.J., Krönke, M., Waldmann, T.A. & Greene, W.C. J. Immun. 133, 1691-1695 (1984).

15. Leonard, W.J., Depper, J.M., Crabtree, G.R., Rudikoff, S., Pumphrey, J., Robb, R.J., Krönke, M., Svetlik, P.B., Peffer, N.J., Waldmann, T.A. & Greene, W.C. Nature (in the press).

16. Uchiyama, T., Broder, S. & Waldmann, T.A. J. Immun. 126, 1393-1397 (1981).

Mantle Zone and Germinal Center B cells Respond to Different Activation Signals

Jeffrey A. Ledbetter, Paul J. Martin, and
Edward A. Clark
Genetic Systems Corporation
3005 First Avenue
Seattle, WA   98121

Introduction

The cross-linking of surface immunoglobulin on resting B lymphocytes by antigen or by anti-Ig antibody leads to proliferation and differentiation to plasma cells (1,2). Helper T cells provide growth and differentiation factors distinct from interleukin 2 (IL-2) that contribute to B cell proliferation (3,4). The proliferation and differentiation process involves multiple steps, including first activation by Ig or antigen. This causes a rapid increase in cell size and an elevation of levels of surface Ia antigens (5,6). These changes result from depolarization of the B cell plasma membrane (7) and can occur without B cell proliferation using low levels of anti-Ig, or using phorbol diesters (8). Anti-Ig activation of B cells also causes expression of receptors for a T cell factor(s) (9). Cells in this stage can proliferate in response to T cell factors alone and have been termed "preactivated" B cells (10,11). The preactivated cells constitute as many as 20% of peripheral blood B cells (12), are IgD$^-$, proliferate in response to pokeweed mitogen (PWM) and are less dense than resting B cells (10,13). The third stage of B cell differentiation depends upon T cell derived differentiation factors (14) that may also be involved in isotype switching.

197

From tissue section studies, it has long been known
that germinal centers are B cell areas that are T cell
dependent and are formed in lymphoid tissues after
antigen stimulation (15). Germinal centers are formed in
secondary follicles after the primary Ab response (15)
and contain a population of B cells that are rapidly
dividing and are different from mantle zone B cells in
Ig, Ia and Bp32(B1) antigen densities (16-18). Germinal
centers are thought to be involved in memory B cell
formation (15) and may be involved in isotype switching
(19).

In this report we examined human germinal center and
mantle zone B cell populations from reactive lymph nodes
and tonsils for surface phenotypes using two color
immunofluorescence and for their responsiveness to activation signals. In addition, we measured quantitative
levels of antigen expression on a series of B cell CLLs
and B cell lymphomas and draw some correlations between
the B cell malignancies and normal stages of B cell
differentiation.

Results and Discussion

Germinal center and marginal zone B cells are
distinguishable in suspension by two color immunofluorescence. This was shown in the mouse by a high level of
peanut agglutinin (PNA) binding in germinal centers
(18). Surface IgM was much lower in the germinal center
while Ia levels were higher. In the human, the Bp32
antigen is expressed at about 10 fold higher levels on a
B cell subpopulation that also expresses low levels of
IgM (Figure 1). These cells have the phenotype of
germinal center B cells. The reciprocal population of B
cells with high levels of IgM and low levels of Bp32
corresponds phenotypically to mantle zone B cells.

To determine whether these two populations identified
by two color immunofluorescence in suspension (Figure 1)
correspond to germinal center and mantle zone populations, we separated the tonsil lymphocytes on discontinuous density gradients. Germinal center B cells are
rapidly dividing blast cells and should be of lower
density than resting B cells. We found that the
IgM^{dull}, $Bp32^{bri}$ population was highly enriched at

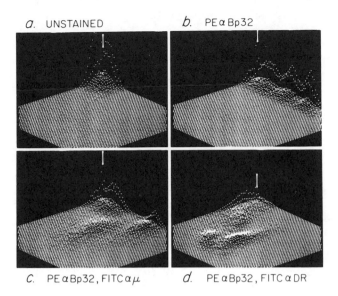

a. UNSTAINED   *b*. PEαBp32

c. PEαBp32, FITCαμ   *d*. PEαBp32, FITCαDR

Figure 1. Two distinct populations of tonsillar B cells
are detected using two color immunofluorescence with
phycoerythrin (PE)-conjugated anti-Bp32 versus
fluorescein-conjugated anti-μ (panel c) or versus
fluorescein-conjugated anti-DR (panel d). Unstained
cells are positioned at the back (panel a) and each panel
shows data from 40,000 cells on a 64 x 64 grid representing 4 $\log_{10}$ units in the red (right) and green
(left) dimensions.

the top of the gradient while the IgM^{bri}, $Bp32^{dull}$
population was highly enriched at the botton of the
gradient. In addition, the $IgM^{dull}Bp32^{bri}$ cells were
all IgD^- (data not shown). Thus, the two color system
appears to distinguish the proliferating germinal center
population (low density cells) from the resting mantle
zone population (high density cells).

We next separated the tonsillar B cell populations on
discontinuous density gradients to study their responsiveness to activation signals. The IgM^{bri} $Bp32^{dull}$

Table I.

Tonsillar Mantle Zone and Germinal Center B Cells Respond
to Different Activation Signals.

	Mean Specific Proliferation After Stimulation With:[a]		
Cell Density[b]	T cell factors	sepharose anti-μ	PWM
Unfractionated	20,763±927	3,656±383	20,763±707
High Density (Germinal Center Cells)	33,968±1,527	884±200	23,558±1,018
Low Density (Mantle Zone Cells)	1,656±85	13,903±91	1,073±274

[a] Mean cpm ± SE of quadruplicate samples of tonsillar
lymphocytes after 4 days in culture. Nonspecific
background counts of unfractionated cells (2,451
cpm), high density cells (7,826 cpm) and low density
cells (1,034 cpm) were subtracted from totals.

[b] Cells were separated on discontinuous percoll
gradients as described. (10)

high density population required anti-Ig to proliferate,
whereas the IgM^{dull} Bp32^{bri} low density population
proliferated in response to T cell factors alone and to
PWM (Table I). Thus the IgM^{dull} Bp32^{bri} cells in the
germinal centers correlate functionally with a population
of "preactivated" B cells found in peripheral blood (10,
13). Some germinal center cells may be capable of
recirculation (20), although germinal center B cells in
general appear to be noncirculating and lack a surface
glycoprotein involved in lymphocyte recirculation (21,22).

Although mouse germinal centers were reported to
express higher levels of Ia antigens than mantle zone B
cells (18), human germinal centers and mantle zone appear
equal in DR expression (16,17). In fact, mantle zones
often appear to have higher levels of DR. We confirmed
that these populations are about equal in DR, DC, and SB
antigen levels using the two color system. Therefore,

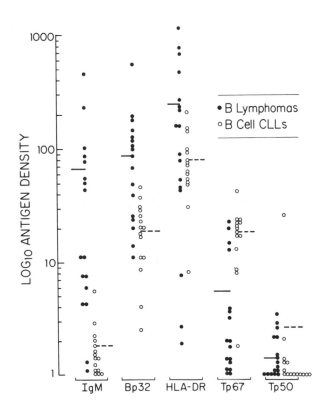

Figure 2. Antigen densities of CLL and B cell lymphomas
is expressed as a ratio of mean brightness of stained
cells/mean brightness of unstained cells (autofluores-
cence). A value of 1 therefore represents no staining
above background. The mean value of all CLLs is shown
with a dashed line and the mean value of all B cell
lymphomas is shown with a solid line.

while Bp32 is a good marker for distinguishing germinal
center and mantle zone B cells, DR is not.

Both mantle zone and germinal center cells showed a wide range of DR antigen levels that were substantially higher than the levels found on B cells in peripheral blood (data not shown). Thus, although germinal center B cells and preactivated B cells in peripheral blood are functionally similar in that both populations can respond to T cell factors, they probably represent distinct populations of B cells rather than a single recirculating population.

We examined a panel of B cell CLLs and lymphomas to measure the quantitative levels of Bp32, IgM, DR, Tp67, and Tp50 antigens (Figure 2) on each. Each of the antibodies was directly labeled with fluorescein, and the brightness of binding is a reflection of antigen density.

There was extensive heterogeneity within each group for mean levels of antigen expression. For example, CLLs varied extensively from one another in DR antigen density. In spite of the variation, several differences between CLLs and lymphomas were apparent. The mean DR levels were higher on lymphomas than on CLLs whereas the mean IgM levels were lower. The Bp32 levels tended to be higher on lymphomas than on CLLs, and the Tp67 (10.2) antigen was higher on CLLs. Most lymphomas did not express Tp67 (Figure 2). We were surprised to find that the Tp50 antigen (E rosette receptor) was expressed on several B cell malignancies (Figure 2) confirming earlier studies of Gugliemi (23).

In addition to within group heterogeneity, the two color immunofluorescence system showed extensive hetero-geneity in antigen expression by individual malignan-cies. The CLLs that we examined fall into one of sever-al patterns for Bp32 versus DR expression illustrated in Figure 3. These ranged from $DR^{bright}Bp32^{+/-}$ (CLL-14 and CLL-12) to $DR^{+/-}Bp32^{bright}$ (CLL-3). In each of these CLLs there were cells expressing only one of these two antigens (Figure 3). This may be evidence for continuing differentiation within the B cell neoplasm, similar to that reported by others (reviewed in 24).

The Tp67 antigen (25) is the evolutionary homologue of murine Ly1 (26) and both are expressed on normal T cells and B cell malignancies. Ly1 is also expressed by

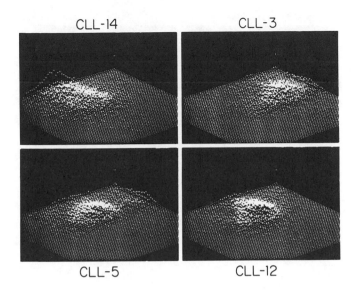

Figure 3. Two color phenotypes of representative CLLs.
Each panel shows PG—conjugated anti—Bp32 (to the right)
versus fluorescein—conjugated anti—DR (to the left). The
data was collected and positioned as described in the
legend to Figure 1.

a subset of normal B cells (27,28). The expression of
Tp67 on normal human B cells has been harder to detect,
although it was reported to be expressed on some B cells
in tonsils (29). We have not detected Tp67 on B cells
from reactive tonsils or lymph nodes. However, we do
find Tp67 expressed in low density on some circulating B
cells (Figure 4). Thus, the Tp67 antigen also distinguishes the B cells in peripheral blood from the mantle
zone and germinal center B cells.

Immunoglobulin production can occur without germinal
center formation. In fact, antibody—antigen complexes
are bound to Fc receptors on dendritic reticulum cells in
a C3 dependent process during germinal centers formation
(30). C3 is also required for generation of memory B
cells (31). Germinal centers are likely to be involved

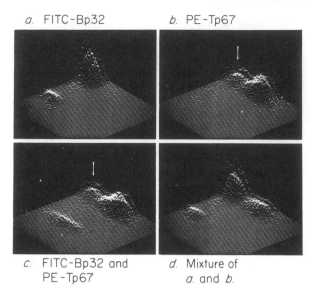

a. FITC-Bp32   *b.* PE-Tp67

c. FITC-Bp32 and   *d.* Mixture of
    PE-Tp67   *a.* and *b.*

Figure 4.   Expression of Tp67 by peripheral blood B
cells.   Fluorescein–conjugated   anti–Bp32   and
PE–conjugated anti–Tp67 were used alone (panels a and b)
or in combination (panel c) to show Tp67 expression on
peripheral B cells.

in memory B cell formation (15) and may be important
sites of immunoglobulin class switching (19). Our
functional studies show that germinal cells proliferate
in response to T cell factors and PWM, suggesting that
they are similar to "preactivated" B cells in peripheral
blood.   However, these two populations are different in
several ways: a) germinal center B cells express higher
levels of DR than peripheral blood B cells; b) germinal
center cells are Tp67$^-$ while some peripheral blood B
cells are Tp67$^+$, and c) germinal center B cells do not
appear to recirculate (22).

     In summary, using a combination of methods including
quantitative two color flow cytometry, density gradient
separation, immunolochemical and functional assays, we
have been able to distinguish at least 3 distinct B cell

subpopulations: mantle zone, germinal center, and circulating.

This work was supported in part by Genetic Systems Corporation and by grants AI-20432 and CA-34199 from the National Institute of Health.

REFERENCES

1. Kishimoto, T., Miyake, T., Nishizawa, Y., Watanabe, T., and Yamamura, Y. J. Immunol. 115, 1179-1185 (1975).
2. Parker, D.C. Nature (London) 258, 361-363 (1975).
3. Maraguchi, A., Kasahara, T., Oppenheim, J.J., and Fauci, A.S. J. Immunol. 129, 2486-2489 (1982).
4. Howard, M., Farrar, J., Hilfiker, M., et al. J. Exp. Med. 155, 914-921 (1982).
5. DeFranco, A.L., Raveche, E.S., Asofsky, R., and Paul, W.E. J. Exp. Med. 155, 1523-1531 (1982).
6. Mond, J.J., Seghal, E., Kung, J., and Finkelman, F.D. J. Immunol. 127, 881-886 (1981).
7. Monroe, J.G., and Cambier, J.C. J. Exp. Med. 158, 1589-1599 (1983).
8. Cambier, J.C., Monroe, J.G., and Niedel, J.E. Fed. Proc. 42, 416-419 (1983).
9. Yaffe, L.F., and Finkelman, F.D. Proc. Natl. Acad. Sci. USA 80, 293-297 (1983).
10. Kuritani, T., and Cooper, M.D. J. Exp. Med. 155, 1561-1566 (1982).
11. Andersson, J., Schrcier, M.H., and Melchers, F. Proc. Nat. Acad. Sci. USA 77, 1612-1616 (1980).
12. Lanzavecchia, A. Eur. J. Immunol. 13, 820-824 (1983).
13. Kuritani, T., and Cooper, M.D. J. Immunol. 131, 1306-1311 (1983).
14. Isakson, P.C., Pure, E., Vitetta, E.S., and Krammer, P.H. J. Exp. Med. 155, 734-742 (1982).
15. Thorbecke, G.J., Romano, T.J., and Lerman, S.P. Prog. Immunol. II, Vol. 3, 25-34 (1974).
16. Bahn, A.K., Nadler, L.M., Stashenko, P., McCluskey, R.T., and Schlossman, S.F. J. Exp. Med. 154, 737-748 (1981).
17. Giorno, R.C. Immunohistology and Histocytochemistry of the Lymphoid System. C.C. Thomas, publisher. Springfield, Ill. (1984).

18. Butcher, E.C., Rouse, R.V., Coffman, R.L., Notten-
    burg, C.N., Hardy, R.R., and Weissman, I.L. J.
    Immunol. 129, 2698–2707 (1982).
19. Kraal, G., Weissman, I.L., and Butcher, E.C. Nature
    298, 377–379 (1982).
20. Opstelten, D., Stikker, R., Deenan, G.J., Bos, L.,
    and Nieuwenhuis. Cell Tissue Res. 218, 59–67 (1981).
21. Parrott, D.M.V. In Germinal Centers in Immune
    Responses. H. Cottier, ed. Springer-Verlag, New York
    168–175.
22. Reichert, R.A., Gallatin, W.M., Weissman, I.L., and
    Butcher, E.C. J. Exp. Med. 157, 813–827 (1983).
23. Gugliemi, P., Preud'homme, J.L., and Brouet, J.C. J.
    Immunol. 13, 641–646 (1983).
24. Godal, T., and Funderud, S. Adv. Cancer Res. 36,
    211–255 (1982).
25. Martin, P.J., Hansen, J.A., Nowinski, R.C. and Brown,
    M.A. Immunogenetics 11, 429–439 (1980).
26. Ledbetter, J.A., Evans, R.L., Lipinski, M., Cunning-
    ham-Rundles, C., Good, R.A., and Herzenberg, L.A. J.
    Exp. Med. 153, 310–323 (1981).
27. Hayakawa, K., Hardy, R.R., Parks, D.R., and Herzen-
    berg, L.A. J. Exp. Med. 157, 202–218 (1983).
28. Monhar, V., Brown, E., Leiserson, W.M., and Chused,
    T.M. J. Immunol., 129, 532–538 (1982).
29. Caligaris-Cappio, F., Gobbi, M., Bofill, M., and
    Janossy, G. J. Exp. Med. 155, 623–628 (1982).
30. White, R.G., Henderson, D.C., Eslami, M.B., and
    Nielson, K.H. Immunology 28, 1–21 (1975).
31. Klaus, G.G.B., and Humphrey, J.H. Immunology 33,
    31–40 (1977).

DEVELOPMENT OF T CELLS WITHIN THE THYMUS

J.J.T. OWEN AND E.J. JENKINSON

DEPARTMENT OF ANATOMY, MEDICAL SCHOOL,

UNIVERSITY OF BIRMINGHAM, BIRMINGHAM, U.K.

INTRODUCTION

There are many unanswered questions concerning the role of the thymus in the generation of T lymphocytes. Questions about the influence of the thymus on the generation of the T cell receptor repertoire are particularly pertinent following recent rapid progress in knowledge of the genetic control and structure of the receptor[1]. Although it is not clear whether the recombination of germ line V-, D- and J- gene segments which forms the basis for coding diverse variable regions of T cell receptors occurs during lymphocyte maturation within the thymus[2] or at an earlier pre-thymic stem cell stage,[3] there is considerable evidence that the thymus shapes the T cell receptor repertoire. Thus T cells show major histocompatibility (MHC) antigen restriction in their response to foreign antigens and tolerance to "self" MHC antigens which maps to the MHC haplotype of the thymus within which they develop[4]. In particular, MHC antigens expressed on thymic stromal cells may select for survival lymphocytes which express the appropriate receptors. This notion is supported by the high rate of cell death within the thymus, presumably of non-compatible cells, although non-productive rearrangements of T cell receptor genes might occur at high frequency resulting in cell death[5].

In this paper, we discuss recent experiments which provide information about the roles of thymic stromal cells in the induction of immunological tolerance to "self".

MHC ANTIGEN EXPRESSION ON THYMIC STROMAL CELLS

Class I MHC antigens are expressed on all thymic
stromal cells, but the expression of class II MHC antigens
is limited to two cell types. Thymic epithelial cells
express class II antigens from an early stage of ontogeny[6].
These cells are derived from epithelium of the pharyngeal
pouches; they are held tightly together by desmosomal
connections with associated pre-keratin tonofilaments.
They form the major component of the stroma of the cortex
of the thymus and so are intimately associated with the
proliferating population of thymocytes in the outer cortex.[7]
The closeness of the association between epithelial cells
and cortical thymocytes is exemplified by epithelial "nurse"
cells which envelop groups of thymocytes.[8] However, the
functional significance of this arrangement is unkown. Not
all thymic epithelial cells express class II MHC antigens,
although in the normal thymus the majority of cortical
epithelial cells do so. In nude mice, none of the epithelial cells of the alymphoid thymus express class II
antigens.[6]

The second population of cells expressing class II MHC
antigens consists of a network of dendritic cells located
in the thymic medulla[9]. The precursors of these cells
migrate into the thymus from foetal liver and bone marrow.
In irradiated animals recolonized by bone marrow cells,
it has been shown that class II antigens expressed on thymic
epithelial cells are of host haplotype, whereas thymic
dendritic cells express class II antigens of donor haplotype
thus demonstrating the independent synthesis of class II
antigens by epithelial and dendritic cells[9]. Like epithelial cells, thymic dendritic cells are closely associated
with lymphocytes. Clusters of lymphocytes are frequently
seen around dendritic cells isolated from the thymus.
Whether or not there are differences between lymphocytes
associated with distinct stromal populations is not clear.

There are other minority populations of thymic stromal
cells; for example, cells which express a GQ ganglioside
characteristic of neuro-endocrine cells can be identified
in clusters throughout the thymus by means of a monoclonal
antibody (A2B5). These cells probably do not express
class II MHC antigens.[10] Their functional role is obscure.

FUNCTIONAL SIGNIFICANCE OF MHC ANTIGENS EXPRESSED ON THYMIC
STROMAL CELLS

It has proved difficult to disentangle the relative
contributions of MHC antigens on thymic epithelial and
dendritic cells in the development of the T cell receptor
repertoire. Experiments aimed at answering this question
by constructing chimaeric thymuses with epithelial and
dendritic cells of different MHC haplotypes have been
difficult to interpret because the techniques used - thymus
grafts with or without irradiation and bone marrow injection
- do not succeed in eliminating all donor lymphoid and
dendritic cells.[11] We have shown that deoxyguanosine,
elevated blood levels of which have been implicated in the
T-cell immunodeficiency of purine nucleoside phosphorylase
deficient individuals, completely eliminates lymphoid cells
from organ cultures of embryonic thymus but spares the
epithelial framework.[12] The alymphoid epithelial lobes can
be recolonized in vitro by the addition of thymic stem cells
or in vivo by host lymphoid stem cells following transplantation of the lobes under the kidney capsule.

It was during the course of the latter experiments that
we noted that deoxyguanosine-treated thymic grafts were not
rejected following transplantation to adult allogeneic
recipient mice, whereas untreated grafts were promptly
rejected.[13] Moreover, deoxyguanosine-treated lobes become
fully lymphoid after colonization by host stem cells and
show considerable growth equivalent to that found following
transplantation to syngeneic recipients. Successful allogeneic transplantation was possible despite continued
expression of class I and class II MHC antigens on donor
thymic epithelial cells. However, it is unlikely that
recipients of allogeneic thymic epithelial grafts are tolerant to donor MHC antigens because graft lymphocytes and
host spleen cells are fully responsive to stimulator cells
of donor haplotype in mixed lymphocyte culture.[13]

Of various possible explanations for the survival of
deoxyguanosine-treated thymus in allogeneic recipients, we
favour the notion that thymic epithelium is not immunogenic
to unprimed recipients. Several recent studies have shown
that reduction of class II MHC antigen-expressing cells
lowers the immunogenicity of tissue grafts.[14,15] Our results
show that survival of deoxyguanosine-treated grafts is not
due to an absence of class II MHC antigen expression suggesting

that immunogenicity also depends on the cell type on which class II antigens are expressed. In this context it is significant that deoxyguanosine eliminates dendritic cells, perhaps by blocking the proliferation of dendritic cell precursors, as well as lymphoid cells from thymus organ cultures.[10] Several other studies have suggested that dendritic cells are important immunogens in tissue grafts.[17] Our studies extend this idea and we propose that donor dendritic cells are essential to the immunogenicity of thymus grafts, although we cannot exclude the possibility that lymphocytes are also immunogenic. Furthermore, host dendritic cells, which populate the medulla of deoxyguanosine-treated grafts, do not present class I and class II MHC antigens of donor cortical epithelial cells to the immune system of unprimed hosts. Even when donor and host are MHC compatible, host dendritic cells do not present minor histocompatibility antigens of epithelial cells to the host's immune system, since deoxyguanosine-treated thymus survives and grows when transplanted between mice differing only for minor antigens.[13]

On the basis of these results, we conclude that epithelial cells of the thymus are neither immunogenic nor tolerogenic. Host lymphocytes developing within deoxyguanosine-treated thymus grafts, whilst responding to MHC antigens on stimulator cells showing the donor epithelial haplotype, do not respond to antigens of host haplotype i.e. MHC antigens expressed on the lymphocytes themselves and on dendritic cells populating the grafts.[13] We have obtained similar results in deoxyguanosine-treated thymus colonized by stem cells in vitro.[18] Differentiating lymphocytes are not responsive to MHC antigens expressed by the colonizing dendritic cells. If mixtures of stem cells of different MHC haplotypes are used to colonize deoxyguanosine-treated thymus in vitro, the resulting lymphoid cells are mutually tolerant, perhaps because the thymus contains dendritic cells of both haplotypes.[18] These results point to the importance of class II MHC antigen-expressing thymic dendritic cells in tolerance induction in maturing lymphocytes. They also allow for the possibility of dendritic cells maintaining tolerance in peripheral lymphoid organs following migration of T cells from the thymus.

CONCLUSIONS

We conclude that, although both thymic epithelial and

dendritic cells express class I and class II antigens, only
dendritic cells are involved in tolerance and immunogenicity.
Reasons why dendritic cells should render maturing cells
tolerant, but immunize recipients of transplants are unclear.
We propose that dendritic cells are essential for the immunogenicity of thymus grafts to non-primed recipients. We have
evidence that the situation is different in primed animals
where deoxyguanosine-treated thymus grafts are rejected.
Thus T cells with low affinity receptors for alloantigen in
non-primed animals may respond to histocompatibility antigens
only when they are an integral part of dendritic cell
membranes. However, primed T cells with high affinity
receptors for alloantigen can respond to donor histocompatibility antigens acquired by host dendritic cells, or
perhaps directly to histocompatility antigens on other
tissues.

REFERENCES

1. Williams, A.F. Nature 308, 108-109 (1984)
2. Acuto, O., Hussey, R.E., Fitzgerald, K.A., Protentis, J.P.,
        Meuer, S.C., Schlossman, S.F. and Reinherz, E.L.
        Cell 34, 717-726 (1983).
3. Morrisey, P.J., Kruisbeek, A.M., Sharrow, S.O. and
        Singer, A. Proc. Natn. Acad. Sci. U.S.A. 79, 2003-
        2007 (1982).
4. Zinkernagal, R.M. Immunol. Rev. 42, 224-270 (1978)
5. Kavaler, J., Davis. M.M. and Chien, Y-H, Nature 310,
        421-423 (1984).
6. Jenkinson, E.J., van Ewijk, W. and Owen, J.J.T. J. Exp.
        Med. 153, 280-292 (1981)
7. Owen, J.J.T. and Jenkinson, E.J. Progr. Allergy 29,
        1-34 (1981)
8. Kyewki, B.A. and Kaplan, H.S. J. Immunol. 128, 2297-2294
        (1982)
9. Barclay, A.N. and Mayrohofer, G.J. Exp. Med. 153,
        1660-1671 (1981)
lo. Jenkinson, E.J., Kingston, R. and Owen, J.J.T. Eur. J.
        Immunol. (in the press).
11. Longo, D.L. and Davis, M.L. J. Immunol. 130, 2525-2527
        (1983)
12. Jenkinson, E.J., Franchi, L.F., Kingston, R., and
        Owen, J.J.T. Eur. J. Immunol. 12, 583-587 (1982)
13. Ready, A.R., Jenkinson, E.J., Kingston R., and Owen, J.J.T
        Nature 310, 231-233 (1984)

14. Lafferty, K.J. Transplantation 29, 179-182 (1980)
15. Morrow, C.E., Sutherland, D.E.R., Steffes, M.W.
        Najarian, J.S. and Bach, F.H. Transplantation 36,
        691-694 (1983)
16. Owen, J.J.T and Jenkinson, E.J. Am. J. Anat (in the
        press).
17. Hart, D.N.J., Newton, M.R., Reece-Smith, H., Fabre, J.W.
        and Morris, P.J. Transplantation 36, 431-435
        (1983).
18. Jenkinson, E.J., Jhittay, P., Kingston, R and Owen, J.J.T.
        Transplantation (in the press).

SECTION IV

SELECTIVE RECOGNITION BY T AND B CELLS

INTRATHYMIC DIFFERENTIATION AND THE T CELL REPERTOIRE

Roland Scollay

The Walter & Eliza Hall Institute of Medical

Research, P.O. Royal Melbourne Hospital,

Victoria 3050, Australia.

In the 1960's immunologists realised that the thymus was of critical importance in the development of the immune system. Without the thymus, T cell numbers were considerably reduced. In the 1970's, immunologists went beyond this concept of a quantitative influence on peripheral T cell numbers, and there was a rush of enthusiasm for the idea that the thymus played an important role in determining the specificity of the cells produced.[1,2] The recent rapid advances in our understanding of the molecular nature of the T cell receptor and its associated molecules, may mean that the 80's will give us a clearer picture of the mechanisms involved in this determination of the T cell repertoire. But while we await these revelations, it may be worth stepping back a little and taking a look at what our current knowledge of thymocyte subpopulations and kinetics tells us, and to see how the recent advances can best be applied.

Leaving aside the questions of how and where the thymus does things (i.e. positive vs. negative selection, cortex vs. medulla etc.), we can regard the thymus as a black box and simply ask, what does it do? Is receptor diversity generated in the thymus, or earlier in the bone marrow? Are the two T cell lineages separated in the thymus or earlier in the bone marrow? Are self tolerance and restriction determined only in the thymus or elsewhere as well? Is restriction to both MHC classes determined in the thymus, or only to one? Is functional maturity attained within

215

the thymus or after export to the periphery? Do non-
thymic or environmental antigens influence events inside
the thymus? In my view, most of these questions cannot
be definitively answered at this stage, but let us consider some of them in more detail.

Generation of Diversity:

Ideally one would approach this question by taking
purified pro-thymocytes from bone-marrow and measuring
the expressed repertoire in functional tests, (assuming
the cells could be stimulated at this early stage) or
by looking for rearrangement of the receptor genes. However at the present time, the nature of the bone-marrow
pro-thymocyte is still unknown, so this approach is not
possible. An alternative would be to use the approach of
Lepault et al,[3] and inject labelled bone-marrow cells
intravenously into irradiated mice, and to purify the
few labelled cells which go specifically to the thymus
over the next few hours. However, these cells are rare,
and although their purification from the thymus in any
number is possible, the technique presents many difficulties. In addition, there is no hard evidence that the
cells observed by Lepault et al. are in fact pro-thymocytes; they did not demonstrate the ability of these cells
to give rise to thymic lymphocytes, although they did
show a progression from T cell marker negative to T cell
marker positive soon after their arrival in the thymus.[4]

Perhaps the best method at the present time would be
identification within the thymus of possible stem or precursor cells on the basis of the known phenotypic markers,
and to look for genetic rearrangement among them. By
analogy with the B cell system, we might expect some
rearrangement before the cells become identifiably "T"
cells. We have recently identified several possible early
thymocyte populations, including those negative for both
Ly 2 and L3T4,[5] but also Ly 1 and Thy 1. These and the
population isolated from thymic nurse cells are being
analysed at the present time in our laboratory.

The second way to look at the question of the generation of diversity is to ask whether the rate of stem cell
input into the thymus is high enough to provide a large
repertoire if the repertoire was generated prethymically.
This question has been examined in considerable detail

over the last 20 years, but remains controversial (reviewed
in ref. 6), largely because there is no good system for
measuring it. However, several papers have shown that
repopulation of each lobe of an irradiated adult thymus
can be by very small numbers of cells (perhaps as few as
one).[7-9] Other studies have suggested that 100-1000 cells
repopulate an irradiated thymus, although these results
depend on a degree of extrapolation and several assumptions
which leave room for considerable error.[10-11] Thus the
estimates of the number of cells required to repopulate an
irradiated thymus are generally low, varying from 1-1000.
Although this does not say much about the rate of stem cell
input into normal thymuses over long periods, it does
apparently say that the thymus can be entirely populated by
very few cells. Whether in such cases the normal range of
receptor specificities is expressed remains unknown, but
experiments to test this are now feasible.

The rate of stem cell input into normal adult thymuses
is even less clearly established. If bone-marrow cells are
injected into normal mice, they do not give rise to significant numbers of thymocytes.[6,12] Experiments with para-
biotic mice and half-body irradiated mice (reviewed in
detail in ref.6) give conflicting results; the parabionts
suggest no thymic stem cell turnover, the half body irradiated mice suggest a slow turnover rate. None of the data
suggest a rapid and continual replacement from extrathymic
sources. Again one is left with the impression that the
number entering is negligible or at least relatively low,
perhaps in the order of 100's or 1000's. It may also be
that the input rate is much higher during the early
developmental stages of the thymus, or in extreme cases of
depletion, such as in thymus grafts or irradiated thymuses.
In this case one might postulate that diversity during the
steady state adult period, is maintained by a pool of
intrathymic stem cells which had diversified at an early
stage in ontogeny and had entered the thymus in large
numbers at that time.

Although it seems unlikely that the pro-thymocyte
repertoire can be probed in the usual way, by assaying
function, several groups have attempted to look at
tolerance in pro-thymocytes. Experiments with thymus
grafted, chimeric mice have suggested that tolerance to
MHC antigens is, or can be, generated prethymically.[13,14]

These studies have been carefully controlled, but there
may be artefacts hidden in these complex non-physiological
systems, so the results should be treated cautiously.
Nonetheless, taken at face value they imply that receptors
for MHC antigens are expressed on pro-thymocytes. The
anti-MHC repertoire need not be more than a few hundred,
so this may not be in conflict with the stem cell data
mentioned above. Prethymic tolerance to non-MHC antigens
(the size of this repertoire and its relationship to the
anti-MHC repertoire is uncertain) has also been analysed.
Tolerance to non-MHC alloantigens appears to occur intra-
or post-thymically,[15] while it has been claimed that
tolerance to foreign protein antigens can occur in pro-
thymocytes.[16] However, in this latter case, excluding
antigen carryover is very difficult. Finally studies with
nude mice,[17] also suggest MHC tolerance can be generated
pre-thymically. Taken together, and putting aside the
possible complication of suppressor mechanisms,[18] these
data lead one to keep in mind the possibility that at
least the anti-MHC repertoire could be expressed prethymically, necessitating a stem cell contribution of at
least hundreds to the thymocyte pool in the models studied.

The Onset of Maturity

     Although the relative maturity of the cells emerging
from the thymus has been somewhat controversial over the
years, I think it is now clear that, at least in the adult,
cells leave the thymus in a relatively mature state. They
are phenotypically mature[19] (with minor exceptions[20]), and
respond as well as lymph node T cells to Con A and alloantigen.[21] Thus, the major maturation events occur inside
the thymus. The critical question about the cells leaving
the thymus concerns their restriction. A careful analysis
of the restriction and tolerance profile of thymus
emigrants compared to peripheral T cells in general, would
answer many of the questions about intra- and extrathymic
processing. Studies of this kind are now possible[21] and
are in progress in our laboratory. They are essential to
allow us to distinguish between post thymic modification
of an intrathymically generated repertoire and extrathymic repertoire generation.

The effect of peripheral events on intrathymic different-iation

There are several cell kinetic studies which suggest that cell production by the thymus is not subject to feed-back controls based on peripheral T cell numbers[22-24] (reviewed in 6). In addition, our own studies, in which emigration rate was directly measured,[25] did not find a change in migrant numbers after administration of antigen peripherally. Thus, there is no evidence that migration rates from the thymus are significantly affected by peri-pheral events. However, this in no way excludes a change in specific cells among migrants, since a 100-fold increase in antigen specific cells (e.g. from 0.1% to 10% of migrants), would not affect the numbers of total migrants in a measurable way.

On the other hand, it is quite clear that the thymus is affected by peripheral events. For example, there are marked changes in subpopulation distribution following high dose peripheral antigen,[26] and peripheral immunisa-tion to minor histocompatibility antigens results in increases in the frequency of intrathymic CTL directed against those antigens.[27] Furthermore there is evidence that both antigen[28] and activated cells,[29] can enter the thymus. What role these play in the usual intrathymic events remains unknown. Finally the data of Matzinger et al,[30] which show that in mice carrying two antigenic-ally different thymus grafts, peripheral T cells (most which have presumably come from only one of the grafts) are tolerant to both types of thymic antigen. This latter point (again ignoring for the moment the possibil-ity of suppressor mechanisms) can be added to the others mentioned above in indicating that the thymus is by no means an isolated, antigen-free, autonomous organ, but must interact with the extrathymic environment in ways which are not yet understood.

Extrathymic T cell differentiation

The facts that neonatal thymectomy leads to a severe T cell deficit and that thymus-less nude mice have no T cells, have led to the general view that all T cells are thymus processed. However, it is clear that some T cells develop in older nude mice[31] (although only a small proportion of them are fully immunocompetent[32]), and this slow accumula-

tion of thymus independent cells could happen in normal
mice but be difficult to detect. Furthermore, there is the
possibility of T cells which are thymus-dependent but not
thymus processed. These would be T cells which develop in
the periphery in response to thymic factors or, more likely
perhaps, in response to cells (or their soluble products)
which have been through the thymus. Thymus-dependent cells
of this type would be difficult to distinguish from true
thymus processed cells, since they would also not appear in
thymectomised animals. However in certain experimental
situations, namely chimeras and thymus-grafted chimeras,
these extrathymic T cells should show different restriction
patterns from cells which had been through the thymus. The
early experiments of Zinkernagel et al.[1] showed that T
cells in the spleen were fully restricted to the MHC antigens of the thymus, leaving little room for extrathymic
differentiation. However, since that time, many papers
have shown that restriction to thymic MHC type is at best
partial,[2,33] and indeed, it now seems likely that responses
restricted to MHC class I antigens can be restricted to
both thymic and extrathymic antigens.[34-36] On the other
hand, responses restricted to class II MHC antigens do
appear to be restricted only by intrathymic antigens,[34]
although recent data (Golding & Singer, reported at this
meeting, see workshop reports) suggests that even some Ia-
restricted CTL (but not Ia-restricted helper cells) can be
determined extrathymically. All these experiments show
that cells can exist in the periphery that are restricted
to antigens not present (i.e. not demonstrably present) in
the thymus. This certainly does not prove that the cells
have not been through the thymus, but it clearly leaves
this open as a possibility. These data are really the best
(and only?) evidence for a significant extrathymic pathway.

Conclusions

Conclusion may well be a misnomer for this final
section, since no firm conclusions are possible. However
we may well ask at this stage whether the concept of the
thymus as the autonomous and singular controller of T cell
production and specificity is valid. From the data we have
mentioned above, it seems that some repertoire generation
may occur prethymically, that T cell production may occur
extrathymically, and that both tolerance induction and
restriction can occur outside the thymus. It remains to
be seen whether these extra-thymic events are limited to

certain lineages or functions, and whether they contribute
significantly to the peripheral T cell pool in normal
animals. It may be that the thymus has no unique role in
determining T cell specificity, but simply represents the
place where T cells grow best and hence the organ from
which most T cells come. If a T cell is tolerised or
restricted by whatever environment it happens to differentiate in, it would then still be true that the cells
developing in the thymic microenvironment would dominate T
cell populations. The apparent absolute restriction to
thymic antigens observed for Ia-restricted helper cells
might then be a result of the requirement of this particular class for growth conditions provided only by the
thymus, not because only the thymus can induce Ia restriction. Even the extremely high rate of cell division and
cell death in the thymus (reviewed in 6) may not signal
anything unique about this tissue, since the same thing
could be happening elsewhere on a much smaller scale.
By this argument, the high rate of attrition could be
characteristic of growing T cells (faulty rearrangements
perhaps, like among B cells?) rather than a reflection of
a unique intrathymic selection procedure. We should however emphasise that T cell growth outside the thymus in
normal mice must be occurring on a fairly small scale
since cells of thymic cortical phenotype are uncommon
in other tissues.[37]

Thus we may well ask at this stage whether there is
anything unique about the thymus other than its quantitative success. Analysis of the genetic rearrangements in
various thymocyte subpopulations should help resolve this
question. These experiments are under way.

References

1.   Zinkernagel, R.M., Callahan, G.N., Althage, A.,
         Cooper, S., Klein, P.A. & Klein, J. J.exp.Med.
         147, 882 (1978).

2.   Fink, P.J. & Bevan, M.J. J.exp.Med. 148, 766 (1978).

3.   Lepault, F. & Weissman, I.L. Nature 293, 151 (1981).

4.   Lepault, F., Coffman, R.L. & Weissman, I.L. J.Immunol.
         131, 1 (1983).

5.   Scollay, R., Shortman, K. & Bartlett, P. Immunol.Rev.
      in press (1984).

6.   Scollay, R. & Shortman, K. In Recognition and Regula-
      tion in cell mediated immunity (Watson &
      Marbrook, eds.). Marcel Dekker, N.Y. (1984).

7.   Wallis, V., Leuchars, E., Chwalinski, S. & Davies,
      A.J.S. Transplant 19, 2 (1975).

8.   Micklem, H.S., Ford, C.E., Evan, E.P. & Ogden,
      D.A. Cell Tissue Kinet. 8, 233 (1975).

9.   Ezine, S., Weissman, I.L. & Rouse, R.V. Nature
      309, 629 (1984).

10.   Kadish, J.L. & Basch, R.S. Cell Immunol. 30, 12
      (1977).

11.   Boersma, W., Betel, I., Daculsi, R. & Van der
      Westen, G. Cell Tissue Kinet. 14, 179 (1981).

12.   Micklem, H.S., Clarke, C.M., Evans, E.P. & Gray, J.
      Transplant 6, 299 (1968).

13.   Bradley, S.M., Morrissey, P.J., Sharrow, S.O. &
      Singer, A. J.exp.Med. 155, 1638 (1982).

14.   Morrissey, P.J., Kruisbeck, A.M., Sharrow, S.O.
      & Singer, A. Proc.Natl.Acad.Sci.U.S.A. 79,
      2003 (1982).

15.   Morrisey, P.J., Bradley, D., Sharrow, S.O. &
      Singer, A. J.exp.Med. 158, 365 (1983).

16.   Cohn, M.L. & Scott, D.W. J.Immunol. 123, 2083
      (1979).

17.   Besedovsky, H.O., de Rey, A. & Sorkin, E.
      J.exp.Med. 150, 1351 (1979).

18.   Stockinger, B. Proc.Natl.Acad.Sci.U.S.A. 81,
      220 (1984).

19.   Scollay, R. J.Immunol. 128, 1566 (1982).

20. Scollay, R., Wilson, A. & Shortman, K. J.Immunol.
    132, 1089 (1984).

21. Scollay, R., Chen, W.-F. & Shortman, K. J.Immunol.
    132, 25 (1984).

22. Vaughan, W.P. & McGregor, D.D. J.Cell Physiol.
    80, 13 (1972).

23. Wallis, V.J., Leuchars, E., Chandhuri, M. &
    Davies, A.J.S. Immunol. 38, 163 (1979).

24. Leuchars, E., Wallis, V.J., Doenhoff, M., Davies,
    A.J.S. & Kruger, J. Immunol. 35, 801 (1978).

25. Scollay, R. & Shortman, K. Amer.J.Anat. in press
    (1984).

26. Durkin, H., Carboni, J. & Waksman, B. J.Immunol.
    121, 1075 (1978).

27. Fink, P., Bevan, M. & Weissman, I. J.exp.Med. 159,
    436 (1984).

28. Raviola, E. & Karnovsky, M.J. J.exp.Med. 136,
    466 (1972).

29. Naparstek et al. Eur.J.Immunol. 13, 418 (1983).

30. Matzinger, P., Zamoyska, R. & Waldmann, H. Nature
    308, 738 (1984).

31. Hunig, T. Immunol.Today 4, 84 (1983).

32. Chen, W.-F., Scollay, R., Shortman, K., Skinner,
    M. & Marbrook, J. Amer.J.Anat. in press
    (1984).

33. Blanden, R.V. & Andrew, M. J.exp.Med. 149, 535
    (1979).

34. Bradley, S.M., Kruisbeck, A. & Singer, A.
    J.exp.Med. 156, 1650 (1982).

35. Kruisbeck, A., Sharrow, S. & Singer, A. J.Immunol.
          130, 1027 (1983).

36. Kruisbeck, A., Sharrow, S., Mathieson, B.J. &
          Singer, A. J.Immunol. 127, 2168 (1981).

37. Scollay, R. & Shortman, K. Thymus 5, 245 (1983).

Molecular Nature of T Cell Recognition of Antigen

Emil R. Unanue, Paul M. Allen, and Evelyn A. Kurt-Jones

Department of Pathology, Harvard Medical School

Boston, Massachusetts 02115

This presentation summarizes two of our recent lines of research on antigen presentation by macrophages. The first deals with the issue of antigen processing, the second with the role of interleukin-1. Recently published papers have dealt with these two issues (1, 2, 3). The reader is referred to them for full presentation of the data, discussion, and references.

Antigen Processing: Numerous studies have indicated that the determinants in globular protein antigens recognized by B cells and T cells are different (reviewed in 4, 5). The antigenic determinants recognized by B cells are represented in the intact tertiary configuration of the protein. In contrast, most T cell reactivity is directed to determinants found in the unfolded, denatured molecule. These results strongly indicate that the B cells selected by protein antigens recognized the protein before extensive degradation by the host, while the protein recognized by the T cells had to suffer alterations during handling. We all accept the statement that, in order for T helper cells to be stimulated, they must recognize antigen in the context of an antigen-handling or -presenting cell (APC) which must express on their membranes the class II histocompatibility molecules (the Ia glycoproteins). Our studies have examined antigen handling by macrophages and have brought evidence for a processing event during antigen presentation.

The first studies indicating an intracellular handling step for antigen presentation employed the intracellular pathogenic bacteria Listeria monocytogenes (6,
7). Macrophages were briefly exposed to heat-killed
bacteria and then washed. Listeria-immune T cells were
added to the culture. The T cells rapidly established
contact with the macrophage surface but only following a
lag period of time during which the bacteria was internalized and partially catabolized. Two further manipulations were of key importance. If, during this lag
period of internalization the macrophages were treated
with lysosomotropic drugs, then no presentation took
place. In contrast, the drugs had no effect if added
following the period of handling. The logical conclusion
was that the drugs were targeting an acid compartment
required for the presentation of the antigen. A second
significant manipulation was the use of mild fixation by
paraformaldehyde. Fixation of the macrophages during the
lag period impaired antigen presentation but not following
it. Thus, after the intracellular stage, the plasma membrane contained all the elements required for T cell
recognition. In fact, T cells not only recognized Listeria antigens on the surface of fixed macrophages but
were stimulated to vigorously proliferate. The scenario
that we envisioned from these series of observations was
that the bacteria was internalized and that it was processed through an acid-labile intracellular compartment in
which some of the immunogens were processed and then recy-
cled to the plasma membrane and there presented in the
context of Ia. Once on the membrane, there was no further
need of a live, active cell.

Our subsequent studies have examined the handling of
the well-defined protein hen egg-white lysozyme (HEL) by
the mouse macrophage (1, 2, 8). The major observations
confirm the results with the bacterial antigens and give
us further insights into defining processing in biochemical terms. The basic system was to develop monoclonal T
cells to HEL. The T cell hybridomas were evaluated for
the production of interleukin-2 following interaction with
macrophages or B cell lymphomas pulsed with HEL. We have
found that:

1. The presentation of native HEL was highly sensitive to chloroquine. Chloroquine did not impair the rate

of uptake of HEL, nor did it have non-specific, deleterious effects on the T cells.

   2. Following a fifteen-to-thirty-minute period of handling, macrophages could be fixed and still were able to stimulate the T cells.

   3. Macrophages treated with chloroquine, pulsed with HEL, and then fixed did not present HEL.

   4. Macrophages fixed before pulsing with antigen (prefixed macrophages) and then given HEL did not present the antigen. These four observations clearly indicate that our T cell hybrids are not recognizing the native HEL displayed on the membrane. Rather, the HEL requires a further step sensitive to chloroquine.

   The use of denatured and tryptic peptides of HEL allowed us to dissect some of the biochemical events, particularly because we have two sets of T cell hybrids which recognize the processed HEL in different forms. Thus, macrophages pulsed with denatured HEL (carboxymethylated or CM-HEL), which binds to the macrophages, were shown to require a chloroquine-sensitive step for one T cell hybrid (hybrid 2A11) but not for another (hybrid 3A9). Moreover, prefixed macrophages pulsed with antigen would present only to those T cells that did not require the intracellular processing (3A9). The tryptic peptides could be presented to both by live macrophages treated with chloroquine or by prefixed macrophages. Hence, the two T cell clones are defining processing for us; processing involved two biochemical events: 1) an unfolding of the molecule which, took place normally in acid vesicles —when the denatured molecule was administered, it was recognized by one set of clones (3A()), and no further intracellular handling was then required; and 2) a proteolytic step following denaturation.

   The structure of the tryptic peptide recognized by both clones has now been identified. Both recognize the same peptide bearing the sequence 46-61 of HEL (Asn-Thr-[]-Asp-Gly-Ser-Thr-Asp-Tyr-Gly-Ile-Leu-Gly-Ile-Asn-Ser-Arg). This peptide has different amino acids from human and mouse lysozye, which are not immunogenic at positions 46, 47, 48, 50, and 56. The 46-61 peptide has now been

synthesized by Drs. G. Matsueda and E. Haber and found to
be as immunogenic as the native peptide. Through the use
of various synthetic peptides and their derivatives, we
have now shown that, although 2A11 and 3A9 T cells are
stimulated by the same tryptic fragment, they are, in
fact, recognizing different antigenic determinants.

    In essence, our T cell clones are indicating some of
the key structural features in the antigen-handling event.
Clearly, native HEL is not the structure that selects for
T cell reactivity since none of about thirteen hybrids
studied so far react with it. The hybrid recognizes only
native HEL when the molecule is subsequently handled by
the APC in an acid intracellular compartment. Processing
is required for a globular protein like HEL to be presented and involves two separate handling events. One
involves only the unfolding of the molecule. Indeed, a
set of T cell clones recognizes the unfolded molecule
without any need of proteolysis (unless the proteolysis
takes place on the surface, for which we have no evidence). A second form involves actual breakdown of the
molecule. Indeed, the prototype clone 2A11 does not even
recognize denatured HEL but only small fragments of it.
We believe that processing reveals small hydrophobic
sequences in a protein which allow their interaction with
relevant structures on the plasma membrane of the APC,
most likely with the Ia antigens. Studies examining this
issue are now in progress.

A Membrane Form of IL-1

    We were puzzled by the results showing that fixed,
antigen-bearing macrophages, that were incapable of IL-1
secretion, stimulated growth of T cell lines and clones.
Either IL-1 was not required (9), or an IL-1-like molecule
was present on the membranes of the fixed macrophages. We
have evidence for the latter (3). The basic observations
are:

    1. Macrophages fixed in formaldehyde, after a brief
period of culture on dishes, stimulated the growth of thymocytes as well as of an IL-1-dependent T cell clone (10).
This clone proliferated to Con A only in the presence of
IL-1 and could be used, therefore, to assay for and ti-
trate IL-1.

2. The stimulation of growth did not depend on Ia expression by the macrophage, i.e., Ia-positive and Ia-negative macrophages were effective.

3. Membranes from culture, unfixed macrophages, likewise, stimulated thymocytes and the cloned T cell.

4. The growth-promoting activity of the membranes was not altered by fixation; it was removed from the membranes only by non-ionic detergents, while high salt, changes in pH, and EDTA did not remove the activity. Hence, the activity behaved as an integral membrane protein.

5. A goat anti-IL-1 made by Steven Mizel (11) blocked the proliferation of T cell lines and clones to fixed antigen-pulsed macrophages; this effect was neutralized by adding an excess of purified, soluble IL-1. The antibody also impaired the activity of the isolated membranes. Hence, the T cell lines and clones raised in our laboratory by David Beller are all IL-1 dependent. The fixed macrophage stimulates these cells, in the absence of IL-1 secretion, because it bears this molecule or an IL-1-like molecule on its membrane.

6. The expression of membrane and secreted IL-1 could be dissociated in culture. The macrophages freshly harvested from the spleen or peritoneal cavity did not bear membrane IL-1. Brief contact with the dish stimulated its membrane expression as well as its secretion. After a twenty-four-to-forty-eight-hour period of culture, there was no further production of either form. However, if such macrophages were then challenged with bacteria or endotoxin, there was a marked appearance of membrane IL-1 without secretion of IL-1.

7. Lastly, the observation that freshly harvested macrophages do not bear IL-1 allowed us to probe if secreted IL-1 could be adsorbed to the macrophage and then cross-linked by formaldehyde. No such results were found.

Hence, IL-1 or an IL-1 molecule is present on the surface of the macrophage. This membrane IL-1 is biologically active, behaves as an integral membrane protein, and can be regulated differently from the secreted form.

Membrane IL-1 is required for the growth of some T cell
lines and clones and is expressed only under conditions of
stimulation of the APC. We are now investigating whether
a similar molecule is found on B cells and other APC.

References

1. Allen, P. M. & Unanue, E. R. J. Immunol. 132, 1077-
    1079, 1984
2. Allen, P. M., Strydom, D. J. & Unanue, E. R. Proc.
    Natl. Acad. Sci. USA 81, 2489-2493, 1984.
3. Kurt-Jones, E. A., Beller, D. I. & Unanue, E. R.
    Proc. Natl. Acad. Sci. USA, in press, 1985.
4. Unanue, E. R. Ann. Rev. Immunol. 2, 395-428.
5. Benjamin, D. C., Berzofsky, J. A., I. J. East, et al.
    Ann. Rev. Immunol. 2, 67-117, 1984.
6. Ziegler, K. & Unanue, E. R. J. Immunol. 127, 1869-
    1985, 1981.
7. Ziegler, K. & Unanue, E. R. Proc. Natl. Acad. Sci.
    USA 79, 175-178, 1982.
8. Allen, P. M. & Unanue, E. R. Am. J. Anat., 170, 483-
    490.
9. Beller, D. I. Eur. J. Immunol., 14, 138-143.
10. Kaye, J. & Janeway, C. A., Jr. Lymphokine Res. 3,
    175-195, 1984.
11. Mizel, S. B., Dukovich, M. & Rothstein, J. J. Immu-
    nol. 131, 1834-1839, 1983.

RECOGNITION OF THE VIRAL NUCLEOPROTEIN BY INFLUENZA A

SPECIFIC CYTOTOXIC T CELLS

A.R.M.TOWNSEND, A.J.MCMICHAEL, G.G.BROWNLEE

NUFFIELD DEPT. OF MEDICINE,

JOHN RADCLIFFE HOSPITAL, OXFORD. OX3 9DU

Summary. The conclusions of the following paper may be summarised as follows:
1/. A minority population of cytotoxic T cells (CTL) from C57BL/6 mice are described which recognise target cells infected with certain subgroups of influenza A viruses. By the use of recombinant A viruses it is shown that recognition by these CTL is determined by the A virus nucleoprotein (NP) gene. Nucleoprotein is is not an integral membrane protein. 2/. Transfection experiments with L cells, using a cDNA copy of the A/NT/60/68 (H3N2) NP gene, show that this subpopulation of CTL recognise L cells expressing the NP gene in the absence of any other viral protein. 3/. The transfection technique demonstrates that a major population of fully A virus crossreactive CTL also recognise transfected nucleoprotein. 4/. Experiments with L cells transfected with A/PR/8/34 (H1N1) haemagglutinin (an integral membrane glycoprotein of the virus) confirm that a subpopulation of CTL exists that recognise haemagglutinin (HA), and show that some crossreactivity in CTL recognition exists between H1 (1934) and H2 (1957), but not between H1 and H3 (1968) haemagglutinins. Thus no fully crossreactive CTL were detected that recognise HA. 5/. Comparative experiments with L cells transfected with either nucleoprotein or haemagglutinin show that in the polyclonal CTL raised against A virus infected cells, a much greater proportion are directed at NP than at HA. 6/. CTL recognition of NP transfected L cells was efficient despite the fact that only

low level of nucleoprotein was expressed (as revealed by
monoclonal antibodies), and NP was not detectable at the
transfected cell plasma membrane. 7/. The mechanisms by
which CTL may recognise NP are discussed. It is suggested
that CTL may recognise "processed"nucleoprotein fragments.
The implications of these results for CTL recognition of
other viruses and minor histocompatibility antigens and in
the design of influenza vaccines is briefly discussed.

Since the definition of the cytotoxic T cell as a
differentiated T lymphocyte (1), the identity of the viral
and minor histocompatibility molecules recognised by these
cells has remained surprisingly elusive (reviewed in refs
2,3). The work of recent years has revealed several
generally applicable facts which are worthy of note before
proceeding to describe our experiments. When a CTL response
is raised to a member virus from a family related by
sharing type specific antigens, but split into subtypes by
the possession of glycoproteins which are serologically
distinct, the majority of CTL crossreact in a manner that
parallels the type specific antigen (reviewed in ref 2). All
CTL recognise virus determined antigens in conjunction with
Class I major histocompatibility (M.H.C.) gene products, and
specificity for the latter is so refined that certain
single amino acid changes are sufficient to abolish CTL
recognition (reviewed in ref 4). Attempts to inhibit CTL
recognition with antibodies have shown that those to the
appropriate MHC molecules reproducibly block CTL recognition
of an infected target cell , whereas antibodies to viral
proteins only rarely inhibit (reviewed in ref 2). Finally,
it is generally accepted that direct contact between CTL
and target is required for delivery of the lytic signal, and
assumed therefore that recognition occurs at the plasma
membrane of the target cell (5).
All these generalisations are exemplified in the CTL
response to influenza viruses. The majority of type A
virus specific CTL are fully crossreactive between all A
subtypes, do not recognise influenza B virus, are Class I
M.H.C. restricted, and are not generally inhibited in
their recognition by antibodies to virus proteins (reviewed
in ref 6).
In addition to the majority of influenza specific CTL
which crossreact between A virus subtypes, a minority
population can be isolated which differentiate between
certain subgroups of A viruses. Recognition by CTL with this
property can be investigated by the use of recombinant A
viruses to infect target cells (7-10). Recombinant A

viruses are produced by mixed infection in vitro with two
A viruses of different subtype. During infection the eight
RNA segments from each parent virus segregate and recombine
to form new viruses which can be isolated and typed for the
parental origin of each of their RNA segments (11). Such
typed recombinant A viruses can then be used to map CTL
recognition to one of the segregating RNA segments. As
each segment codes for only one or two proteins, this
approach is able to pin point the viral proteins
responsible for recognition by the minority population of
CTL that can differentiate between the A virus subtypes used
as parental viruses.

The experiments which directed our attention to the NP
gene were done using C57BL/6 mice (10,12). Cloned CTL
raised against the recombinant A virus X31 (see Table 1 for
the genotype of each recombinant), only lysed target cells
which shared the NP gene (RNA segment 5) with X31. This NP
gene was derived from the wild type virus A/PR/8/34. Wild
type viruses isolated at different dates were either
clearly recognised (H1N1 viruses isolated between 1934-1943)
or clearly not recognised (all A viruses isolated between
1946-1968). These results were extended by selecting
polyclonal CTL by stimulation with the recombinant virus
E61-13-H17, which differs from X31 only by containing the
NP gene from A/HK/8/68 (Table 1). The latter CTL showed the
exact opposite specificity of the clone raised to X31 (13). Only
recombinant viruses sharing a post 1968 NP gene were
recognised. Recognition of natural isolates was also
appropriate : H1N1 viruses isolated between 1934-1943 were
now not recognised, whereas all A viruses isolated after
1946 were recognised (results summarised in tables 1 and 2).
It should be noted that the latter subgroup of A viruses
contains representatives of H1N1, H2N2 and H3N2
serologically defined subtypes. The timing of this antigenic
change detected with CTL, coincides with an antigenic
change in NP detected with rabbit antisera (14) and certain
monoclonal antibodies (15).

These findings indicated that the A virus NP gene played
a role in determining the specificity of the CTL response in
vitro of C57BL/6 mice. However, this approach could not
examine directly the specificity of fully A virus
crossreactive CTL, and also left open the possibility of
complex interactions between nucleoprotein and other viral
proteins, such as haemagglutinin, which could account for
its action.

In order to approach these questions the segment 5 RNA

TABLE 1

Recognition by influenza A specific CTL from C57BL/6 mice is determined by

the nucleoprotein gene.

TEST VIRUS	PARENTAL H3N2 VIRUS	PB1	PA	PB2	HA	NA	NP	M	NS	A3.1	B	C
										ACTIVITY OF CTL LINES		
E6113H17	A/HK/8/68				+	+	+			0	59	52
X31	A/Aichi/2/68				+	+				82	5	66
X47	A/Vic/3/75	+			+	+	+			1	71	36
X61	A/Texas/1/77	+			+	+				34	1	39
X45	A/Scot/840/74	+		+	+	+	+			2	71	38
X57	A/Vic/112/76	+		+	+	+				76	2	61
A/Aichi/68		+	+	+	+	+	+	+	+	0	63	57
A/PR/8/34										67	2	67

CTL clone A3.1 is specific for the 1934 NP from X31(12),CTL line B is
specific for the 1968 NP from E61-13-H17(13),and CTL line C is a
crossreactive control produced by stimulating E61-13-H17 primed spleen
cells with X31(13). The numbers are % specific ^{51}Cr release at a
killer:target ratio of 2.5:1. EL4 was used as target cell.All the
recombinant viruses tested were derived from mixed infections with
A/PR/8/34 (H1N1) and post 1968 H3N2 viruses.The genotype of each is
shown by representing genes derived from the H3N2 parent by + ,and
those derived from A/PR/8/34 as blanks.PB1,PA,PB2,genes coding for
polymerase proteins;HA haemagglutinin;NA neuraminidase; NP
nucleoprotein;M matrix protein;NS non structural proteins.

TABLE 2

Natural influenza A viruses isolated between 1934-1979 fall into two groups

defined by the CTL described in table 1.

TEST VIRUS	SUBTYPE	A3.1	B	C
		ACTIVITY OF CTL LINES		
A/PR/8/1934	H1N1	75	7	60
A/Eng/1937	H1N1	30	8	54
A/Bel/1942	H1N1	63	9	67
A/Weiss/1943	H1N1	32	7	19
A/Cam/1946	H1N1	0	49	56
A/FM/1/1947	H1N1	0	40	52
A/USSR/90/1977	H1N1	nt	51	58
A/Jap/305/1957	H2N2	nt	39	35
A/Aichi/1/1968	H3N2	0	39	39
A/Bangkok/1/1979	H3N2	nt	50	61
B/HK/8/73		0	5	0

Key as for table 1.

(coding for NP) from A/NT/60/68 was used to make a full
length cDNA, which was then inserted into an expression
vector where the NP cDNA was under the transcriptional
control of the Herpes Simplex virus thymidine kinase
promoter and the SV40 Early poly A addition signal. A
plasmid with this construction (pTKNP2) was made and
kindly donated by J. Davey (manuscript in preparation). As
CTL with specificity for the 1968 NP were available from
C57BL/6 mice (H-2b), we elected to co-transfect L cells
(H-2k) with pTKNP2 in addition to a cosmid (isolated and
kindly donated by A. Mellor (16)) containing the D^b gene
and a dominant selection marker for resistance to the
neomycin analogue G418.

Transfected L cell clones were characterised by
immunoprecipitation, and indirect immunoperoxidase or
immunofluorescence. All clones expressed the D^b protein at
easily detectable levels, exactly analogous to other
examples using a variety of genomic class I M.H.C. gene
clones (17-19). Expression of NP on the other hand was low
in comparison to infected cells. Immunoprecipitation with
monoclonal or polyclonal anti NP antibody revealed a faint
NP band on SDS polyacrylamide gels at 56 kD from some but
not all clones which were lysed by NP specific CTL. Indirect
immunoperoxidase staining was more sensitive and detected
NP at a stainable level in less than 10% of nuclei in
transfected L cell clones, in comparison to greater than
80% in L cells infected for 5 hours with A/NT/60/68 (this
and all the remaining data are submitted for publication).
Indirect immunofluorescence and analysis on the Ortho
Cytofluorograf failed to detect any nucleoprotein at the
transfected cell surface, and attempts to sort positive cells
on the basis of surface fluorescence failed.

In spite of the low level of NP expression, cotransfected
L cell clones, which expressed both D^b and NP, were lysed
efficiently by D^b restricted CTL that had NP specificity
defined by the use of recombinant A viruses (Table 3).
This result formally showed that no other viral proteins
other than NP were required in the target cell for
recognition by these highly selected CTL.

We were now in a position to test polyclonal CTL from
mice responding to a variety of A viruses for their ability
to recognise the NP transfected L cells. Such CTL show full
crossreactivity between serologically defined A virus
subtypes (reviewed in ref 6). The earlier results described
above, combined with the knowledge that the NP amino acid
sequence is 94% conserved between 1934 and 1968 (20),

TABLE 3

L cells cotransfected with D^b and 1968 NP are recognised by C57BL/6 CTL.

CTL CLONE		TARGET CELLS		
	K:T	L/D^b+X31	L/D^b+E6113H17	L/D^b/NP14
C4	5:1	6	62	43
C8	3:1	6	71	69
D4	3:1	4	38	13
D7	3:1	4	54	40
E10	1:1	7	53	40
F5	4:1	8	67	61
F6	4:1	2	36	16

CTL clones were isolated by limiting dilution from polyclonal CTL lines
produced by repeated stimulation of primed C57BL/6 spleen cells with
E61-13-H17 virus(13).L/Db+X31 = L cells transfected with Db and infected
with X31 virus;L/Db+E61-13-H17 = L/Db cells infected with E61-13-H17 virus;
L/Db/NP14 = L cells cotransfected with both Db and NP genes.

TABLE 4

A virus crossreactive CTL from C3H mice (H-2k) recognise transfected NP.

CTL CULTURE			TARGET CELLS		
	L/Db	L/Db+NT60	L/Db+PR8	L/Db/NP14	L/Db+BHK
A/PR/8/34(H1N1)	2	65	80	55	15
A/NT/60/68(H3N2)	8	76	81	61	17
B/HK/8/73	7	8	7	7	88

Secondary in vitro cultures raised against A/PR/8/34 (H1N1),A/NT/60/68
(H3N2), or B/HK/8/73 were set up as described previously (13),and
tested at a K:T ratio of 2.5:1.For remaining key see tables 1 and 3.

made the NP molecule an attractive candidate as a target
for crossreactive CTL. Polyclonal secondary in vitro
cultures were set up from C3H mice (H-2k) primed with either
A/PR/8/34 (H1N1) or A/NT/60/68 (H3N2) or B/Hong Kong/8/73
as a specificity control. Table 4 shows that CTL from mice
responding to either A/PR/8/34 or A/NT/60/68 lysed control
L cells infected with either A virus, demonstrating the
crossreactivity of these CTL. The same CTL lysed the NP
transfected target very efficiently. The specificity of
the effect was shown by the CTL raised to influenza B virus
which lysed only L cells infected with B virus; neither the
A virus infected nor the NP transfected cells were lysed.
These results revealed the presence of a major population
of fully A virus crossreactive CTL which recognised
nucleoprotein transfected L cells. We have since repeated
these experiments using the NP gene from A/PR/8/34 with
the same result (data not shown). Using L cells transfected
with NP but not D^b we were also able to demonstrate that
CTL recognition of transfected cells was characteristically
M.H.C. restricted (Table 5).

In view of the fact that nucleoprotein is not an
integral membrane protein, unlike the haemagglutinin (HA),
it was of interest to compare the CTL responses to these
two viral proteins directly. An expression vector was made
in which a full length DNA copy of segment 4 RNA (coding
for haemagglutinin) from A/PR/8/34 (H1) was under the
transcriptional control of the SV40 Early promoter and
poly A addition signals. In addition the vector carried the
dominant selection marker for G418 resistance, and the 69%
transforming section of bovine papilloma virus. The latter
was included with the aim of allowing the plasmid to
replicate extra chromosomally in transfected cells. However,
this strategy was not successful and the plasmid integrated
into high molecular weight DNA. Expression of HA was
detected by immunoprecipitation and indirect
immunofluorescence. L cells expressing high levels of HA
were selected twice on the Ortho Cytofluorograf and cloned.
These clones were found to be unstable in their expression
of HA, and required resorting for bright cells about every
4 weeks. However, recently sorted cells were found to
express between 1/3 - 1/2 the amount of HA molecules at the
cell surface as L cells infected for 5 hours with A/PR/8/34.
This was comparatively a much higher level of expression
than the NP transfected cells, presumably because we were
able to select for high expressing variants on the Ortho
Cytofluorograf.

TABLE 5

CTL recognition of transfected nucleoprotein is H-2 restricted.

CTL	K:T	TARGET CELLS		
		L/D^b/NP1 (Db+NP)	L/D^b (Db alone)	L/NP24 (NP alone)
Clone F5.	8:1	46	7	4
C3H anti A/PR/8/34 polyclonal.	10:1	65	4	55

Key as for tables 1 and 3.L/Db/NP1 = a second clone of L cells cotransfected with Db and 1968 NP.L/NP24 = L cells transfected with 1968 NP but not Db.

TABLE 6

Direct comparison of CTL recognition of nucleoprotein and haemagglutinin.

TARGET CELLS	C3H CTL CULTURES K:T10/5:1	A/PR/8/34 (H1N1)	A/JAP/305/57 (H2N2)	A/NT/60/68 (H3N2)
L/BPV		13/7	19/12	19/10
L/BPV/HA1		42/30	32/20	24/13
L/BPV+PR8		86/85	84/86	79/81
L/Db		13/8	19/11	17/9
L/Db/NP		84/75	83/76	80/75

Secondary in vitro cultures were set up as described (13).L/BPV = L cells transfected with the BPV containing vector lacking the HA gene;L/BPV/HA1 = L cells transfected with the BPV vector containing the A/PR/8/34 (H1) HA gene;remaining key as in tables 1 and 3.

Table 6 compares the recognition of HA transfected with NP transfected L cells by polyclonal CTL from C3H mice (H-2k), responding to representatives of the three pandemic strains of human influenza A virus. It shows that a subpopulation of CTL in the response to A/PR/8/34 (H1N1) were able to recognise the H1 haemagglutinin on transfected L cells. This result confirmed earlier work that demonstrated an HA specific component in the CTL response (7,8). The response to A/JAP/305/57 (H2N2) also had a detectable level of CTL which crossreacted on H1 haemagglutinin. Such CTL crossreactivity for H1 and H2 haemagglutinins, demonstrated by the use of the transfection technique, has also recently been desribed by Braciale et al (21). However, we were not able to detect CTL in the response to A/NT/60/68 (H3N2) that were able to recognise the H1 haemagglutinin, and thus could find no evidence for fully A virus crossreactive CTL that recognised HA. This pattern of HA recognition is compatible with the amino acid sequence relationships of the three haemagglutinins; H1 and H2 are more closely related to each other than either is to H3 (22). In comparison, all three responding CTL cultures contained a major population of CTL that recognised the NP transfected L cell target. On a cell to cell basis the CTL response to NP was at least ten fold stronger than that to HA, even in the A/PR/8/34 culture tested on L cells expressing the homologous HA (an approximate calculation based on the killer : target ratios in these experiments).

An interesting aspect of our results is the efficient recognition of NP transfected L cells by CTL despite the low level of NP expression (as detected by antibodies), and the apparent absence of NP at the cell surface. One explanation for this could be that NP was "processed" in the transfected cell, resulting in the presentation of peptide fragments which were recognised by CTL in conjunction with appropriate class I M.H.C. molecules, but which no longer retained enough of the tertiary structure of the native NP to bind the antibodies we tested. This suggestion would have to predict that CTL generally recognise presented protein fragments and that many different cell types, including fibroblasts, can process and present protein antigens provided they are manufactured inside the cell concerned. It would also go some way to explaining the lack of blocking effect on CTL recognition found with antibodies to native viral proteins, described earlier. However, other explanations cannot be ruled out.

It is possible that CTL may be able to recognise very low
levels of native NP at the cell surface (as suggested by
Yewdell et al (23)), or even that the NP molecule induces
or alters a cell protein which is subsequently recognised
at the cell surface.

Whatever the mechanism may be, these results show that
non-transmembrane proteins can be responsible for
stimulating CTL, and are analogous in many respects with
the work on SV40 large T antigen (24). The implication is
that other CTL antigens, such as 'LYDMA' of Epstein Barr
virus and minor histocompatibility gene products, need
not be transmembrane glycoproteins and thus they may be
very difficult to identify at the cell surface with
antibodies.

Finally, our results have practical implications for
influenza vaccine design. Killed virus and sub-unit
vaccines are generally poor inducers of crossreactive CTL
(25,26), and evidence is accumulating that crossreactive
CTL may play a role in the cross-protective immunity
observed after infection with serologically distinct A
viruses (28). If the NP molecule could be presented to the
immune system in a form appropriate for CTL stimulation
(such as in a recombinant vaccinia virus (27)), it is
possible that a cross-protective CTL response could be
induced.

References.
1.MacDonald, H.R. Immunology Today, 3, 183-187.(1982).
2.Zinkernagel, R.M. and Rosenthal, K.L. Immunological
Reviews.58, 131-155. (1981).
3. Simpson,E. Ann. Immunol. (Inst.Pasteur). 135C, 410-
   413. (1984).
4. Melief, C. Immunology Today. 4, 57-61. (1983).
5. Henney, C.S. Immunology Today. 1, 36-41. (1980).
6. Askonas, B.A., McMichael, A.J., and Webster, R.G. In
Basic and Applied Influenza Research. A.S.Beare, editor.
CRC Press Inc. Florida. 159-188. (1982).
7.Zweerink, H.J., Askonas, B.A., Millican, D., Courtneidge,
S.A. and Skehel, J.J. Eur. J. Immunol. 7, 630-635. (1977).
8.Braciale, T.J., Andrew, M.E. and Braciale, V.L. J. Exp.
Med. 153, 910-923. (1981).
9. Bennink, J.R., Yewdell, J.W., Gerhard, W. Nature. 296,
75-76. (1982).
10. Townsend, A.R.M., Skehel, J.J. Nature, 300, 655-657.
(1982).
11.Palese, P. Cell. 10, 1-10. (1977).

12. Townsend, A.R.M., Skehel, J.J., Taylor, P.M., Palese, P. Virology. 133, 456-459. (1984).

13. Townsend, A.R.M., and Skehel, J.J. J. Exp. Med. (in the press). (1984).

14. Schild, G.L., Newman, R.W., Webster, R.G., Major, D.and Huishaw, V.S. Devl. Cell Biol. 5, 373-384. (1980).

15. van Wyke, K.L., Huishaw, V.S., Bean, W.J. and Webster, R.G. J. Virol, 35. 24-30. (1980).

16. Flavell, R.A., Grosveld, F., Busslinger, M., de Boer, E., Kloussis, D., Mellor, A.L., Golden, L., Weiss, E., Hurst, J., Bud, H., Bullman, H., Simpson, E., James, R., Townsend, A.R.M., Taylor, P.M., Schmidt, W., Ferluga, J., Lebel, L., Santamaria, M., Atfield, G. and Festenstein, H. Cold. Spring Harb. Symp. Quant. Biol. 47, 1067-1077. (1983).

17. Mellor, A.L., Golden, L., Weiss, E., Bullman, H., Hurst, J., Simpson, E., James, R.F.L., Townsend, A.R.M., Taylor, P.M., Schmidt, W., Ferluga, J., Leben, L., Santamaria, M., Atfield, G., Festenstein, H. and Flavell, R.A. Nature. 298, 529-534. (1982).

18. Evans, G.A.. Margulies. D.H.. Camerini-Olero. R.D.. Ozato. K. and Seidman. J.G. Proc. Natl. Acad. Sci. U.S.A. 79, 1994-1998. (1982).

19. Goodenow, R.S., McMillan, M., Nicolson, M., Sher, T.B., Eakle, K., Davidson, N. and Hood. L. Nature. 300. 231-237. (1982).

20. Huddleston. J.A. and Brownlee, G.G. Nucleic Acids Res. 10, 1029-1038. (1982).

21.Braciale, T.J., Braciale, V.L., Henkel, T.J., Sambrook, J. and Gething, M.J. J. Exp. Med. 159, 341-354. (1984).

22.Winter, G., Fields, S. and Browmlee, G.G. Nature, 242, 72-75. (1981).

23.Yewdell, J.W., Frank, E., and Gerhard, W. J. Immunol. 126, 1814-1819. (1981).

24. Tevethia, S., Tevethia, M., Lewis, A., Reddy, V. and Weissman, S. Virology. 128, 319-330. (1983).

25.Webster, R.G. and Askonas, B.A. Eur. J. Immunol. 10, 396- 401. (1980).

26. McMichael, A.J., Gotch, F.M., Cullen, P., Askonas, B.A. and Webster, R.G.ClinExpImmunol. 43, 276-284. (1981).

27.Smith. G.L.. Murphy. B.R. and Moss. B. Proc. Natl. Acad. Sci. U.S.A. 80, 7155-7159, (1983).

28. McMichael, A.J., Gotch, F.M., Noble, G.R. and Beare, A.S. New. Eng. J. Med. 309, 13-17, (1983).

THE CHEMISTRY OF ANTIGEN-ANTIBODY UNION

Elizabeth D. Getzoff, John A. Tainer,
and Richard A. Lerner

Department of Molecular Biology
Research Institute of Scripps Clinic
La Jolla, California 92037 U.S.A.

A complete understanding of the cellular immune response requires a detailed knowledge of the structural basis for protein antigenicity at a molecular level that approaches atomic resolution. Both site-specific anti-peptide antibodies[1,2] and monoclonal anti-protein antibodies against proteins of known three-dimensional structure[3] allow examination of the molecular and chemical basis for antigen-antibody interaction. Our experiments suggest that antigenic recognition can be divided into at least three stages: 1) precollision orientation by electrostatic forces, 2) local antibody-antigen recognition involving the interaction of specific residues, and 3) induced fit accomplished by local rearrangments of epitope and paratope structure. Here we report on experiments concerning precollision orientation and induced fit, as the influence of specific residues on antigenic recognition is well documented elsewhere[3].

PRECOLLISION ORIENTATION

Electrostatic forces have been implicated in a variety of biologically important intermolecular interactions including drug orientation by DNA[4], macromolecular assembly[5], substrate binding and catalysis[6-8] and macromolecular complementarity with inhibitors, drugs and hormones[9-12]. To define the possible role of electrostatic forces in orienting molecules prior to their actual collision, we have developed a new method for both the analysis and color-coded computer graphics display of the three-dimensional electrostatic vector field surrounding a macromolecule[13]. We calculate both the electrostatic potential and field from partial charges assigned to each of the atoms of the protein, thus enabling the contributions of specific residues to be identified.

Using this approach, we are currently examining the electrostatic molecular surface and electrostatic field of the variable region of phosphorylcholine bound mouse immunoglobulin Fab M603[14] (updated atomic coordinates from Gerson Cohen and David Davies, personal communication). The electrostatic potential of this protein's molecular surface complements the charges of the bound phosphorylcholine hapten. We find that the electrostatic field surrounding the hapten binding site appears to guide the dipolar hapten into the orientation found in the crystallographic coordinates of the docked complex. To quantitate the contributions of each of these residues, we mathematically neutralized their partial charges and examined the resultant electrostatic field. Our initial results indicate that arginine 52 and glutamic acid 61 of the heavy chain, in conjunction with aspartic acid 1 of the light chain, are influential in aligning the field to direct the hapten toward the binding region. Lysine residues 57 and 67 from the heavy chain and 36 from the light chain also contribute to a lesser extent. Electrostatic alignment should be significant because the overall electrostatic potential energy between the antibody and the hapten exceeds thermal energy, even when the hapten is located over 12 Å from its binding site. Our calculations also confirm and quantitate the local electrostatic stabilization of the hapten suggested in the crystal structure analysis[15]: heavy chain arginine 52 interacts with the phosphate, and heavy chain glutamic acid residues 35 and 61 are located near the positively charged choline. We find that aspartic acid 97 of the light chain also influences local electrostatic interactions. Work is in progress on an automated docking algorithm based upon the electrostatic forces between the partial charges of the hapten and the three-dimensional electrostatic field of the protein.

SITE MOBILITY AND INDUCED FIT

To evaluate the role of induced fit in antigen-antibody interaction, we have studied antigenic sites of proteins for which both the three-dimensional structure and the relative flexibility of the different parts of that structure are known. If induced fit is an important feature of antigenic recognition, then highly ordered areas should be less antigenic than mobile areas having low energy barriers between different conformations. We analyze the relationship of atomic mobility to the antigenicity of sites in proteins by direct experimental work using anti-peptide antibodies representing sites in the protein myohemerythrin and by retrospective studies on insulin and cytochrome *c*.

Mobility of Protein Surfaces

Besides identifying the atomic positions, refined high resolution x-ray crystal structures of molecules provide empirically determined information about the relative mobility of different atoms. This information is termed the atomic temperature factor and can be given by the equation $B = 8\pi^2\overline{u^2}$, where the mean square displacement $\overline{u^2}$ is averaged over time and the crystal lattice[16]. Temperature factors can provide important data about the lower frequency concerted motions of groups of atoms, indicating the relative conformational variability of different regions[17,18]: high temperature factors indicate shallow potential wells allowing access to multiple conformations at biological temperatures. For convenience in discussing peptides representing regions of a protein, we will use the terminology "hot" and "cold" to refer to highly mobile (high temperature factors) and well-ordered regions (low temperature factors), respectively. In addition to dynamic conformational variation, temperature factors incorporate a variety of factors that affect the measured x-ray scattering intensity: primarily static disorder in the crystal, error in the absorption corrections, improper scaling, and errors in the interpretation of the electron density. By examining the overall pattern of atomic temperature factors for a highly refined protein structure which has been solved independently in different crystal systems, the differential mobility of various regions of the molecule can be isolated from these other factors[19].

Computer graphic analysis of the differential mobilities of protein surfaces suggested that crystallographic temperature factors might be relevant to the understanding of antibody-antigen recognition and could be examined experimentally through the use of anti-peptide antibodies[20]. For this experimental study we needed a protein whose structure was known to sufficient resolution to provide accurate thermal parameters. We avoided proteins with considerable sequence homology to rabbit proteins (thereby eliminating immunological tolerance) and the proteases (since they could complicate the immunoassays). Among the remaining proteins, we looked for the following features: well-refined temperature factors, a wide range of mobility at the molecular surface, and contiguous regions of the amino acid sequence characterized by by either high or low mobility. On the basis of this analysis, the protein myohemerythrin was chosen for immunological study. The crystal structures of myohemerythrin and the related protein hemerythrin are unique in having temperature factors empirically corrected for crystal contacts[21].

Myohemerythrin Peptides

The selection of peptides from the myohemerythrin sequence was based on the main-chain temperature factors averaged by residue, since the main-chain mobility reflects the global conformational variability of the protein. Both helical and non-helical peptide regions were selected for synthesis. Three of the hot peptides were chosen to include residues liganding the irons; in the native protein the mobility of these sequences is limited to conformations which do not disrupt the metal ligand geometry. The 12 peptides synthesized include 83 of myohemerythrin's 118 residues (70% of the sequence). Of the exposed molecular surface area of myohemerythrin (5846 Å^2), the peptides synthesized account for 4005 Å^2 (69%). The four peptides synthesized for each of three categories encompass roughly equal parts of the protein surface area: hot (23.0%), cold (19.3%), and hot/contact (hot after correction for crystal contacts, 26.2%). All the peptides chosen have large areas of exposed molecular surface available for interaction with antibodies.

Highly exposed amino acid residues tend to be less hydrophobic and, due to their external, relatively unconstrained position, more highly mobile than internal residues[22,23]. Peptides were specifically chosen to minimize differences in average exposed area and hydrophobicity per residue. Although there is some correlation of exposed area and mobility among the selected peptides, this is much stronger for side-chain than for main-chain atoms. In fact, peptides with very similar average exposed areas may either be cold (peptides

22–35, 26–35, and 96–109) or hot (7–16, 42–51, and 57–66). There is very little correlation between temperature factor and average hydrophobicity per residue for the peptides chosen.

Regions of High Mobility are Most Antigenic

To define the possible role of molecular surface mobility in the antigenic recognition of the native protein by anti-peptide antibodies, polyclonal antibodies to each selected sequence were raised against synthetic peptides in pairs of rabbits (Table 1). The anti-peptide antisera were originally assayed for reactivity against the homologous immunizing peptide by enzyme-linked immunoabsorbant assay (ELISA). All but one of the synthetic peptides were immunogenic; their relative immunogenicity is not correlated with their mobility. The anti-peptide antisera were next assayed for reactivity with myohemerythrin (Table 1). The same results were obtained when the ELISA assay was performed under less denaturing conditions (the protein was not dried or methanol-fixed to the plate). All anti-peptide antisera raised against cold peptides (22–35, 26–35, 96–109, and 100–109) gave negative or low reactivity with the protein, while all anti-peptide antisera raised against hot peptides (excluding peptide 42–51, which did not raise any anti-peptide antibodies) gave higher reactivity against the protein. Of the antisera against hot peptides, those with the lowest reactivity to myohemerythrin (57–66 and 63–72) also had the lowest reactivity against their respective homologous immunizing peptides. The relative averaged avidity[25] of the anti-peptide antisera against the protein (peptide 3–16 > 7–16 > 37–46, > 57–66 > 63–72, 69–82, 73–82, 96–109) matched the pattern of relative antigenicity; antisera with higher titers generally showed greater avidity.

Antigenicity studies were repeated in immunoprecipitation assays under conditions preserving the native structure of myohemerythrin. Retention of the characteristic visible spectrum with a 338 nm peak[26] due to the iron center verified that the ligand environment remained unchanged, indicating that the protein was largely in its native conformation under the assay conditions. The results of these immunoprecipitation studies (Table 1) were consistant with the ELISA analyses: antisera against hot peptides react more strongly with myohemerythrin, than do antisera against cold peptides.

TABLE 1

Reactivity of MHr Anti-Peptide Antisera

Sequence Position	ELISA titers†		Immunoprecipitation	
	αPeptide vs. Peptide	αPeptide vs. MHr	^{125}I-MHr c.p.m.*	% Inhibition by Peptide‡
Hot/Contact				
3-16	640-1280	12800	14849	97.1
7-16	640-1280	3200	7384	92.6
37-46	640-1280	9500	4026	100.0
42-51	—	—	0	0.0
Hot				
57-66	160-320	600	7277	80.0
63-72	160-320	375	2543	77.6
69-82	>2560	1050	3774	91.3
73-82	>2560	1400	2154	62.0
Cold				
22-35	1280-2560	—	180	0.0
26-35	320-640	60	0	0.0
96-109	1280-2560	200	2617	22.5
100-109	320-640	—	0	0.0

Data from Tainer, et. al.[24].
† ELISA titers are expressed as the reciprocal of antibody dilution extrapolated to bind 50% of 50 pmole antigen per well.
* Average of two independent experiments, after correction for non-specific binding.
‡ 100.0% minus percent of activity remaining in the presence of the peptide.

To confirm the specificity of the anti-peptide antisera, immunoprecipitation was also done in the presence of homologous and heterologous peptides (Table 1). The anti-myohemerythrin reactivity of antisera raised against the hot peptides was strongly inhibited by incubation with the corresponding homologous peptide, whereas incubation with the irrelevant heterologous peptide (synthesized from a sequence from influenza virus haemagglutinin) did not inhibit anti-myohemerythrin reactivity, thus confirming the specificity of the antisera. Interestingly, antisera against cold peptides that showed low reactivity with the protein (22–35, 96–109) were, at most, only slightly inhibited by incubation with the corresponding homologous peptides suggesting that the anti-myohemerythrin reactivity measured for the antibodies raised against these cold peptides may largely represent non-specific binding.

A strong correlation was seen in both types of immunoassay between mobility and antigenicity. Of the cold peptides, only antibodies to peptide 96–109 have reactivity with intact myohemerythrin; this peptide has 4 residues with higher temperature factors on its N-terminal end. Of the hot peptides, the N-terminal loop peptide 3-16 has both the highest mobility and the highest antigenicity. Reduced mobility due to structural constraints in myohemerythrin resulting from the metal liganding may modulate the degree of antigenicity. In the immunoprecipitation assays, antisera against the shorter of the two nested peptides containing two metal ligands in the intact myohemerythrin (73–82) has the lowest anti-protein reactivity of any hot peptide. All of these results appear to support the correlation of antigenicity and mobility.

MAPPING ATOMIC MOBILITY AND ANTIGENICITY

Sufficient data do not exist to rigorously analyze the correlation of structural mobility and antigenicity in many proteins. However, most of the available data supports this correlation. The relatively mobile N and C-terminal residues[27] are often antigenic determinants: the N-terminal regions of both bovine pancreatic ribonuclease[28] and mammalian cytochrome c[29] bind antibodies raised in rabbits against the intact molecule, for example. Antigenic determinants involving active site regions known to be mobile are also common: monoclonal antibodies bind in the active site regions of neuraminidase[30], carboxypeptidase A[31], and hexokinase[32], as well as in the NADPH binding regions of dihydrofolate reductase and glucose-6-phosphate dehydrogenase[33].

Although the antigenicity of proteins appears to be influenced by evolutionary variance[34], surface exposure[3], and hydrophilicity[35], these factors may all be related to site mobility. Due to the phenomenon of immunological tolerance, antibodies may not be elicited against those regions of the antigen which share structural or chemical properties with self-molecules of the host[36,37]. However, since natural selection favors mutations that do not perturb the overall conformational stability of a protein, polymorphism in evolutionarily variant proteins is related to polypeptide chain flexibility. Indeed, amino acid sequence variability is most likely to persist in those regions of the molecule where local changes in conformation can be tolerated. In addition, such changes are most likely to occur on the surface regions of the molecule and be accessible to contact with the B cell immunoglobulin receptor. Hydrophilicity (or hydrophobicity) indices[38-40] have been in wide use in recent years to predict the exposed surface regions of proteins and consequently the potential antigenic sites. Regions of the polypeptide chain that are highly exposed often have few interactions with the rest of the protein and are therefore also relatively mobile.

We have examined patterns of mobility and antigenicity in detail for 8 proteins: insulin, cytochrome c, myoglobin (together with hemoglobin, and leghemoglobin), lysozyme, lactate dehydrogenase, ribonuclease, snake and scorpion neurotoxins, and ferredoxin. Here we summarize the patterns of antigenicity and mobility for insulin and cytochrome c which are representative of our current findings.

Insulin

The two disulfide bound polypeptide chains of the peptide hormone insulin form a hydrophobic core and two predominantly hydrophobic surfaces which are involved in dimeric and hexameric contacts[41,42] and may be important in the binding of the active monomeric hormone to receptor[43]. Most hydrophilic residues are on the surface exposed by the hexameric form of the molecule. The sequences of more than 28 species have been determined[44] and indicate that the disulfide bridges and hydrophobic core of the monomer are invariant. The most highly variable residues for most mammals are residues 8 to 10 on the A chain and residues 29-30 on the B chain. These evolutionarily variable residues are thought to have little effect on the ability of the monomer to bind to its receptor[43], but have been shown to be important in the antigenicity of the molecule. Epitopes involving residues A4, the A-chain loop (residues A8 - A10), B3, and residues B28-B30 have been identified in studies using a panel of 18 monoclonal antibodies raised in mice

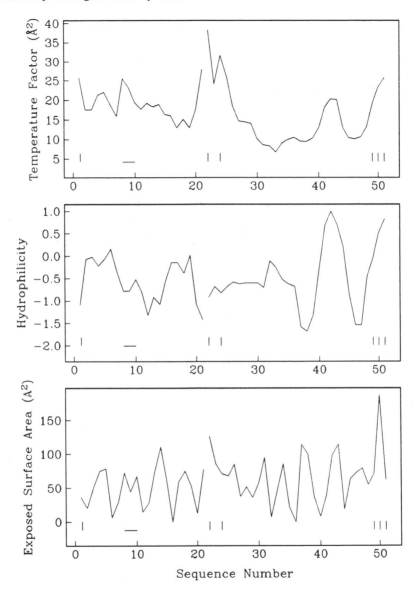

Fig. 1: Plots of the linear relationship of temperature factor, hydrophilicity and exposed area to sequence position in the insulin A and B chains. A chain residues are numbered 1-21, B chain residues are numbered 22-51. Contiguous determinants are shown as horizontal bars; discontiguous (conformational) determinants as vertical bars. Temperature factors are taken from ref. 48, hydrophobicity values from ref. 49, and algorithm for exposed area calculation from ref. 50.

to bovine and human insulin[45,46]. Studies with insulin derivatives shortened at the N-terminal end indicate the importance of B1 in antigenic recognition[47]. All of these antigenic determinants occur in local temperature factor maxima along the sequence (Fig. 1) and cluster in a stripe of high mobility on the molecular surface. In insulin, antigenicity shows a better correlation with mobility, than with hydrophilicity or exposed surface area (Fig. 1).

Cytochrome c

The amino acid sequence of cytochrome c, an electron carrier in the respiratory chain, has been determined for more than 75 eukaryotic species[44,51]. Fine specificity immunological studies by Margoliash and others[52-57] with these evolutionarily variant cytochromes have identified three important sites of antigenicity which can be mapped onto the known three-dimensional crystal structures[58-60]. The first antigenic site includes residues 89 and 92 at the N-terminal end of the C-terminal α helix, the second occurs near residues 60 and 62 at the N-terminal end of a distorted helix, and the third involves residue 44, which is located in a beta turn. Two of the three immunodominant regions, residues 44 and 89/92 show high mobility (Fig. 2-3) as measured by average main-chain temperature factors in the tuna structure[48,59,60]. The third immunodominant region, residues 60/62, shows high mobility in molecular dynamics calculations[64]; its lower crystallographic mobility appears to result from a crystal packing contact. More recently, fine specificity studies using antipeptide antibodies raised in rabbits against the C-terminal cyanogen bromide fragment (residues 81-104) from horse cytochrome c identified residues 100 and 103 as a fourth determinant[65]. C-terminal residue 103 has the highest average main-chain temperature factor in the entire molecule (Fig. 3).

SUMMARY AND IMPLICATIONS

The detailed information now available on both antigen and antibody structure allows antigenic recognition to be chemically analyzed. We suggest that antigenic recognition is not simply a lock and key fit based upon random collision of antigen and antibody, but instead involves both precollisional orientation by electrostatic

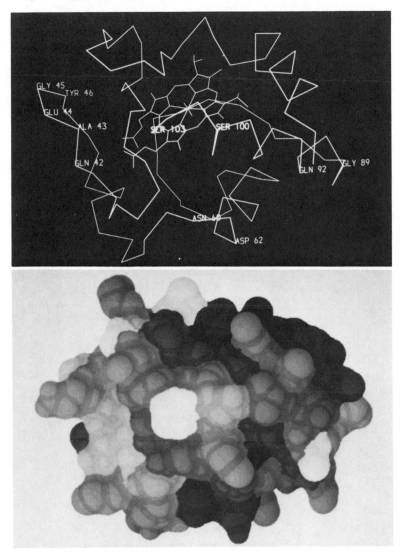

Fig. 2: Computer graphics views showing cytochrome c alpha carbon backbone with residues involved in antigenic determinants labeled (top) and solid external molecular surface (bottom) in the same orientation. The backbone is displayed using the general purpose graphics language GRAMPS[61] and the molecular modeling program GRANNY[62]. The external surface was calculated using M. L. Connolly's program RAMS[63] and coded by the average main-chain temperature factors using a radiating body brightness scale (highest white to lowest black). Except for areas in crystal contacts, the antigenic determinants are associated with the most highly mobile regions.

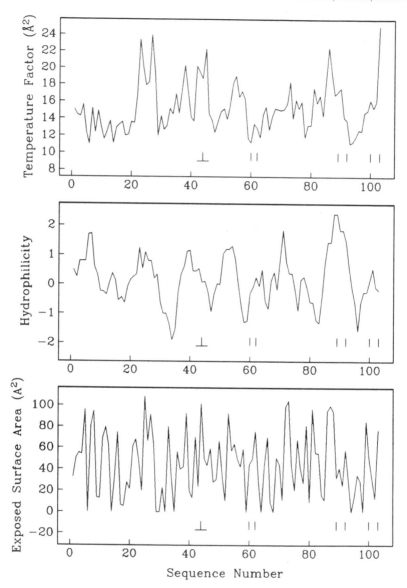

Fig. 3: Plots of temperature factor, hydrophilicity and exposed area versus sequence position in cytochrome c (see legend Fig. 1).

forces and a degree of induced fit to achieve the final complementarity between the corresponding epitope and paratope.

Electrostatic forces generated by the arrangement of atomic charges appear to have a role in orienting molecules prior to their actual collision. These orienting forces may influence the kinetics of antigen-antibody interaction, since the electrostatic energy is sufficient to affect the orientation of the phosphorylcholine hapten more than 12 Å from its binding site on M603. Further elucidation of the role of electrostatic forces in the antigen-antibody union awaits additional x-ray structural data.

Examination of local flexibility or mobility and antigenicity of sites in proteins suggests that mobility is a major factor in the recognition of the native protein by anti-peptide antibodies and in the antigenicity of contiguous determinants in proteins. The relationship of mobility and antigenicity for conformational determinants is more complex and needs further study. Currently, we find that anti-peptide antibodies against contiguous, highly mobile regions react strongly with the native protein, while anti-peptide antibodies from well-ordered regions do not. In addition, we have found a high correlation between mobility and antigenicity in a number of proteins by combining previously observed immunological data with high resolution crystallographic results. Mobility is unlikely to be the only intrinsic factor involved in determining the degree of antigenicity. However, the realization that mobility is a parameter effecting antigenicity has implications for any model of antigenic recognition in that it implies a multiple step process rather than single collision resulting in simple lock and key complementarity.

We thank S. Sheriff and W. Hendrickson for sharing their results on myohemerythrin temperature factors prior to publication, Y. Paterson, H. Alexander and A. Olson for useful discussions, and M. Connolly for the use of AMS [63a] and RAMS [63b].

1. Lerner, R.A. *Nature* **299**, 592–596 (1982).
2. Arnon, R. in *Impact of Protein Chemistry on the Biomedical Sciences* (eds Schechter, A. N., Dean, A. & Goldberger, R. F.) 187–198 (Academic, Orlando, 1984).
3. Benjamin, D. C., Berzofsky, J. A., East, I. J., Gurd, F. R. N., Hannum, C., Leach, S. J., Margoliash, E., Michael, J. G., Mil-

ler A., Prager, E. M., Reichlin, M., Sercarz, E. E., Smith-Gill, S. J., Todd, P. E. & Wilson, A. C. *Ann. Rev. Immunol.* **2**, 67–101 (1984).

4. Dean, P. M. *Br. J. Pharmac.* **74**, 39–46 (1981).
5. Perutz, M. F. *Science* **201**, 1187–1191 (1978).
6. Hayes, D. M. & Kollman, P. A. *J. Am. Chem. Soc.* **98**, 7811–7816 (1976).
7. Sheridan, R. P. & Allen, L. C. *J. Am. Chem. Soc.* **103**, 1544–1550 (1981).
8. Warshel, A. & Levitt, M. *J. Mol. Biol.* **103**, 227–249 (1976).
9. Blaney, J. M., Weiner, P. K., Dearing, A., Kollman, P. A., Jorgensen, E. C., Oatley, S. J., Burridge, J. M. & Blake, C. C. F. *J. Am. Chem. Soc.* **104**, 6424–6434 (1982).
10. Weiner, P. K., Langridge, R., Blaney, J. M., Schaefer, R. & Kollman, P. A. *Proc. Natl. Acad. Sci. U.S.A.* **79**, 3754–3758 (1982).
11. Pullman, B., Lavery, R. & Pullman, A. *Eur. J. Biochem.* **124**, 229–238 (1982).
12. Friend, S. H., March, K. L., Hanania, I. H. & Gurd, F. R. N. *Biochemistry* **19**, 3039–3047 (1980).
13. Getzoff, E. D., Tainer, J. A., Weiner, P. K., Kollman, P. A., Richardson, J. S. & Richardson, D. C. *Nature* **306**, 287–290 (1983).
14. Segal, D. M., Padlan, E. A., Cohen, G. H., Rudikoff, S., Potter, M. & Davies, D. R. *Proc. Natl. Acad. Sci. U.S.A.* **71**, 4298–4302 (1974).
15. Padlan, E. A., Davies, D. R., Rudikoff, S. & Potter, M. *Immunochemistry* **13**, 945–949 (1976).
16. Debye, P. *Annl. Phys.* **43**, 49 (1914).
17. Swaminathan, S., Ichiye, T., van Gunsteren, W. & Karplus, M. *Biochemistry* **21**, 5230–5241 (1982).
18. Holbrook, S. R. & Kim, S. -H. *J. Mol. Biol.* **173**, 361–388 (1984).
19. Artymiuk, P. J., Blake, C. C. F. Grace, D. E. P., Oatley, S. J., Philips, D. C. & Sternberg, M. J. E. *Nature* **280**, 563–568 (1979).
20. Tainer, J. A., Getzoff, E. D. & Olson, A. J., *Proc. of the Conference on Molecular Dynamics and Protein Structure* (ed. Hermans, J.) (Univ. of N. C., Chapel Hill, in press).
21. Sheriff, S., Hendrickson, W. A., Stenkamp, R. E., Sieker, L. C. & Jensen, L. H. (in preparation).
22. Huber, R. & Bennett, W. S., Jr. *Biopolymers* **22**, 261–279 (1983).
23. McCammon, J. A. & Karplus, M. *Acc. Chem. Res.* **16**, 187–193

(1983).
24. Tainer, J. A., Getzoff, E. D., Alexander, H., Houghten, R. A., Olson, A. J., Lerner, R. A. & Hendrickson, W. A. *Nature* (in press).
25. Farr, R. S. *J. Infect. Dis.* **103**, 239–262 (1958).
26. Klippenstein, G. L., Van Riper, D. A., & Oosterom, E. A. *J. Biol. Chem.* **247**, 5959–5963 (1972).
27. Thornton, J. M. & Sibanda, B. L. *J. Mol. Biol.* **167**, 443–460 (1983).
28. Chavez L. G. & Scheraga H. A. *Biochem.* **18**, 4386–4395 (1979).
29. Jemmerson, R., Morrow, P. R., Klinman, N. R., Paterson, Y. *Proc. Natl. Acad. Sci. U.S.A.* (in press).
30. Jackson, D. C., Nestorowicz, A. & Webster, R. G. *Proc. Int. Workshop Mol. Biol. Ecol. Influenza Virus* (ed. Laver, W.G.) 87 (Elsevier, New York, 1983).
31. Solomon, B., Moav, N., Pines, G., & Katchalski-Katzir, E. *Mol. Immunol.* **21**, 1–11 (1984).
32. Lawrence, G. M., Walker, D. G. & Trayer, I. P. *Biochim. Biophys. Acta.* **743**, 219–225 (1983).
33. Katiyar, S. S., Porter, J. W. *Proc. Natl. Acad. Sci. U.S.A.* **80**, 1221–1223 (1983).
34. Jemmerson, R. & Margoliash, E. *J. Biol. Chem.* **254**, 12706–12716 (1979).
35. Hopp, T. P. & Woods, K. R. *Proc. Natl. Acad. Sci. U.S.A.* **6**, 3824–3828 (1981).
36. Burnet F. M. *Selection Theory of Acquired Immunity* (Cambridge University Press, Cambridge, 1959).
37. Nossal G. J. V. *Ann. Rev. Immunol.* **1**, 33 (1983).
38. Fraga, S. *Can. J. Chem.* **60**, 2606–2610 (1982).
39. Hopp, T. P. & Woods, K. R. *Mol. Immunol.* **20**, 483–489 (1983).
40. Kyte J. & Doolittle R. F. *J. Mol.Biol.* **157**, 105–132 (1982).
41. Isaacs, N. W., Agarwal, R. C. *Acta Crystallogr.* **A34**, 782 (1978).
42. Blundell, T., Dodson, G., Hodgkin, D., Mercola, D., *Adv. Protein Chem.* **26**, 279–402 (1972).
43. Blundell, T. L. & Wood, S. P. *Nature* **257**, 197–203 (1975).
44. Dayhoff, M. O. & Eck, R. V. *Atlas of Protein Sequence and Structure* (Nat. Biomedical Research Foundation, Washington, D.C., 1982).
45. Schroer, J. A., Bender, T., Feldmann, R. J., & Kim, K. J. *Eur. J. Immunol.* **13**, 693–700 (1983).
46. Bender, T. P., Schroer, J. & Claflin, J.L. *J. Immunol.* **131**, 2882–

2889 (1983).

47. Lai, K., Dong, B., Xie, D. & Yuan, H. *Shengwu Huaxue Yu Shengwu Wuli Xuebao* **15**, 457–462 (1983).

48. Bernstein, F. C., Koetzle, T. F., Williams, G. J. B., Meyer, E. F., Brice, M. D., Rodgers, J. R., Kennard, O., Shimanouchi, T. & Tasumi, M. *J. Mol. Biol.* **112**, 535–542 (1977).

49. Eisenberg, D., Weiss, R. M., Terwilliger, T. C. & Wilcox, W. *Faraday Symp. Chem. Soc.* **17**, 109 (1982).

50. Connolly, M. L. *Science* **221**, 709–713 (1983).

51. Borden, D. & Margoliash, E. in *Handbook of Biochemistry and Molecular Biology, Proteins, VIII* (ed. Fasman, G. D.) 268 (The Chemical Rubber Co., Cleveland, 1976).

52. Jemmerson, R. & Margoliash, E. in *Immunobiology of Proteins and Peptides I* (eds Atassi, M. Z. & Stavitsky, A. B.) 119 (Plenum, New York, 1978).

53. Nisonoff, A., Reichlin, M. & Margoliash, E. *J. Biol. Chem.* **245**, 940–946 (1970).

54. Urbanski, G. J. & Margoliash, E. *J. Immunol.* **118**, 1170–1180 (1977).

55. Urbanski, G. J. & Margoliash, E. in *Immunochemistry of Enzymes and their Antibodies* (ed. Salton, M. J. R.) 203–225, (John Wiley & Sons, New York, 1977).

56. Jemmerson, R. & Margoliash, E. *Nature* **282**, 468–471 (1979).

57. Eng, J. & Reichlin, M. *Mol. Immunol.* **16**, 225–230 (1979).

58. Dickerson, R. E., Takano, T., Eisenberg, D., Kallai, O. B., Samson, L., Cooper, A. & Margoliash, E. *J. Biol. Chem.* **246**, 1511–1535 (1971).

59. Swanson, R., Trus, B. L., Mandel, N., Mandel, G., Kallai, O. B. & Dickerson, R. E. *J. Biol. Chem.* **252**, 759–775 (1977).

60. Takano, T., Trus, B. L., Mandel, N., Mandel, G., Kallai, O. B., Swanson, R. & Dickerson, R. E. *J. Biol. Chem.* **252**, 776–785 (1977).

61. O'Donnell, T. J. & Olson, A. J. *Computer Graphics* **15**, 133 (1981).

62. Connolly, M. L. & Olson, A. J. *Computers & Chem.* (in press).

63a. Connolly, M.L. *J. Appl. Crystallogr.* **16**, 548–558 (1983).

63b. Connolly, M.L. *J. Mol. Graphics,* (in press).

64. Northrup, S. H., Pear, M. R., McCammon, J. A. & Karplus, M. *Nature* **286**, 304–305 (1980).

65. Wang, K.M. & Reichlin, M. *Mol. Immunol.* **19**, 729–736 (1982).

PEPTIDES AS POTENTIAL VACCINES AGAINST FOOT AND MOUTH DISEASE

F. Brown

Wellcome Biotechnology Ltd.

Langley Court, Beckenham, Kent BR3 3BS

SUMMARY

Synthetic peptides corresponding to the immunogenic site of foot-and-mouth disease virus elicit levels of neutralizing antibody which can protect experimental animals and cattle against challenge infection with high levels of virus. This has allowed us to study the chemical basis for antigenic variation which is a major problem in controlling the disease by vaccination. Comparison of the sequences of the immunogenic sites of viruses belonging to different serotypes and subtypes shows that single amino acid changes in the immunogenic site can alter the antigenic spectrum of the virus. Moreover peptides with appropriate amino acid substitutions have been made which have a wider antigenic spectrum than peptides with the "natural" sequence. Combining this approach with molecular modelling should allow the "tailoring" of peptide vaccines with more useful antigenic characteristics.

VACCINATION AGAINST THE DISEASE

Foot-and-mouth disease is the most economically important virus disease of farm animals. It occurs worldwide and its control is important, not only because of the loss of productivity it causes but because of the

effect on trading.   In general countries free from the
disease do not import farm animals or meat and meat
products from those areas where the disease is present.

Control is usually by vaccination in those countries
where the disease is endemic.   This involves frequent
prophylactic vaccination, as many as 3 injections being
given each year in some countries.

Vaccination is complicated by the occurrence of the
virus as seven distinct serotypes.   In practical terms
this means that an animal which has been infected with
virus of one serotype, although then immune to re-infection
with viruses of the same serotype, is still susceptible
to infection with viruses of other serotypes.   In
addition there is sufficient variation within serotypes to
cause problems in the selection of vaccines to combat
field outbreaks.   Selection of vaccines to be used in any
particular outbreak is made on the basis of the serological
relationship between the viruses used for preparing the
vaccines used in the prophylactic programmes and the virus
causing the outbreak.

By far the greatest proportion are killed vaccines
prepared by inactivating the fluid harvested from tissue
culture cells infected with the virus.   Inactivation
is usually achieved by incubating the virus with an imine
or, to a diminishing extent, formaldehyde.   The record of
innocuity is good but there are occasional problems with
inactivation procedures.   In practice only about 0.01%
of a batch of vaccine is tested directly for innocuity and
reliance that the procedure is satisfactory depends also
on previously established kinetics of inactivation.

Protection against the disease is measured by a PD50
test in which animals are challenged 21 days after primary
vaccination with 100,000 ID50 of infectious virus injected
into 10 sites on the tongue.   Protection can be correlated
with the level of neutralizing antibody elicited by the
vaccine.   In general an animal with a serum which can be
diluted 100 fold and still neutralize 100 ID50 of the
homologous virus will be protected against challenge.

STRUCTURAL REQUIREMENTS FOR A GOOD VACCINE

The structural features which determine the efficacy of foot-and-mouth vaccines have been determined by a prolonged series of experiments. The first step was to recognise the particular components of the virus harvest which elicited an immune response.

The virus harvest contains four virus specific particles.

1) the infectious virus particles, diameter c 25nm, sedimenting at 146S and consisting of one copy of a single stranded RNA, mol wt c 2.6 x 10^6 and 60 copies of four proteins, mol wt c 24 x 10^3 for VP1-VP3 and c 10 x 10^3 for VP4.
2) the so-called empty particle, with the same diameter as the infectious particle but sedimenting at 75S. The particle does not contain any RNA but possesses the same proteins although VP2 and VP4 are covalently linked as VP0.
3) a protein sub unit, mol wt c 350 x 10^3 consisting of 5 copies of each of VP1-VP3.
4) the RNA polymerase, mol wt c 56 x 10^6.

The major part of the immunizing activity is associated with the virus particle. This particle is very fragile below pH7, being disrupted into the infectious RNA, an aggregate of the protein VP4 and the 12S pentameric unit of VP1-VP3. This mixture has very low immunizing activity.

The observation that virus particles which have been treated with trypsin have a much reduced infectivity and ability to elicit neutralizing antibody provided an important clue about the structural features required to evoke an immune response. The only detectable difference between the untreated and treated particles is the cleavage of VP1, indicating that this protein contains the immunodominant site on the virus. This conclusion was supported by the observation that the isolated VP1, but not VP2, VP3 or VP4, will also elicit neutralizing antibody, although this is at a very low level compared with that evoked by the intact particle. Combined with the observations with the 12S particle, it becomes apparent that the configuration of the immunodominant site of VP1

differs in the isolated protein,when it is part of the
12S particle and when it forms part of the virus particle.
Indeed the neutralizing antibody induced by both the
12S sub unit and the isolated VP1 differs from that
elicited by the 146S particle.   Whereas the neutralizing
activity of the anti VP1 and anti 12S antisera are
absorbed by the two antigens, the neutralizing activity
of the anti 146S antiserum is not absorbed by either
VP1 or the 12S sub unit.

IDENTIFICATION OF IMMUNOGENIC SITES

        Further information about the immunodominant site on
VP1 has been gained from Strohmaier's work on the immune
response to fragments of VP1.   This is an approach used
first by Anderer with tobacco mosaic virus and consists
of isolating active fragments of the protein by either
chemical cleavage of the separated protein or enzymatic
cleavage of the protein in situ.   The location of these
active fragments on VP1 was obtained by comparing limited
amino acid sequences at their N and C termini with the
sequence of the entire VP1 predicted from the nucleotide
sequence of that part of the virus genome coding for it.
By aligning overlapping peptides on the amino acid
sequence of VP1 these workers predicted that residues
146-154 and 200-213 would be included in antigenic sites
eliciting neutralizing antibody.

        As nucleotide sequences for the part of the virus
genome coding for VP1 became available for different
serotypes and subtypes of the virus, it became clear that
considerable sequence variation occurred at residues
42-61, 129-160 and 193-204.   The remainder of the
molecule is highly conserved between serotypes.   Those
regions with amino acid differences would be expected
to correlate with serological differences.   Regions
occurring at the surface of the virus particle are likely
to be hydrophilic in character and when predicted
hydrophilicity plots were superimposed on amino acid
sequence variation plots, it was found that the only
regions of high variability which were hydrophilic were
those between 129-160 and 193-204.   Synthetic peptides
corresponding to these regions elicit neutralizing
antibody in experimental animals.   The 129-160 region
appears to be the immunodominant site because it elicits

much higher levels of neutralizing antibody.   The
level of neutralizing antibody induced by a single
injection of a peptide corresponding to amino acids
141-160 of serotype O virus, linked to keyhole limpet
haemocyanin, protected guinea pigs against challenge with
large amounts of the haemotypic virus.

USE OF PEPTIDES IN STUDYING ANTIGENIC VARIATION

The identification of the immunodominant site has
enabled a more precise study to be made of antigenic
variation within foot-and-mouth disease.   A fortuitous
observation that serum from animals receiving a peptide
corresponding to amino acids 141-160 of a virus of
serotype A12, although containing high levels of
anti-peptide antibody, did not neutralize the corresponding
virus, led us to examine more closely the virus being used
for the neutralization tests.   The sequence of amino acids
in the 141-160 region had been obtained by cloning the RNA
from a virus stock derived by multiple passage in a variety
of host cells from the parental virus used in the
neutralization tests.   Plaquing of the parental virus
revealed that it contained in roughly equal proportions
three viruses which differed at amino acid positions 148
and 153 of the VP1 polypeptide.   Moreover, the virus whose
sequence had been used for the synthesis of the peptide
also had amino acid differences at the same positions.
Neutralization tests performed with antisera from animals
injected with each of the four viruses or the
corresponding 141-160 peptides showed the importance of
amino acids 148 and 153 in determining antigenic
specificity within this group of viruses (Table I).   The
results also demonstrated that antigenic variants may be
present in field isolates of the virus.   Provided
subsequent passage of the virus for the purpose of
preparing vaccines does not select variants, the vaccine
should perform well in controlling the disease.
Retrospective analysis of the performance of some
foot-and-mouth disease vaccines which has been worse than
anticipated indicates that selection of antigenic
variants may have occurred during passage of the virus
for vaccine production.

TABLE I   Neutralization of viruses containing different amino acids at positions 148 and 153 of VP1 with homologous and heterologous anti virion and anti peptide sera.

Serum	Serum dilution	Log_{10} virus neutralized by 0.015ml serum			
		A	B	C	D
		Ser 148 Leu 153	Leu 148 Pro 153	Ser 148 Ser 153	Phe 148 Pro 153
Antivirion A	1/200	3.3	1.3	1.7	0.7
Antipeptide A	1/1	2.5	1.1	1.5	0.9
Antivirion B	1/200	0.9	3.7	0.9	2.1
Antipeptide B	1/1	Nil	3.2	0.5	2.2
Antivirion C	1/2000	1.9	0.5	2.5	0.5
Antipeptide C	1/1	1.5	0.1	2.6	1.5
Antivirion D	1/200	1.3	2.5	1.1	3.7
Antipeptide D	1/1	Nil	2.0	Nil	2.7
Antipeptide Leu 148 Leu 153	1/1	0.3	0.9	0.5	0.7
Antipeptide Phe 148 Leu 153	1/1	Nil	0.4	0.4	0.3

PRIMING WITH PEPTIDES

Recent work by Wimmer and his colleagues with poliovirus has shown that rabbits which have received injections of synthetic peptides corresponding to different regions of one of the capsid proteins gave a very high level of neutralizing antibody when injected with an amount of poliovirus particles which did not evoke a response in unprimed animals.   Although we have not been able to repeat these observations with the structurally similar foot-and-mouth disease virus and the 141-160 peptide, we have found that successive injections of this peptide, coupled to keyhole limpet haemocyanin, in amounts which do not elicit neutralizing antibody in a single injection, evoke high neutralizing antibody levels.   The interval between the injections appears to be important.   No boost of neutralizing antibody was obtained when the injections were given 14 days apart and the optimal boost was at about 42 days.   The boost in neutralizing antibody titre was apparently specific,not being obtained when the animals received the 200-213 KLH linked peptide or KLH alone as the first injection.

The neutralizing antibody level of animals which had received small doses of virus particles was also boosted by a second injection of the 141-160 KLH linked peptide.   In addition to its potential application in vaccination procedures, this approach should allow the antigenic site of the virus to be defined more precisely.

BONE MARROW DIFFERENTIATION

J.G. Sharp, University of Nebraska Medical
Center, Qmaha, Nebraska, U.S.A.
Ellen E.E. Jarrett, University of Glasgow
Veterinary School, Glasgow, Scotland.

This workshop covered diverse topics which were nomin-
ally related in that they included the characterisation and
regulation of differentiation of pluripotent hematopoietic
stem cells and their progeny into B cells, mast cells and
other leucocytes.

Barlozzari et al, (Frederick) reported that natural
killer (NK) cells in the rat inhibited day 9 spleen colony
(CFU-S) formation by exogenously administered colony forming unit enriched bone marrow cells. Prior administration
of anti-asialo GMl antibody increased the number of colonies
observed. Pisa et al (Karolinska) observed that in both the
human and the mouse, NK cells inhibited the growth of granulocyte-macrophage progenitors in agar. In both of these
situations the stem-progenitor cell targets are presumably
proliferating. As both groups of authors pointed out, these
observations may have relevance to the phenomenon of hybrid
resistance against bone marrow grafts. However, in the
physiological situation, the majority of CFU-S are not proliferating and it is more difficult to assign a role for NK
cells in normal hematopoiesis. Furthermore, the mechanism(s)
of the in vivo effects are most uncertain in that it is not
known if the target cells are killed, altered in their
seeding efficiency for the spleen or suppressed by other
mechanisms. The inhibition of hematopoietic precursors by
NK cells has now become established phenomenology but its
significance remains elusive. The morphological similarities between large granular lymphocytes and mucosal mast

cells described by Jarrett et al later in this session were
striking. Although morphological correlations can be misleading, it would appear to be a worthwhile endeavour to
determine the NK/NC activity of developing mucosal mast
cells, perhaps more particularly the latter, given the effect of interleukin 3, (IL-3) in augmenting NC activity (1).

    The HL-60 human promyelocytic cell line was employed
by Chiao et al, (New YOrk), Nunn et al, (London) and
Sullivan and Shemetek (Montreal) to study myeloid differentiation. The latter authors have developed a variant which
lacks myeloperoxidase and fails to mature to metamyelocytes
on stimulation with dimethylsuphoxide or retinoic acid.

    Schlick et al, (Frederick) described some potential
applications of biological response modifiers to augment
hematopoiesis and immune function following treatment of
mice with cyclophosphamide. In addition to the effect of
these modifiers acting on hematopoiesis via the production
of several types of colony stimulating factor, there appeared to be an anti-tumor effect of CSF. Effects on NK
cells appeared later and potentially as a consequence of
increased γ-interferon levels. This in turn might augment
NK cytotoxicity and have an additional anti-tumor effect.
The overall efficacy of such biological response modifiers
might well vary significantly with tumor type depending on
the primary effector mechanisms (macrophages, NK cells,
T cells) involved in killing a particular tumor cell type
and the survival of these effector cells after therapy.
Anaemia in response to BCG reported by Milon (Paris) might
also be modulated either by stem cell competition in response to elevated CSF levels or perhaps by augmented NK/NC
killing of hematopoietic precursor cells as a consequence
of stimulation of γ-interferon levels. Perhaps these observations have relevance to the anaemia sometimes seen in
chronic infections and malignancies (2).

    Leonore Herzenberg and colleagues (Stanford) described
a minor subpopulation (1-2% in the adult) of splenic B cells
in the mouse which carries the Ly-1 antigen. (The recom-
mendation was made to return to the original designation of
this antigen as Ly-1 (3) rather than Lyt-1 because it is
clearly not a T cell restricted antigen). Such B cells constitute a significant proportion of Ig positive cells in
the spleen of 3-5 day old mice and they are found in large

numbers in peritoneal lavages, particularly in Balb/c and
NZB mice. Their numbers are low in SJL mice. These cells
are slightly larger and more adherent than other B cells
and non-phagocytic. Many peritoneal macrophage preparations may contain significant numbers of such cells. Increased levels of this cell population are observed in
autoimmune mice and it appears to be associated with autoantibody production. The Ly-1 antigen is expressed by a
number of B cell tumors in the mouse and its equivalent(T-1)
in some B cell tumors in man. Although Ly-1 B cells appear
to be responsible for much of the IgM autoantibody production in autoimmune mice, the marker is not found on normal
plasma cells. Surprisingly many Ly-1 positive tumor cells
express the lambda light chain which is rare in the mouse.
A most interesting correlate to these observations was reported at the 8th International Germinal Centers Conference
by Plater-Zyberk et al (4) who demonstrated that almost 20%
of circulating surface Ig positive cells in patients with
rheumatoid arthritis were T-1 positive compared to about 1%
in controls. The origins of Ly-1 B cells are uncertain but
Dr. Herzenberg suggested on the basis of very preliminary
evidence that they may not be replaced readily in bone
marrow chimeras. In this regard Kubai and Auerbach (5) have
reported an omental origin of lymphoid cells in the mouse.
Additionally, the ileal Peyer's patch in lambs and pigs
appears to have some characteristics of a primary B lymphoid
tissue (6,7). One wonders if these observations might be
related. Clearly the role of Ly-1 B cells in autoimmunity
in the mouse which appear to correlate with those in man
raise many questions as to the involvement of this newly
described B cell sub-set in autoimmune disease.

Ratcliff et al (London) described the re-population of
cyclophosphamide depleted chicken bursal follicles by the
injection of immunoglobulin allotype marked bursal stem cells.
Virtually all follicles carried one allotype marker suggesting that the repopulating stem cells were already committed
to the synthesis of a particular allotype at the time of
entry into the follicle. Thus each follicle can be considered to be the clonally derived progeny of a single Ig
positive committed precursor cell. Studies presented elsewhere (8) have indicated that bursectomy does not prevent
the maturation of T and B cells although it reduces the size
of the B cell pool. One suspects however that the available
repertoire of B cells may have been altered in a manner

which is perhaps somewhat analogous to the influence of
thymectomy or the nude gene on the T cell repertoire in the
mouse. Clearly Ig gene rearrangement occurs in B cell
progenitors more primitive than the pre-B cell populations
which have been extensively studied to date. The bone
marrow culture system described by Dexter et al (9) and
modified by Witte and associates (10) might provide a system in which rearrangement can be studied. This type of
culture system together with the availability of IL-3 and
related preparations has lead recently to exciting development in our understanding of the differentiation of mucosal
mast cells.

    Jarrett and colleagues (Glasgow) showed studies of
progressively developing mast cells in rat bone marrow cultures stimulated with conditioned medium from antigen-
activated T cells. In various respects, e.g. lack of hepar-
in, low content of histamine and high content of the serine
protease RMCPII (11) these cells resemble mucosal mast cells
rather than mature connective tissue mast cells. The
progenitors of these cells are present in considerably
greater numbers in the bone marrow of Nippostrongylus
brasiliensis infected than in uninfected rats, a finding
which led to a debate about the "normality" of haemopoiesis
in SPF laboratory animals given that most animals in the
field are "normally" parasite infected. Although the differentiation of mucosal mast cells is T cell-dependent -
requiring the addition of T cell-produced factors in nude
rat bone marrow cultures - the increase in progenitor cell
frequency does occur in infected nude rats indicating a T
cell-independence at this stage.

    Courtoy et al (Liege) using mouse bone marrow cultures
showed beautiful transmission and scanning EM pictures of
groups of mast cells attached by membrane folds to cytoplasmic protrusions on the surface of large adherent cells
(LAC). This contact was critical for mast cell development.
The LAC were positive for Thy1, Lyt-1 and Lyt-2 and differed
morphologically from macrophage and fibroblasts. This report must be seen in context with another report of the importance of adherent cells in the development of mast cell
granulation (12) and the growing recognition that molecules
produced by stromal cells have crucial activities in haemopoiesis (13). Clearly there is still much to be learned
about the regulatory molecules produced by stromal cells in
various parts of the body.

Perhaps one question regarding the basophil/mast cell conundrum has been answered by Stadler and colleagues (Bern) and that is that distinct T cell-derived factors and not just more of the same cause a selective proliferation of one cell type or the other. Two factors were purified from lectin-stimulated human PBL, a basophil promoting activity (M.W. 20-35K, pI 5.8-7.5) and a mast cell promoting activity (M.W. 15-19K, pI 5.2-6.0) which copurified with IL3. Both this paper and the communication from Rimmer and Horton (London), who join the growing band of people to grow mast cells from human haemopoietic tissues, emphasise a new recognition of mast cell heterogeneity not only between but also within species. It is clear that the days are passed when rat peritoneal mast cells were regarded as exponents of the type.

References

1. Lattine, E.C., Pecoraro, G.A. & Stutman, O. J. exp. Med. 157, 1070-1075 (1983).
2. Hansen, N.E. Scand. J. Haematol. 31, 397-402 (1983).
3. Cantor, H. & Boyse, E.A. in Biological Activity of Thymic Hormones (ed. van Bekkum, D.W.) 77-85 (Kooyker Scientific Publishers, Rotterdam, 1975).
4. Plater-Zyberk, C., Lam, K., Kennedy, T.D., Maini, R.N. & Janossy, G. in Proc. Morphological Aspects of the Immune System (ed. Klaus, G.G.B.) (in press) (Plenum, New York, 1984).
5. Kubai, L., & Auerbach, R. Nature 301, 154 (1983).
6. Reynolds, J.D. & Morris, B. Eur. J. Immunol. (1983) 13, 627-635.
7. Binns, R.M. & Licence, S.T. in Morphological Aspects of the Immune System (ed. Klaus, G.G.B.) (in press) (Plenum, New York, 1984).
8. Ewert, D.L., Oats, C. & Chen, C. in Morphological Aspects of the Immune System (ed. Klaus, G.G.B.) (in press) (Plenum, New York, 1984).
9. Dexter, T.M., Allen, T.D., & Lajtha, L.G. J. Cell Physiol. 91, 335-344 (1977).
10. Whitlock, C.A., Robertson, D. & Witte, O.N. J. Immunol. Methods 67, 353-369 (1984).
11. Woodbury, R.G. & Neurath, H. in Metabolic Interconversions of Enzymes (ed. Holzer, H.), 145-158 Springer Verlag Berlin (1981).

12. Davidson, S., Mansour, A., Gallily, R., Smolarski, M.,
    Rofolovitch, M. & Ginsburg, H.   Immunology 48,
    439-452 (1983).
13. Dexter, T.M.   This symposium (1984).

ROLE OF CELL SURFACE MOLECULES IN T CELL TRIGGERING

P.C.L. Beverley[1] & J.P. Revillard[2]

[1] ICRF Human Tumour Immunology Group

University College London, Faculty of Clinical Sciences

University Street, London WC1E 6JJ

[2] Hopital Edouard-Herriot

Lyon cedex 08, France

The workshop illustrated how the use of antibodies to investigate cell function has changed in recent years. When reliable alloantisera and then monoclonal antibodies were produced many investigators used them to separate cell populations and show that cells with a particular phenotype could carry out a given range of functions. More recently monoclonal antibodies and monoclonal cell populations have been used to investigate the function of the molecules identified by the antibodies.

Several papers dealt with the first aspect of lymphocyte biology, reporting new rat subpopulations defined by monoclonal antibodies[6] specific membrane lectins of human T suppressor cells[7] or the use of Helix pomatia A haemagglutinin to separate subpopulations of human T cells.[11] However, a major part of the workshop was taken up by studies which used monoclonal antibodies in attempts to define more closely the role of surface molecules in T lymphocyte function.

Five reports dealt mainly with the regulation of interleukin-2 (IL-2) receptor expression, studied in cloned IL-2 dependent T cells. Murine GAT-specific helper cell

273

clones showed two different patterns of response when restimulated after reaching a (resting) state in which IL-2 receptors were undetectable with a rat monoclonal antibody.[2]   One clone could be induced to proliferate and express high levels of IL-2 receptor by either antigen presented by accessory cells or cloned human IL-2. Another clone could only be restimulated by antigen and accessory cells.   In this clone however viability of "resting" T cells was maintained when IL-2 was present in the medium, suggesting that IL-2 may have a trophic effect on some T cells which have not recently encountered antigen whereas recently antigen and accessory cell restimulated cells respond by active proliferation.

In cytolytic murine clones the requirements for restimulation by antigen were examined.[8]   Both antibody to target H-2 antigen or anti-Lyt-2 could block the acquisition of IL-2 responsiveness.   Addition of blocking antibodies at varying times after addition of antigen showed that only a short period of contact (<3 hours) with antigen is required.   These cytolytic clones exemplify the necessity for antigenic restimulation since even in the presence of IL-2 there is a decline in pro-liferation rate and expression of IL-2 receptors unless the cells are restimulated with antigen.   The decline in receptor expression precedes slow down in proliferation and loss in viability.

Attempts have been made to substitute for antigen/ accessory cell stimulation by other stimuli.   Thus IL-2 receptor expression can be increased by phorbol esters in both fresh lymphocytes[1] and T cell clones whereas PHA or anti-T3 antibody[3] do not stimulate human long term cultured clones.

A consensus view is thus that T cell clones require periodic restimulation with antigen and accessory cells and cannot be repeatedly stimulated with IL-2.   Those clones which become 'addicted' to IL-2 generally have chromosomal aberrations.   Following stimulation with antigen or IL-2 there is an initial rise in IL-2 receptor expression followed by a gradual decline.   An additional role for IL-2 may be to maintain viability in cells with low receptor expression (resting cells).

These results raise questions regarding the mechanism by which binding of IL-2 to its receptor leads to a gradual decline in receptor expression. The requirements for restimulation of cells by antigen or mitogen with accessory cells require further definition and it is not clear whether these differ between T cell clones and virgin T cells.

A second series of communications dealt with the effects of antibodies to cell surface antigens on cell function. Antibodies to non-polymorphic determinants of Thy-1 initially showed inconsistent effects when added to mouse mixed lymphocyte or mitogen stimulated cultures.[5] Kinetic analysis showed that antibody added at the commencement of the culture has an early stimulatory effect while antibodies added later are only suppresive. Confirmation that anti-Thy-1 can act on T cell function came from the observation that anti-Thy-1 stimulates the production of macrophage activating factor by a cytolytic clone.[9] Ligand binding to both polymorphic and non-polymorphic determinants of Thy-1 can therefore trigger various effects in resting or activated lymphocytes by a pathway independent of the T cell receptor complex. Thy-1 does not appear to be analogous to the T3 molecule of humans since anti-Thy-1 does not block T cell cytolysis and is not directly mitogenic. Furthermore Thy-1 differs biochemically from T3, the mature form consisting of a single species of 25 KD.[4] However the biosynthesis of Thy-1 presents a paradox in that it has so far proved impossible to detect translation products containing the 30 extra amino acids predicted by the sequence of the genomic clone isolated by Silver, compared to the sequence of the protein.

Interestingly anti-HLA antibodies were also shown to have inhibitory effects on the proliferative responses to anti-T3 monoclonal antibodies[10] but not PHA. The mechanism of this effect appears to be at the level of induction of IL-2 receptors since antibodies added to IL-2 receptor expressing cells in the presence of IL-2 did not prevent proliferation. Two out of three antibodies to non-polymorphic determinants of HLA class I and anti-β2 micro-globulin antibody could mediate this effect while the third anti-HLA monoclonal had no effect. It is not yet clear whether the effect operated at the level of responding or accessory cells.

As yet the significance of many effects of monoclonal antibodies is obscure.   There is increasing evidence however that several molecules at the T cell surface interact with accessory or target cells in triggering T cell function including T_i, LFA-1, Lyt-2 or L3T4.   The data presented here suggest that Thy-1 and HLA class I may also deliver signals to T cells.   What remains to be determined is whether these molecules interact with each other in the cell surface or whether signals delivered by them are integrated at a post receptor, intracellular level.

References

1. Ando, I., Crawford, D.H., Hariri, G., Wallace, D. & Beverley, P.C.L. Immunobiology Vol. 167, Abstract No. 124, p. 81 (1984) (16th International Leucocyte Culture Conference) (Gustav Fischer Verlag Stuttgart).

2. Bismuth, G., Dautry, A., Duphot, M. & Theze, J. Immunobiology Vol. 167, Abstract No. 126, p. 82 (1984) (16th International Leucocyte Culture Conference) (Gustav Fischer Verlag Stuttgart).

3. Bolhuis, R.L.H., van Krimpen, B.A. & van de Griend, R.J. Immunobiology Vol. 167, Abstract No. 127, p. 82 (1984) (16th International Leucocyte Culture Conference) (Gustav Fischer Verlag Stuttgart).

4. Bron, C. & Leuscher, B. Immunobiology Vol. 167, Abstract No. 135, p. 88 (1984) (16th International Leucocyte Culture Conference) (Gustav Fischer Verlag Stuttgart).

5. Hollander, N. Immunobiology Vol. 167, Abstract No. 132, p. 86 (1984) (16th International Leucocyte Culture Conference) (Gustav Fischer Verlag Stuttgart).

6. Joling, P., Tielen, F.J., Vaessen, L.M.B. & Rozing, J. Immunobiology Vol. 167, Abstract No. 133 p. 87 (1984) (16th International Leucocyte Culture Conference) (Gustav Fischer Verlag Stuttgart).

7. Kieda, C. & Monsigny, M. Immunobiology Vol. 167, Abstract No. 134, p. 87 (1984) (16th International Leucocyte Culture Conference) (Gustav Fischer Verlag Stuttgart).

8. Lowenthal, J.W., Tounge, C., MacDonald, H.R. & Nabholz, M. Immunobiology Vol. 167, Abstract No. 129, p. 84 (1984) (16th International Leucocyte Culture Conference) (Gustav Fischer Verlag Stuttgart).

9.   Macdonald, H.R., Bron, C. & Cerottini, J.-C.
     Immunobiology Vol. 167, Abstract No. 136 p. 89 (1984)
     (16th International Leucocyte Culture Conference)
     (Gustav Fischer Verlag Stuttgart).

10. Turco, M.C., Corbo, L., Morrone, G., Welte, K.,
     Wang, C.Y., Mertelsmann, R., Ferrone, S. & Venuta, S.
     Immunobiology Vol. 167, Abstract No. 135, p. 92
     (1984) (16th International Leucocyte Culture Conference)
     (Gustav Fischer Verlag Stuttgart).

11. Wiken, M., Hellstrom, U., & Perlman, P.   Immuno-
     biology Vol. 167, Abstract No. 144, p. 94 (1984)
     (16th International Leucocyte Culture Conference)
     (Gustav Fischer Verlag Stuttgart).

MECHANISMS OF T CELL SUPPRESSION

G.L. Asherson and E. Culbert

Clinical Research Centre, Harrow, U.K. and
I.C.I. Plc, Macclesfield, U.K.

By way of introduction it was noted that there are several different T suppressor cell circuits and that there are at least four different kinds of linkages between the cells of these circuits.

(1) The link of immunization in which a cell bearing antigen may present it to another cell and induce a T suppressor cell (Ts). In some cases the cell may be a conventional antigen presenting cell perhaps with I-J on its surface. In other cases it is a T cell bearing idiotype on its surface and is sometimes called Ts_1 or a Ts inducer cell.

(2) The link of specific and nonspecific "helper factors". Here specific and nonspecific factors are produced which augment the production of suppressor cells. These factors are formally equivalent to the antigen specific and nonspecific T helper factors involved in the induction, proliferation and differentiation stages of the conventional "positive" immune response. A good example is the induction of Ts-efferent cells in the picryl contact sensitivity system by antigen together with antigen specific T suppressor factor (TsF). The question whether IL-2 is essential for the proliferation of all Ts is unresolved, but T suppressor cell lines have certainly been maintained with crude supernatants containing IL-2.

(3) The link of stimulation (triggering) in which a

primed Ts releases its antigen specific or perhaps nonspecific products after stimulation with antigen (in general
together with MHC related products such as I-J) or with
anti-idiotypic T cell factors. The classical example is the
release of TsF, which is nitrophenyl acetyl (NP) specific,
from Ts_3 after stimulation with the anti-idiotypic TsF_2.

(4) The nonspecific acceptor cell link in which a cell
without relevant immunological specificity is passively
armed by antigen-specific or idiotype-specific TsF (which
behaves like a mobile receptor) and then releases nonspecific inhibitors when exposed to antigen together the
appropriate MHC-linked product, such as I-J (cf. IgE and
the mast cell).

Patient work will be needed to dissect the control
systems first in terms of individual cells and then in
terms of the linkages between the cells. The interaction
of the different circuits with each other must then be
considered. Finally the overlay of contrasuppressor cells
must be added to the picture. The sophistication needed to
handle the large numbers of metazoa, protozoa and micro-
organisms which live in symbiosis or are parasitic on
mammals suggests that the suppressor cell circuits and
their control will be complicated and may have "anti-
intuitive" properties.

The first part of the workshop dealt with the issues
of the relative roles of clonal anergy and suppressor cells
in T cell unresponsiveness and regulation of the size of
the immune response. This led to a consideration of
whether suppressor cells might cause clonal deletion and
the role of suppressor cells in favouring tolerance during
the prenatal and neonatal period. Finally the importance
of considering contrasuppressor cells in regulatory
circuits was discussed.

Until recently there was no positive test for clonal
anergy in the whole animal and its existence was assumed
when suppressor cells could not be demonstrated. [Loblay
pointed out an important experimental detail. It may be
necessary to boost the donor of the suppressor cells with
antigen before undertaking mixture experiments to detect
suppressor cells. This is because memory suppressor cells
need activation by antigen before they act, while their
target cell may become refractory to their action shortly

after exposure to antigen]. However recently Eichmann and others have used limiting dilution assays to give an estimate of the frequency of cytotoxic precursor cells. This approach was used to study mice shortly after a single shot of picrylsulphonic acid--a procedure which causes only partial unresponsiveness. Precursors which occurred in high frequency were activated by mitogen (Concanavalin A) but not by antigen in vitro and could not be demonstrated after tolerance induction. Mixture experiments showed that their absence after tolerance induction was due to suppressor cells. These high frequency precursors were regarded as virgin cells which were sensitive to the effect of suppressor cells. Precursors with much lower frequency were also found. These disappeared after tolerance induction when antigen (but not mitogen) was used. This was not due to suppressor cells. The differential effect of mitogen and antigen suggested that clonal anergy and not clonal deletion was occurring perhaps through a mechanism suggested by the term "receptor blockade". Alternatively the "tolerogen" may have affected high affinity cells. The question whether true clonal anergy or deletion occurs with more prolonged treatment with tolerogen was left unresolved.

The rapid renewal of B and probably T cells implies either that persistent tolerogenic antigen or suppressor cells are needed for prolonged clonal anergy. In this context Waldmann described irradiated mice restored with A bone marrow and then given both an A and an A1 thymus graft. The mice showed tolerance to A1 skin graft although presumably some of the T cells had matured in the A thymus. The implication that suppressor cells were involved was confirmed by demonstrating cytotoxic precursor cells to A1 by limiting dilution. As an approach to the possible role of suppressor cells in causing clonal anergy Asherson described a system in which lymphocytes stimulated in a mixed lymphocyte reaction in the relative absence of IL-2 (caused by nonspecific inhibitor produced by nonspecific T acceptor cells) failed to give a "secondary response" when restimulated with the same alloantigen on day 4. The third party response was intact. The provisional conclusion was that stimulation of lymphocytes in the relative absence of IL-2 causes clonal anergy. The other side of this coin was discussed by Colizzi who showed that the tolerogenic effect of injecting picrylated cells intravenously was converted into an immunogenic effect (contact sensitivity) by the injection of IL-2. The implication was that the degree of

activation of antigen presenting cells and hence of IL-1
and IL-2 production was an important determinant of the
balance between immunity and tolerance.

The classical example of tolerance is neonatal tolerance produced the injection of allogeneic cells. This was
originally attributed to clonal anergy or deletion. However
continued tolerance probably depends on the continued
presence of antigen and suppressor cells can sometimes be
demonstrated. Moreover the induction of tolerance can be
prevented by the injection of IL-2 (Malkovsky).

The importance of tolerance induction to self antigens
before birth gives special interest to the suppressor cells
present in embryonic and early neonatal life as causes of
long lasting unresponsiveness due to clonal anergy and
specific suppressor cells. Globerson argued that if tolerance in the embryo was due to suppressor cells then they
should be demonstrable before T helper cells and should be
nonspecific in their action. In fact mouse embryo liver
contains suppressor cells as early as 10 days at a time
when the thymus is not yet lymphoid. These suppressor cells
lack adult markers including theta but adhere to peanut
agglutinin. They block in vitro immune responses and can be
kept in culture. They disappear from the liver two days
after birth and are then found transiently in the spleen
and thymus.

The late Professor Gershon suggested that the suppressor cell circuits are so important that they must
themselves be subject to special control mechanisms which
may be termed contrasuppressor. In general terms contrasuppressor cells may act
   (1) by inhibiting the suppressor cell itself (suppressor
        of suppressor cell)
   (2) by producing a factor (e.g. IL-2) whose production
        is inhibited by the suppressor cell
   (3) by direct activation of the target cell (e.g. the T
        helper cell) by a method which bypasses or blocks
        the suppressive signal.
Lehner showed that the variation in the dose response curve
of the production of antigen specific T helper and suppressor factors to Streptococcus mutans in vitro in
subjects with different class II (DR) haplotypes could be
attributed to a contrasuppressor cell. This cell bound

antigen, as shown by autoradiography and its affinity for antigen depended on the DR type (4 or w6). This cell blocked the effect of T suppressor cells on the helper cell which makes T helper factor. This was due to a direct effect on the helper cell and not to inactivation of the suppressor cell. The implication was that the contrasuppressor cell bound antigen and presented it directly to the T helper cell.

The second part of the workshop discussed the conditions for the induction of suppressor cells and the genetic restriction in their action. It is known that antigen together with I-J is an induction signal for some but not all suppressor cells. An interesting exception is the ability of cloned T cell lines to induce T suppressor cells. Crispe described how small numbers of cloned helper cells provide help for antibody production while larger numbers induce suppressor cells. Perhaps the number of cells with a particular idiotype has to rise above a critical threshold before Ts are induced. Alternatively the cloned cell line may have a developmental sequence in vitro and may contain some I-J$^+$ cells. The question arises whether this mode of inducing suppressor cells is confined in vivo to those antigens which induce a response with a dominant idiotype.

The cues which enable the immune system to distinguish immunogenic and tolerogenic antigen are still unclear. "Positive" immune responses are usually initiated by factors which activate the antigen presenting cell to acquire class II antigens and to produce IL-1. The equivalent on the suppressor cell side is unknown. Bocchieri raised the question whether the autologous mixed lymphocyte reaction (AMLR) sometimes provided the initial stimulus for suppressor cell activation. In fact most cloned T cell lines derived from the AMLR have the Ly-2$^+$ phenotype characteristic of many suppressor cells and respond to stimulation with autologous non-T cells by producing a factor which suppresses the conventional mixed lymphocyte reaction.

Many suppressor cells are genetically restricted in their action. The I-J restriction has led to the suggestion that both the precursor T cell which is primed by antigen and the effector T cell which is triggered by antigen have a receptor for antigen together with I-J. However some

suppressor cells such as the human gamma globulin specific
T suppressor cells which depress antibody production in
mice do not show I-J or MHC restriction in their action.

There are several possibilities. There may in fact be
no genetic restriction in their action. Alternatively the
injected Ts may release nonspecific inhibitors when exposed
to antigen and appropriate MHC, but the appropriate MHC may
be provided by the injected cell population. Alternatively
the injected cells may serve to present antigen to the
recipient and hence generate second order suppressor cells
which may be genetically restricted. The absence of any
Igh restriction provides some evidence against the view
that the injected Ts induce second order anti-idiotypic
cells. These Ts, like the Ts-efferent cells in the picryl
system, can be purified by adherence to antigen and are
I-J$^+$. However they differ in being unaffected by adult
thymectomy and can be produced in nu/nu mice.

The third part of the workshop dealt with suppressor
factors and their mode of action. Bentwich described the
isolation of cell lines producing thyroglobulin-specific
suppressor factors from patients with autoimmune thyroid
diseases and suggested that antigen-specific suppressor
factors might be important in limiting autoimmune disease.
However despite studies by Bentwich, James and Colizzi
there is still no unequivocal evidence that antigen specific T suppressor factor acts directly on an target cell.
The explanation of Asherson and Zembala that antigen-
specific factors may work by "arming" nonspecific acceptor
cells such as the T acceptor cell or macrophage, which then
release nonspecific inhibitors on exposure to antigen and
I-J is one of several hypotheses which use the concept of a
suppressor cascade. If the current nonspecific suppressor
molecules are indeed the final mediators of suppression
(and do not act by generating further nonspecific factors),
it will be important to know how many different factors
there are, their specificity for different cell types such
as T cells, B cells and antigen presenting cells and their
subsets and their specificity for different types of immune
responses.

Several groups have described nonspecific factors with
apparently broad target specificity with alteration of T
cell, B cell and macrophage function. Two of these factors
were partially purified by immunoaffinity (Oh) or physico-

chemically (Platsoucas). Nevertheless, it is likely that there are families of closely related nonspecific suppressor molecules and it is unclear whether the effects on different cell types are due to one factor or distinct factors present in the mixture. Platsoucas et al have biochemical evidence that their T cell hybridoma-derived suppressor factor differs from other lymphokines with similar activities, such as lymphotoxin and alpha interferon. The functional stability of their hybridoma should enable cloning of the gene shortly.

Some of the suppressor factors may work by blocking the production of important cytokines, rather than by neutralizing their biological activity. Oh's factor inhibits the production of IL-1 by monocytes, and of IL-2 by T cells, but has no effect on the action of IL-1 or IL-2. Similarly the nonspecific inhibitor elaborated by the T acceptor cell described by Asherson and Zembala (which is probably identical to the T suppressor auxiliary cell of Claman) blocks production of IL-2 and its activity is overcome by adding exogenous IL-2. The suppressive effect on B cell responsivensss of Zan-Bar's factor is neutralized by exogenous BCGF. He attributed this to competition between BCGF and the nonspecific factor for the B cell receptor for BCGF. However it is possible that the suppressor factor directly prevents BCGF production by T cells, B cells or NK cells.

Undoubtedly the strongest message from the discussion of what we know about different suppressor factors and their interrelationship is that "we do not know". Clearly, monoclonal sources of suppressor molecules are needed to obtain sufficient homogenous protein for biochemical study and to allow gene cloning. This will provide the starting point for the in vivo studies needed to analyse the interactions within and between the various suppressor and contrasuppressor circuits.

At a practical level T cell hybridization suffers from the problem of functional instability although a few relatively stable clones have been obtained (Platsoucas). Some suppressor cells are IL-2 dependent and can therefore be cloned. However these lines are more difficult to handle than transformed cells. Immortalization of suppressor cells by transforming virus appears a clear winner over hybridomas and factor-dependent cell lines in terms of

stability ease of handling. Murine radiation leukaemia
virus-transformed mouse suppressor cells have proved very
useful sources of antigen specific T suppressor factor and
mRNA (Colizzi). Immortalization of human suppressor cells
by this technique is a real possibility, as
HTLV-transformed human T cells clones have already been
described (see Kishimoto et al; Fauci et al, this
volume).

MECHANISMS OF IMMUNOLOGICAL PERTURBATIONS

Susanna Cunningham-Rundles
Memorial Sloan Kettering Cancer Center
New York, New York

Richard L. O'Brien
Creighton University School of Medicine
Omaha, Nebraska

Immunological Perturbations were discussed in three sections: Pharmacologic Modulation, Acquired Immunodeficiency, and Transplantation.

Pharmacologic Modulation. The discussion focused solely on Cyclosporine A (CsA). There was agreement that:

- CsA is a good in vivo immunosuppressant.

- It inhibits the induction of T cell proliferation by acting early during activation (6-8 hours after mitogens; 1 d in MLC).

- CsA inhibits production of IL-2 and other lymphokines but not the response of primed lymphocytes to IL-2.

Though agreement on the foregoing was reached, several unresolved questions regarding mechanisms of action were raised. Perhaps the most important question is which cells are subject to CsA inhibition of activity.

It was reported that accessory cells are targets for CsA in mitogen-induced responses and that T cells are the subjects of inhibition of antigen-induced

287

responses. Earlier work has suggested that CsA
inhibits antigen presentation to lymphocytes without
identifying which cells are affected, i.e., are
antigen presenting cells prevented from presentation
or are lymphocytes prevented from acceptance of
antigen? The mode of action of CsA is not simple if
it affects more than one of the cell types involved in
the immune response.

Another unresolved question is whether inhibition of
lymphokine production is a key to CsA activity. IL-2
production is inhibited and IL-2 mRNA production is
diminished. This is difficult to interpret because
CsA activity results from early effects at times
before lymphocytes have begun to make IL-2. This
suggests that inhibition of IL-2 production is an
event subsequent to and resulting from an earlier CsA
effect.

The biochemical mechanism of CsA inhibition remains to
be defined. A report submitted but not presented
suggests that CsA has an early effect on membrane
phospholipid turnover in T cells. Another paper
demonstrated that the primary target of CsA action is
a calcium-dependent process of the first few hours
after activation, implicating calmodulin or
calcium-activated enzymes.

Unresolved questions acknowledged but not extensively
discussed include individual variations in
susceptibility to CsA immunosuppression and evidence
that phagocytosis is at least partially inhibited by
CsA.

Because CsA affects different cells, biochemical
studies of CsA action should be performed on purified
cell populations. Studies on heterogeneous
populations do not allow confident conclusions that
observed inhibitions involve cells key to CsA
inhibition of immune function. Further, if different
cell types are inhibited, CsA may inhibit different
functions of different cells. Studies of inhibition
of biochemical functions by CsA are complicated by
cell cooperation in immune responses. If CsA inhibits
a biochemical action of one cell type requiring the

cooperaton of another cell type (which may also be inhibited by CsA), careful sorting of studies on purified and mixed cell populations stimulated by different means will be necessary to arrive at the biochemical mode(s) of action of CsA.

Acquired Immunodeficiency. Several issues were addressed: Are any of the immune perturbations associated with AIDS unique? Is there a definite prodrome? Does the AIDS retrovirus cause immune deregulation? Is AIDS the result of immune deregulation? What determines transmission?

Several immune impairments occur in AIDS, and there have been extensive efforts to identify characteristic markers.

Immune derangements in male homosexuals, not alcohol or drug abusers, include decrease of total T cells and Th cells, inverted Th/Ts ratios, increased serum interferon, and decreased natural killer (NK) activity which were not correlated with clinical AIDS. This stimulated discussion concerning the basis of classification. Some investigators use terms such as "prodrome", AIDS related condition (ARC), generalized lymphadenopathy (LA) to indicate a constellation of symptomatology, presence of risk factors, and abnormal immune response. The meaning of abnormal immune response in risk groups was debated.

Several groups reported that many people who do not fit the CDC definition of AIDS have immune dysfunctions equivalent to those of AIDS. Inverted Th/Ts ratios, serum interferon, reduced NK activity, proliferative response, and circulating immune complexes do not constitute unique markers for AIDS; their relationship to pathogenesis is unclear. New data presented suggest regulatory defects rather than absence (or reduction) of any single function or cell type. Most agreed that data being gathered now will have to be re-examined when it is determined whether AIDS develops in individuals now under study.

Several groups reported simultaneously increased activity of NK cells, activation of interferon production in vitro, and marked alterations of numbers

and ratios of T cells in risk groups. Other data
suggest that hyper-activation may precede the decline
of immune function in AIDS. Loss of IL-2
responsiveness in AIDS and LA patients was reported;
this may be responsible for the lack of effect of IL-2
in clinical trials. The possibility that B cell
dysfunction may be equally as critical to AIDS as T
cell deregulation was suggested by several
abnormalities of B cell function in asymptomatic
homosexuals in a high incidence AIDS region, as well
as adults and children with AIDS.

With respect to etiology it was argued that infection
by any of the several viruses associated with acquired
immunodifiency is not sufficient to cause disease. It
was reported that HTLV-III may effect selective
depletion of Th cells, but that it does not integrate
without a secondary activating signal. The
association between retrovirus infection and
immunologic abnormality in risk groups is not
documented. New information presented suggested that
the retroviruses (HTLV III, LAV, IDAV) associated with
AIDS have multiple integration sites.

A fraction of patients with LA develop malignant
lymphoma characterized by 8/14 translocations.
Interaction of EBV and retroviral disregulation of Ts
activity was discussed. It was generally agreed that
development of AIDS probably requires more than one
event, and that specific manifestations, e.g. Kaposi's
sarcoma, pneumocystis carinii pneumonia, may reflect
different regulatory disorders. The incidence of AIDS
in children suggests that immaturity of the immune
system or pre-existing conditions may contribute to
disease development.

Immune response dysfunctions were also reported in
transient or intrinsic states of immune system
challenge that mimicked AIDS, e.g., trauma, burns,
intrinsic "low" response. These findings suggest that
the hallmark of AIDS is lack of reversibility of
immune functional modulations and in other respects is
similar to other states of acquired deficiency.

The most urgent question in AIDS research is the means
whereby viral transmission occurs. Association of

blood transfusion with cases AIDS positive for retrovirus antibody does not compel a conclusion that virus transmission necessarily leads to AIDS. It was generally agreed, however, that testing blood donors for antibodies against the putative AIDS agent should be carried out.

Transplantation. It was reported that in irradiated mice reconstituted with mixed syngeneic and allogeneic or xenogeneic bone marrow, T cell depletion of the host (syngeneic) marrow resulted in long survival of reconstituted animals without graft-versus-host disease (GVHD) and prolongation of allogeneic skin graft survival. This effect was independent of whether or not the allogeneic or xenogeneic bone marrow was T cell depleted. The mechanism of GVHD prevention is not clear. In other species similar results are difficult to achieve, suggesting that it may be a species specific effect. However the posssibility of tolerance induction is promising and this area of research will be very interesting in the near future.

Another study suggested that macrophage activation is important in GVHD, though the means by which this is accomplished is not clear. A third workshop presentation reported that a rejected allograft from a human patient with primary antitubular basement membrane antibody produced antiTBM antibodies in vitro. It was suggested that the rejection of allograft was the result of the recurrence of the original disease.

(We wish to thank Stanley Jordan and John Kay for their leadership in workshop discussions.)

REGULATION OF T CELL GROWTH

Amnon Altman

Scripps Clinic and Research Foundation

La Jolla, California

Vladimir A. Nesmeyanov

Shemyakin Institute of Bioorganic

Chemistry, U.S.S.R. Academy of Sciences

Moscow, U.S.S.R.

The knowledge accumulated in the last few years on the regulation of T cell growth is a good example of the transformation of a field from its infancy to a highly advanced state as the result of the application of modern biotechnologies. Following the discovery of T cell growth factor, or interleukin 2 (IL2), it became possible to clone and establish long-term lines of functional T cells. The field was further advanced with the establishment of a sensitive IL2 bioassay, and the identification of T cell leukemias and hybridomas secreting large quantities of IL2 (and other lymphokines). Finally, the application of monoclonal hybridoma technology, modern purification methods, and gene cloning techniques resulted in a pure product of a defined primary structure, which can be obtained in virtually unlimited quantities for further probing its structure and function. The fact that the symposium on Growth and Differentiation Factors in this conference did not include a single presentation on

IL2 is a testimony to the rapid progress in this
area.

As a result of this progress, molecular
probes are now available which enable us to determine at which level different regulators of
IL2 production operate. Using such a probe, for
example, made it possible to determine that cy-
closporin A inhibits IL2 production by selectively blocking the transcription of IL2 mRNA (Bleack-
ley).

Thus, several themes which can, and should,
be addressed at this point in time dominated the
workshop. These included: a) The cell surface
molecule which binds IL2 and serves to transduce
its signal(s), i.e., the IL2 receptor on activated T cells and the regulation of its expression;
b) The role of factors other than IL2 in regulating the growth and differentiation of T cells; and
c) The biological effects of IL2 in vivo.

Recent studies made it clear that, in addition to IL2 itself, the other limiting factor determining the growth of T cells is the number and
affinity of IL2 receptors which can be probed
with labeled ligand (IL2) and monoclonal antibodies. This can now be done on a more sophisticated
level by using DNA probes which will undoubtedly
find wide use following the very recent and ele-
gant molecular cloning of the human IL2 receptor
(Leonard).

Optimal expression of IL2 receptors on the
surface of cloned cytotoxic (Havele) and helper
(Reske-Kunz) T cell lines requires stimulation
with antigen. This finding provides an important
element of immunological specificity to the action
of IL2 in a physiological context. Thus, only
antigen-specific T cells that are localized in the
site of antigen stimulation will be stimulated to
display IL2 receptors and, consequently, proliferate in response to it. Although the induction
of IL2 receptors following antigen stimulation is
likely to involve the antigen-specific T cell receptor, its exact mechanism remains to be deter-

mined.

Since the optimal display of IL2 receptors is an essential component in T cell growth, it is obvious that receptor defects could have a profound effect on immune responses. Indeed, defective responses to IL2 were reported in some diseases, although their significance is still unclear. To this can now be added the interesting possibility of genetic factors playing a role in determining levels and/or affinity of IL2 receptors (Pink). With the availability of monoclonal antibodies to the IL2 receptor, it should now be possible to quantitate receptors directly rather than relying on indirect biological assays in order to analyze the potential role of such genetic factors.

Finally, it should be remembered that antigen not only has a positive influence on T cell growth (by inducing IL2 production and expression of IL2 receptors), but can also induce anergy in T cells (1), although this latter aspect was not discussed directly in the workshop. Thus, the intricate interplay of positive and negative influences on T cell growth exerted by antigen needs to be dissected and understood in order for us to control and regulate T cell growth, especially in immunotherapeutic applications in vivo.

Is IL2 exclusively a growth-stimulating molecule, or does it possess additional differentiation-inducing activity for T cells? Results in two different systems strongly suggest that IL2 alone is sufficient to trigger the differentiation of polyclonal CTL from Lyt-2+ precursors in limiting dilution cultures (Vohr), or the induction of cytolytic activity (even in the presence of inhibitors of DNA synthesis) in a CTL clone which has been deactivated by treatment with PMA (Finke). These results are in agreement with some recent studies demonstrating the induction of T cell differentiation by IL2 preparations (2, 3). However, since the IL2 preparations used in most of these studies were not homogeneously pure,

it would be necessary to test formally whether
affinity-purified or recombinant IL2 (rIL2) can
induce differentiation.

If IL2 can indeed activate CTL, as seems to
be the case, it would also be necessary to determine whether this involves interaction with cellular IL2 receptors and modulation of their number, since it was claimed recently that augmentation of NK activity by IL2 does not seem to involve a cellular IL2 receptor (4). Thus, the interesting possibility arises that the prolifera-
tion-inducing activity of IL2 is receptor-depen-
dent, whereas its differentiation-inducing activity is receptor-independent or involves a different receptor. It should be noted that the systems in which IL2 appears to be a sufficient differentiation signal have one common denominator,
namely, they all involve the activation of lytic
function in CTL. This may indicate that memory
CTL requires different (and perhaps less) signals
than T helper cells or early precursors for full
activation.

Other studies presented in the workshop seemed to indicate that factors distinct from IL2 can
act either alone (Finke) or, more frequently, in
association with IL2 (Mannel, Burlington) to induce the differentiation of T cells. In general,
the acquisition of cytolytic activity is the end
point in these assays, although T cell proliferation is also measured occasionally. Evaluation
of these other factors is complicated by the fact
that their cellular sources and chemical nature
are not defined. In some cases, they appear to
be derived from macrophages (Finke), and in others
from T cells. A factor that appears to induce responsiveness to IL2, and acts as a differentiation
signal prior to the action of IL2, termed TCF1,
has now been found to be produced by murine T cell
hybridomas (Mannel). TCF1 acts in concert with
IL2 to stimulate both the proliferation of thymocytes and the development of CTL. In contrast,
purified IL1 (together with IL2) was active only
in the first of these two assays. It is obvious
that a major effort should be invested in the

identification and establishment of permanent lines which secrete large quantities of such factors, enabling their biochemical characterization and molecular cloning.

The mechanism of action of the T cell-tropic differentiation-inducing factors is far from being clear. As noted above, there are some good indications that at least some of them act at a relatively early stage by inducing responsiveness to IL2, as shown directly in a very recent study (5). However, in the majority of cases, differentiation is indicated by the acquisition of cytolytic function. It would, therefore, be necessary to correlate the acquisition of effector function with direct measurements of IL2 receptor levels. Since antigen stimulation is required for expression of IL2 receptors, it would be interesting to ascertain whether the antigen triggers this response directly or via the stimulation of production of soluble mediators which in turn induce IL2 receptors. Secondly, it remains to be determined whether such factors act directly on T target cells or on some intermediary cells (e.g., macrophages) which in turn influence the growth of T cells. In the majority of cases, these differentiation-inducing factors are tested in heterogeneous target cell populations, and elucidation of their mechanism of action would require bioassays which utilize cloned lines of target cells. Relevant to this issue is the demonstration that defined growth factors, i.e., epidermal and platelet-derived growth factors, indirectly stimulate T cell growth by increasing the expression of Ia antigens on antigen-presenting cells (Acres).

To summarize that part of the workshop, there was a general agreement that: a) IL2 is likely to provide a stimulus for differentiation, most probably as a late signal for, e.g., memory CTL; b) Factors distinct from IL2 appear to be required for full functional maturation of T cells. These may represent a group of diverse and unrelated molecules produced by T cells or macrophages (or other cells?) which act on different functional subsets of T cells; c) In at least some instances,

such factors act early by inducing IL2 receptors.
Clearly, steps which were so critical in the ad-
vancement of our knowledge of IL2, i.e., biochemical and molecular characterization and the development of sensitive and well-defined bioassays,
will have to be taken to bring the state of the
art of these other factors to a similar level.

In contrast to several studies which failed
to detect IL2-specific mRNA in resting lymphocytes,
evidence was presented for a pre-existing mRNA,
based on experiments using preincubated rat spleen
cells and inhibitors of RNA or protein synthesis
(Nesmeyanov). Failure to detect IL2-specific
mRNA in other studies may reflect the instability
of mRNA in resting T cells, as reported at another workshop (Kecskemethy). Alternatively, the
mRNA may be associated with a minor subpopulation
of T cells that has been activated in vivo prior
to mitogen stimulation.

Despite the impressive progress in the areas
of T cell growth and IL2, we still know very
little about the physiological role of IL2 and
its behavior in vivo. To date, production of IL2
in vivo has not been demonstrated convincingly.
This may be due to its short biological half-life,
its production in rather small quantities at the
local site(s) of antigen stimulation, or the presence of inhibitory molecules, all of which may
make it very difficult to detect IL2 in body
fluids. Moreover, our knowledge on the growth
and traffic of activated T cells in vivo is scant.
Obviously, these questions have to be resolved
before IL2 (or other lymphokines) or T cell lines
can be used in immunotherapeutic applications in
a rational and effective manner.

Antibodies to IL2 or its fragments may complement the IL2 bioassay, and furthermore may
allow visualization of IL2 in cells, and thus help
elucidate the role of IL2 defects in disease.
Towards this end, antibodies to chemically-synthe-
sized IL2 peptides or whole rIL2 could detect IL2
in biological fluids, and stain mitogen-activated
T cells and lymphoid tissue sections (Altman).

Anti-peptide antibodies of predetermined specificity could also be useful in attempts to map functional sites on the IL2 molecule.

Two presentations dealt with the in vivo effects of IL2. One study raised the intriguing possibility that IL2 may control the balance between tolerance and immunity by demonstrating that antigenic stimulation in the relative lack of IL2 production led to immunologic tolerance, and second, that administration of IL2 corrected this situation and allowed an effective immune response (Asherson). In another interesting study, it was shown that IL2 preparations augmented the ability of adoptively-transferred immune Lyt-1[+] T cell populations to confer resistance to herpes virus infection in mice (Rouse). To make this treatment sufficiently effective, IL2 had to be incorporated in gelatin, which is known to extend the biological half-life of IL2 in serum (6).

Many more studies need to be done in order to evaluate the biological effects and immunotherapeutic potential of IL2 in vivo. The practically unlimited quantities of IL2 produced by recombinant DNA techniques make such studies feasible. Some of the most important questions which need to be solved are how to stabilize IL2 in vivo and prevent its rapid degradation and/or clearance, and secondly, how to target it to the desired anatomical site (e.g., the site of virus infection or tumor growth). Moreover, potentially negative effects in vivo need to be evaluated carefully, since IL2 (including pure rIL2) was recently found to induce non-specific suppressor T cells in vitro (7) or antigen-specific anergy (8). It can be concluded that the methodologies and tools which are now available make it possible for us to elucidate many of the open questions in the area of T cell growth in the near future.

ACKNOWLEDGEMENT: This is publication No. 3699IMM
from the Department of Immunology, Scripps Clinic
and Research Institute. The work performed in
the laboratory of Dr. Amnon Altman is supported
by USPHS grant CA-35299, a grant from Cambridge
Research Laboratories, and a Leukemia Society of
America, Inc., Scholarship Award.

REFERENCES:

1. Lamb, J.R., Skidmore, B.J., Green, N., Chill-
    er, J.M. & Feldmann, M. J. Exp. Med. 157,
    1434-1447 (1983).
2. Lefrancois, L., Klein, J.R., Paetkau, V., &
    Bevan, M.J. J. Immunol. 132,1845-1850 (1984).
3. Reem , G.H. & Yeh, N.-H. Science 225,429-430
    (1984).
4. Ortaldo, J.R., Mason, A.T., Gerard, J.P.,
    Henderson, L.E., Farrar, W., Hopkins, R.F.,
    Herberman, R.B. & Rabin, J. J. Immunol. 133,
    779-783 (1984).
5. Erard, F., Corthesy, P., Smith, K.A., Fiers,
    W., Conzelmann, A. & Nabholz, M. J. Exp. Med.
    160,584-599 (1984).
6. Donohue, J.H. & Rosenberg, S.A. J. Immunol.
    130,2203-2208 (1983).
7. Ting, C.-C., Yang, S.S. & Hargrove, M.E. J.
    Immunol. 133,261-266 (1984).
8. Wilde, D.B., Prystowsky, D.B., Ely, J.M.,
    Vogel, S.N., Dialynas, D.P. & Fitch, F.W.
    J. Immunol. 133,636-641 (1984).

SECTION V

*ACCESSORY CELLS AND
ANTIGEN PRESENTATION*

INDUCER ACCESSORY CELLS AS REGULATORS OF THE IMMUNE RESPONSE

David R. Katz

Bland-Sutton Institute of Pathology,
Middlesex and University College Medical
Schools, London. W1P 7PN

Recently attention has focussed on the molecular
biology of the immunocompetent cell and there are many new
observations concerning the nature of the genes which regulate the proliferation of these cells (1); the gene rearrangements associated with the generation of a response
to antigen (2); and the structure of the surface products
encoded for by these genes (3). A feature of these studies
has been the resemblances observed between the conformation
of T cell and B cell membrane receptors (4).

Studies using both T and B cells reflect events which
occur at the effector cell level; the area of immunology
which has this far not been analysed using molecular biology
as a tool is the inducer phase. Part of the reason for this
is that there continues to be much confusion about certain
basic elements of induction. In order to investigate the
molecular biology of induction properly it is necessary to
have clear answers to questions such as: (1) what are the
cell types involved in induction; (2) are inducer cell lines
and clones available for this type of study; (3) what is the
relationship between the inducer cell and the antigen to
which the response is to be induced; and (4) how surface
class II major histocompatibility complex expression relates
to inducer accessory cell function in any given system.

In collaborative experiments with colleagues at
University College (Drs Czitrom, Feldmann and Sunshine), at
the Basle Institute for Immunology, (Dr M H Schreier and

Ms R Tees) and more recently in the Middlesex/University
College Medical School (Drs McDowell and Nunn and Ms
Cifelli) we have examined these types of questions using
in vitro techniques.

Nature of inducer cells

When these studies were initiated, a question which
had aroused considerable controversy was whether a dendritic cell (5) or a macrophage (6) was the cell responsible
for antigen presentation. Subsequently the B cell itself
was suggested as a possible presenting cell (7) and the
list has now increased to include other cell types including endothelium (8) and epithelium (9) as will be discussed by other speakers in this symposium.

A unifying hypothesis to account for this range of
findings must accept that more than one inducer cell can be
effective. Perhaps the most striking illustrations of this
are the observations made using T cell clones grown in
serum free medium. In these studies we showed that cell
lines similar to those from which clones are derived subsequently will proliferate in response to antigen presented
by both macrophages and dendritic cells. However, some of
the clones will respond selectively to antigen introduced
on macrophages and others to antigen introduced on dendritic cells (10). This type of heterogeneity can also be
illustrated in mitogenic responses; for example, in vitro
concanavalin A induction can also be linked to both cell
types. An aspect of this type of analysis is that we have
consistently used non-dendritic cells from the same preparation (such as 18 hour Fc receptor bearing cells and 2
hour adherent cells) as controls in order to characterise
absolute as well as relative induction effects.

Inducer cells as immune response regulators

If we accept that inducer function should be regarded
as an activity rather than as a single cell event, then
there must be some way in which this capacity to make a
variety of inducer cells is significant.

A framework which could combine the concept of inducer
activity with current concepts of effector cell function is
that the association of antigen with one type of inducer
cell in a single tissue microenvironment generates a

particular type of response; the association of antigen
with another inducer cell generates a different response.
In vivo studies give support for this hypothesis (11).
Two other speakers in this symposium will raise related
questions in comparing T cell proliferation and help (12)
and in discussing the role of the follicular dendritic cell
(13).

In the murine system such a comparative selective
effect was illustrated in the experiments which examined
comparative induction of alloproliferation where dendritic
cells were the most potent inducers (14), and allocytotoxi-
city (15) where both dendritic cells and macrophages were
effective.

A postulated explanation which attempted to combine
the different observations on dendritic cells and macrophages suggested that dendritic cells were non-phagocytic
and lacked lysosomal enzymes; thus they were responsible
for inducing responses to soluble antigens. Macrophages,
on the other hand, were phagocytic and hence responsible
for processing larger foreign antigens and preparing them
for presentation. This suggestion has not been borne out
by in vitro experiments. For example, at the clonal level,
dendritic cells can induce proliferation of red cell
specific clones in the absence of macrophages. Similar
results have been obtained in studies on the presentation
of mycobacteria and mycobacterial digestion products (16).

Human inducer cells as immune response regulators

Recently studies on human tissue derived accessory
cells have produced further evidence which illustrates the
regulatory role of the inducer cells. In these studies a
density gradient system has been used, similar but not
identical to the murine albumin gradient. It is now possible to isolate a low density non-adherent cell without Fc
receptors and with a constitutive high expression of class
II products in its surface. When these cells are pulsed
with concanavalin A they are the most potent inducer cell;
there is much less difference in inducer activity in the
presence of continuous mitogenic stimulation. Thus it is
possible that when the ability to trap and retain the mitogen is a prerequisite for a given response then the human
dendritic cell is more efficient than any other individual
cell type. It is interesting that when the mitogen is

continuously present then a unique inducer is less critical; but that the dendritic cells themselves are distinguished by their failure to respond to any of the known
lymphomedullary mitogens and growth factors.

The human studies also illustrate that quantitative
differences in class II product expression are significant
in assessing inducer activity. Thus the maximum expression of these antigens is found on the dendritic cell. One
of the features of these cells is that the combination of
class II expression and the lack of Fc and C_3 receptors
appears to be a stable phenomenon. In addition even in a
non-restricted response such as that seen to a mitogen,
these antigens are important: although their expression
may be masked in a radio-immunoassay performed immediately
after pulsing, nonetheless the correlation between expression and induction is an extremely consistent feature of our
studies.

Associated products of other murine loci such as the
mls (17) have also been linked to inducer function. As yet
similar products have not been described in the human but
they probably do occur. Even in these mls experiments
class II expression remains an essential feature of the
inducer cells.

Induction of suppression

If inducer cell activity is a major regulatory cell
component in the nature of immune responsiveness then a key
element in this is that induction of suppression should be
related to one or other of the cells which we are discussing. Bypass of normal presentation as a mechanism for
induction of suppression has been shown (18) but a 'positive selection' of suppressor cells by a particular inducer cell has not. In the absence of clear evidence for an
inducer cell for suppression, several other possible routes
of inducer involvement can arise, such as the inducer cell
itself acting as a mediator via prostaglandin release (19);
or for the inducer to be the target for the suppressor cell
(20). The in vivo experiments could also be indicating a
potential mechanism: this is that suppression is in fact
conventional inducer cell independent, but that in this
response T and B cells in their own microenvironment act as
inducers.

New approaches to induction mechanisms

There are now several new approaches to the study of
inducer cells in vitro which we are investigating. The
most straightforward approach is to use monoclonal reagents as cell separation tools; however, as discussed in
the workshop sessions, the precise functional relationships
of most of the reagents directed against cells in the
inducer compartment has not been clearly established.

Another approach is to use fusion-type studies analogous to those which have been used for B and T cells.
Thus far few laboratories (21) have had success with these
protocols. This is particularly so for dendritic cell
fusions; this could be because activation of these cells
prior to fusion has proven extremely difficult. Recent
preliminary collaborative experiments (22) suggest that
retinoids may prove to be dendritic cell activators and
thus provide a suitable source. A report which describes
transfection of macrophages followed by growth in selective
factors has been published recently (23); this method could
be applied to a wider range of inducer cells and induction
mechanisms in the future.

If most inducer cells are of myelomonocytic lineage,
one of the ways to examine comparative behaviour in in
vitro responses could be to modify (differentiate) a precursor cell and monitor at which point inducer function
appears. Several laboratories have described differentiation pathways in the human promyelocytic cell line, HL-60
(24) and aspects of this have already been discussed at a
symposium. Modulation of HL-60 by vitamin D metabolites
has been reported (25); we were interested to see whether
this method could alter alloinducer capacity. We have
established that 1,25 dihydroxycholecalciferol will inhibit
proliferation of the cell line and induce morphological
changes; parallel studies have shown that the compound has
no effect on a control T cell line. Preliminary studies
have confirmed that this is linked to decreased expression
of the c-myc oncogene; and that after 7 days of culture the
cells are differentiated into a type of cell which will act
as an inducer in an allogeneic system. We are currently
investigating other possible genetic events which are
associated with this process.

Conclusions

Inducer activity in an immune response is a property of a group of related cells.

In in vitro studies variations in inducer cell phenotype are associated with functional difference in responder cells. This supports the in vivo microenvironmental studies in favouring the hypothesis that the inducer cell is the regulatory site at which the nature of the subsequent response is determined. Quantitative class II MHC expression is the best characterised feature associated with induction.

Inducer cell heterogeneity and regulatory function has been demonstrated by experiments using effectors such as T helper cells, cytotoxic cells and B cells. To complete the circuit, a satisfactory explanation of the relationship between inducer cells and suppressor T cells has to be found.

To characterise the group of molecular events which are involved in this inducer activity will require a study of several individual cell types. One way to approach this is to use the differentiation pathway of bone marrow precursors; an example of this is seen in a leukaemic cell line where there is preliminary evidence that the induction of alloinducer capacity is associated with decreased endogenous proliferation and to decreased expression of the c-myc oncogene.

Other ways to look at this question must include studies on activation of accessory cells other than macrophages and B cells, and transfection studies on highly purified inducer cell types.

A useful overall hypothesis may be to regard the peripheral lymphoid tissues as similar to the bone marrow: a background network of inducer microenvironments which act either locally, or by releasing soluble mediators in order to induce appropriate responses in the surrounding effector lymphocyte pool.

References

1. Taniguchi, T. et al Nature 302, 305 (1983)
2. Hedrick, S.M. et al Nature 308, 153 (1984)
3. Kappler, J.M. et al J Exp Med 153, 1198 (1981)
4. Saito, H. et al Nature 309, 757 (1984)
5. Steinman, R.M. and Cohn, Z.A. J Exp Med 139,380 (1974)
6. Rosenthal, A.S. and Shevach, E.M. J Exp Med 138, 1194 (1973)
7. Chesnut, R., Colon, S. and Grey, H.M. J Immunol 128, 1764 (1982)
8. Hirschberg, H., Braathen, L.R. and Thorsby, E. Immunol Rev 66, 57 (1982)
9. Bottazzo, G.F. et al Lancet, ii, 1115 (1983)
10. Katz, D.R. et al in Intercellular communications in leucocyte function (ed J Parker) (Wiley) 279, (1983)
11. Humphrey, J.H. and Grennan, D. Eur J Immunol 11, 221 (1981)
12. Ramila, G and Erb, P. Nature 304, 442 (1983)
13. Klaus, G.G.B. et al Immunol Rev 53, 3 (1980)
14. Sunshine, G.H., Katz, D.R. and Feldmann, M. J Exp Med 152, 1817 (1980)
15. Czitrom, A.A., Katz, D.R. and Sunshine, G.H. Immunol 45, 553 (1982)
16. Kaye, P., Chain, B.M. and Feldmann, M (submitted for publication)
17. Janeway, C.A. et al Nature, 306, 80 (1980)
18. Greene, M.I. et al Proc Nat'l Acad Sci USA 76, 6591 (1979)
19. Mertin, J. and Stackpole, A. Nature 294, 456 (1981)
20. Abruzzo, L.V. and Rowley, D.A. Science 222, 581 (1983)
21. Treves, A.J. et al J Immunol 132, 690 (1984)
22. Dryzmala, M. et al in Morphological Aspects of the Immune System (ed G.G.B. Klaus) (Plenum Press) in press (1984)
23. Nagata, Y, Diamond, B and Bloom, B.R. Nature 306, 597 (1984)
24. Breitman, T.R., Selonick, S.E. and Collins, S.J. Proc Nat'l Acad Sci USA 77, 2936 (1980)
25. Reitsma, P.H. et al Nature 306, 492 (1983)

FUNCTIONAL ASPECTS OF ACCESSORY CELL HETEROGENEITY

Erb, P., Ramila, G., Sklenar, I.

and Kennedy, M.

Institute for Microbiology, University

of Basel, Petersplatz 10

CH-4003 Basel/Switzerland.

Introduction

The activation of T cells requires the participation of Ia+ accessory cells (AC) (1-4). Originally, macrophages (Mph) were identified as AC (1,2) but soon, their role as unique AC was challenged by the detection of other, non-Mph cell types which also expressed AC function (5-14). In the meantime, it has been established that all Ia+ cells, be they macrophages or not, can function as AC (1-19). Although this clearly demonstrates AC heterogeneity, the question has not been answered whether any AC type can activate all or only certain T cell functions, ie. whether functional heterogeneity exists.

We have addressed this question by comparing AC of various origins for their potential to activate different T cell functions. In this report we will summarize and evaluate our data, which show that the activity of many AC is restricted to the induction of a limited range of T cell functions.

Materials and Methods

This has been described in detail elsewhere (17,18, manuscript submitted). The AC tested and their characteristics are listed in Table 1. The AC were tested for the following functional parameters: (a) the activation of antigen-specific T cell proliferation (T-prol),

Table 1 : Ia+ accessory cells tested

A) Non-transformed cells
  1) Mph-type: peritoneal exudate cells (PEC)
               splenic adherent cells (SAC)
               bone marrow derived (BMMph)
               Langerhans cells
  2) Non-Mph-type: dendritic reticular cells (DC)
                   mast cell precursor (PB-3c)
B) Transformed cells
  1) Virus-induced leukemias: BC3A, D1B, D2N
  2) B-lymphomas: A20.2J, M12
  3) B-hybridoma: TA3
  4) Mph-tumors: P388D1, WEHI-3, J744.1, IC-21
  5) Mast cell precursor tumor: PB-1

(b) lymphokine-production by T cells (T-lymph), (c) the
induction of antigen-specific T helper cells (T-help) which
help B cells for antibody production, (d) the activation of
T suppressor cells (T-supp) which interfere with antibody
production and (e) their activity in T-B cooperation (T-B).

Results and Discussion
      Several transformed and non-transformed AC of
macrophage or non-macrophage origin were tested for their
ability to activate various T cell functions and to support
T-B cooperation. The results obtained, many of which are
published (17,18) are summarized in a simplified form in
Table 2.

Table 2 : Functional heterogeneity of AC

Ia+ AC used	Functions tested				
	T-prol	T-lymph	T-help	T-supp	T-B
Mph-type	+	+	+	v	+
Non-Mph-type	+	+	−	−	+
Leukemias	+	+	−	+	+
B-lymphomas	+	+	−	+,−	+
B-hybridomas	+	+	−	+/−	+
Mph-tumors	+	+	−	+,−	+
Mast cell tumor	+	+	−	?	+

v=variable: depending on the number of input Mph
+=strong, +/-=weak, -=no response; ?=not known

Table 3 : Differential AC function

T + KLH +	T-prol 125 IUdR uptake / CPM	T-lymph	T-help IgG-AFC/10^6
NIL	730	148	475
PEC 10^4	41995	19233	3838
PB-3c 10^4	42189	20470	323
10^3	30975	16718	399
PB-1 10^4	9194	4473	19
10^3	11212	8417	456
D2N 10^4	43049	17233	722
10^3	41049	22243	684
WEHI-3 10^4	34269	14269	342
10^3	42055	22246	190
J744.1 10^4	13457	3281	418
10^3	30930	10509	570
A20.2J 10^4	38084	13494	76
10^3	24086	13067	171
M12-4-1 10^4	52756	8222	152
10^3	48246	18094	266

T-prol : 3×10^5 purified lymph node T cells were incubated
for 2d with KLH (50µg/ml) and 2 doses of AC, 8h before
termination 125-IUdR (0,25µc/well) was added. The lymph
nodes were from BALB/c mice primed with KLH-CFA 10 days
previously.
T-lymph : 100µl of supernatants of the T-prol cultures were
incubated with 5×10^3 CTL/L cells for 24h. Pulsing was done
as above.
T-help : 8×10^5 splenic T cells were incubated with KLH
(5µg/ml) and 2 doses of AC. After 4d 5×10^4 T cells were
added to 4×10^5 DNP-primed B cells and TNP-KLH (0.05µg/ml)
and incubated for 5d. The anti-DNP-antibody forming cells
(AFC) were determined in a Cunningham plaque assay. The
spleens were from BALB/c mice primed with KLH-CFA 2 months
previously.

It was found that all Ia+ AC tested so far, induced
antigen-specific T cell proliferation or the release of
lymphokines by T cells, although to a variable degree. Some
AC, eg. DC, TA3 were more potent than others, eg. PEC. Some
AC , eg. P388D1, WEHI-3, IC-21, required the preincubation

with ConA sup (which is supernatant of spleen cells
incubated with ConA for 24 to 48h) in order to reliably
function as AC. The AC-T cell interaction is MHC-restricted
and can be blocked by adding appropriate anti-Ia antibodies
into the cultures.
In contrast, only the non-transformed macrophages
(PEC,SAC,BMMO) or the macrophage-like Langerhans cells were
able to induce antigen-specific T helper cells (17-19). All
the other AC tested, including DC and various tumor cell
lines of B cell or macrophage origin did not activate Thc.
A typical example comparing PEC and different tumor cell
lines as AC is shown in Table 3. Many conditions were tried
to exclude technical errors, such as antigen titrations, AC
titrations, using antigen-pulsed AC, preincubation of AC
with ConA sup, using lymph node or spleens as source of T
cells. The failure of the AC to generate Thc was also not a
factor problem as adding ConA sup to the Thc induction or
T-B cooperation cultures did not result in antibody
production (17).

However, other groups reported that some tumor cell
lines or DC reconstituted the anti-sheep erythrocyte (SE)
response of AC-depleted spleen cells (14,20,21). These data
indicated that the AC tested were involved in antibody
production and thus, contradicted our results. We therefore
performed similar reconstitution experiments and found,
that all our AC also reconstituted the antibody response of
recently primed (last immunization 2 weeks ago) AC-depleted
spleen cells to soluble (DNP-CGG, TNP-KLH) or to
particulate antigens (SE) (ref. 19 and Table 2). Moreover,
the same AC also reconstituted the response if instead of
AC-depleted spleen cells highly purified Thc (eg.
repeatedly in vitro with KLH and PEC restimulated T cells)
and highly purified (T cell and AC-depleted) TNP-primed B
cells were used and if TNP-KLH-pulsed AC were added instead
of AC and antigen (manuscript submitted). The failure to
induce Thc but the efficiency of these AC in T-B
cooperation seems to be a contradiction. However, this
discrepancy is resolved by the fact that for Thc activation
memory T cells (which were primed in vivo a long time ago)
were used which required the in vitro restimulation with
antigen and AC in order to become functional helper cells,
while in the T-B cooperation cultures functional Thc (ie.
recently in vivo primed or in vitro restimulated) were
already present.

Our results suggest that the functional role of AC in
Thc induction and in T-B cooperation is different. The role

of AC in T-B cooperation is not to restimulate Thc to
enable them to cooperate with B cells but rather to
activate T cells to produce B cell stimulatory factors
and/or to produce such factors themselves, factors which
are required for B cell stimulation beside the specific
helper signal provided by Thc. This thesis is supported by
the fact that ConA sup, which is known to contain various T
cell and B cell stimulatory factors, replaces AC in T-B
cooperation provided functional Thc and antigen are present
(manuscript submitted).

Why are a number of tumor cell lines or DC unable to
activate Thc, but induce other T cell functions or work in
T-B cooperation? The answer to this question might either
reside at the AC level or at the T cell level. The
following pathways have to be taken into consideration:
1) The Ia+ tumor cells or DC may induce suppression:
Indeed, we found that some tumor lines activated T
suppressor cells (Tsc) which non-specifically inhibited
antibody formation. However, other tumor cell lines induced
only weak Tsc or none at all, as did the DC (Table 2, ref.
17,18). Moreover, although some Ia+ tumor lines activated
Tsc, suppression was not the reason for the failure to
demonstrate helper activity. This was demonstrated by
constructing antigen-specific T cell long term cultures
(LTC) either with PEC or some tumor cell lines as AC. While
the PEC generated LTC provided help to B cells, the tumor
cell line-generated LTC did not, but suppressed helper
activity if added into T-B cooperation cultures (18).
Pretreatment of these LTC with anti-Lyt2 and complement
which kills suppressor cells, abolished their suppressive
activity, but the remaining cells did not help.
2) Activation of different Thc populations: It has been
indicated that two types of Thc exist (22,23). One type
cooperates with B cells through linked recognition and
requires low amounts of antigens, the other type interacts
with B cells without the need for linked recognition but
requires high amount of antigens. It has been suggested
that the nylonwool purification step of T cells depletes
the T cell population involved in non-linked recognition
interactions (23). It is possible that the tumor cells or
DC activate this type of Thc. To test this hypothesis T
cells purified with and without nylonwool filtration were
incubated with KLH and either PEC or DC as AC. Table 4
demonstrates that DC did not induce Thc independent of
whether a nylonwool purification step was performed or not.

Table 4 : Failure of DC to induce Thc

T cells (8x10^5) incubated with	A) T cell purification		B) Non-linked recognition IgG-AFC/10^6
	with NW	without NW	recognition
NIL	57	0	n.d
KLH (5µg/ml)	19	19	n.d
KLH + PEC 10^5	3876	1121	1121
5x10^4	1406	836	874
10^4	228	684	38
KLH + DC 10^4	0	38	0
5x10^3	38	0	19
10^3	38	190	n.d

A) T cell purification was done with or without nylonwool column filtration (NW) (other purification steps were treatment with anti-Ia+complement and adherence, ref.17,18). The KLH-immune T cells were tested for help as described in Table 3.
B) The KLH-immune T cells were added to DNP-primed B cells and incubated with KLH (100µg/ml) + DNP-OVA (0.05µg/ml) for 5d.

Interestingly, the non-nylonwool purified T cells expressed always less helper activity after incubation with KLH and PEC, indicating that the nylonwool treatment might remove a suppressor cell. The PEC or DC and KLH activated T cells were also tested for cooperation with B cells through a non-linked recognition interaction by adding an high dose of KLH (20ug/culture) and the wrong hapten-carrier conjugate (DNP-OVA) into the cultures. No plaque-forming response was obtained if DC-activated T cells were tested, suggesting that DC did not induce Thc which stimulate B cells by non-linked recognition (Table 4B).
3) Difference in antigen-handling and presentation: The failure of AC to activate Thc might be due to a different antigen-uptake, handling and/or presentation. There are quite different views on whether antigen-handling is a cell surface or an intracellular phenomenon (24-26). As DC and many other tumor cell lines, eg. of B cell origin have pinocytic but not phagocytic capacity (27-29) it is

possible that their antigen-uptake and/or processing is
different from macrophages. Thus, Thc activation might
require intracellular processing of antigen by AC, while
for the induction of other T cell function , eg.
proliferation, surface handling of antigen is sufficient.
This would explain why DC and the tumor lines induce many T
cell functions but not Thc. However, this hypothesis does
not explain why the Ia+ tumor cell lines of macrophage
origin which we tested did not induce Thc.
4) The amount of Ia on a per cell basis or the ratio of Ia
to the immunogenic fragment on AC might be important. There
is indeed evidence that the induction of optimal
proliferative responses in vitro depends on the optimal
'product' of Ia and antigen concentrations (30). As DC and
perhaps many of the tumor cell lines have more Ia than
other AC, in the presence of equivalent concentrations of
antigen the excess of Ia-antigen might be less stimulatory
for help. The mechanims of this effect is not known, but it
could be due to immunological tolerance, which has been
recently shown to be MHC restricted (31,32). Tolerance
induction of helper function at the level of a single clone
requires approximately one hundred times less antigen than
necessary to tolerize proliferation (ref.19, Lamb and
Feldmann, personal communication). Thus, DC and the tumor
cells could in principle be non-stimulatory for help but
stimulatory for proliferation based on tolerance
thresholds.
5) Differences at the T cell level: Thc might differ in
their receptor repertoires from proliferating or lymphokine
producing T cells and therefore either see antigen in a
different way or require different antigen-presentation.
Although this possibility is less likely from a
conceptional point of view, there are a few observations in
support of it. Thus, it is easy to block T cell
proliferation by adding appropriate anti-Ia antibodies into
the cultures (17), but it is not possible to block Thc
induction by this way (33). In addition, the potential of T
cells to proliferate or to produce lymphokines does not
correlate with helper activity (18,34-36) and it is
possible to select T cell lines or clones expressing one or
the other function (18,34). An example is shown in Table 5
in which T cell were activated with KLH and graded numbers
of PEC. The T cell which provided optimal help to B cells
were inefficient in lymphokine-production and vice versa.

Table 5 : Low correlation between help and lymphokine
           production

T cells (8×10^5) incubated with	Functions tested	
	T-lymph ^{125}IUdR uptake/CPM	T-help IgG-AFC/10^6
NIL	715	266
KLH (5μg/ml)	1114	247
KLH + PEC 10^5	3978	3382
5×10^4	4322	1501
10^4	10334	247

Purified T cells (obtained from the spleens of CBA mice
primed with KLH-CFA 2 months previously) were incubated
with or without KLH and graded numbers of PEC for 4d. The T
cells were tested for helper activity as explained in Table
3.
Supernatants of the Thc cultures were taken on day 3 and
tested for lymphokines as described in Table 3.

Concluding remarks
    The results presented and discussed here not only
confirm the existence of AC heterogeneity but also
demonstrate functional heterogeneity. Thus, in vitro many
AC can only activate some but not all T cell functions.
Various Ia+ tumor cell lines tested independent of whether
they were of B cell or macrophage origin, and the DC were
unable to induce Thc, although they were fully active in
the stimulation of other T cell functions. Despite this
marked differences in AC activity these results at this
stage do not imply that only normal macrophages or
macrophage-like cells are able to activate Thc. As the
number of tumor cell lines so far tested is small, it is
possible that in regard to Thc activation the wrong lines
were used in our experiments. Only the testing of many more
different tumor cell lines will provide the answer. The
existence of Thc inducing permanent AC lines would greatly
ease the difficult task to study the mechanisms of
antigen-processing and presentation by AC as well as the
mechanisms of T cell activation.
    The differential T cell activation might be of

biological significance. One could postulate that the role
of AC expressing (a high amount of) Ia constitutively might
be to activate and expand certain types of antigen-reactive
T cells, eg. lymphokine producing T cells. The lymphokines
produced would induce Mph to express the right amount of Ia
in order to activate and expand Thc which stimulate B cells
for antibody production or initiate the cytotoxic pathway.

In a variety of circumstances, Ia can be expressed on
epithelial, endothelial and fibroblastic cells. The role of
Ia antigens on these cells is not clear. Perhaps they are
also involved in antigen presentation. Under certain
conditions they might even present self antigen and thus
initate a major step in the chain of events leading to
autoimmune reactions. The Thc activating potential
restricted to Mph might guarantee that not every Ia+ cells
in the body can activate Thc and therefore reduce the risk
of autoimmune induction.

Acknowledgment
This work was supported by the Swiss National Science
Foundation, grant nr. 3.112.0.81.

References

1. Rosenthal, A.S. and Shevach, E.M. J.Exp.Med. 138 :
    1194, (1973).
2. Erb, P. and Feldmann, M. 1975. J.Exp.Med. 142 : 460,
    (1975).
3. Miller, J.F.A.P., Vadas, M.A., Whitelaw, A. and Gamble,
    J.G. Proc. Natl. Acad. Sci. USA. 72 : 5093, (1975).
4. Weinberger, O., Herrmann, S.H., Mescher, M.F.,
    Benacerraf, B. and Burakoff, S.J. Proc. Natl.Acad.Sci.
    USA. 77 : 6091, (1980).
5. Steinman, R.M. and Cohn, Z.A. J.Exp.Med. 137 : 1142,
    (1973).
6. Schrader, J.W. and Nossal, G.J.V. Immunol. Rev. 53 :
    61, (1980).
7. Kakiuchi, T., Chesnut R.W., and Grey, H.M. J.Immunol.
    131 : 109, (1983).
8. Stingl, G., Katz, S.I., Clement, L., Green, I., and
    Shevach, E.M. J. Immunol. 121 : 2005, (1978).
9. Fontana, A., Fierz, W., and Wekerle, H. Nature 307 :
    273, (1984).
10. Hirschberg, H., Bergh, O.J., and Thorsby, E. J.Exp.Med.
    152 : 249, (1980).
11. McKean, D.J., Infante, A.J., Nilson, A., Kimoto, M.,

Fathman, C.G., Walker, E., and Warren, N. J.Exp.Med.
$\underline{154}$: 1419, (1981).

12. Cohen, D.A., and Kaplan, A.M. J.Exp.Med. $\underline{154}$: 1881,
(1981).

13. Glimcher, L.H., Kim, K.J., Green, I., and Paul, W.E.
J.Exp.Med. $\underline{155}$: 445, (1982).

14. Walker, E.A., Lanier, L.L., and Warner, N.L. J.
Immunol. $\underline{128}$: 852, (1982).

15. Buchmueller, Y., Mauel, J., and Corradin, G. Adv.
Exp.Med.Biol. $\underline{155}$: 557, (1982).

16. Schwarzbaum, S., and Diamond, B. J. Immunol. $\underline{131}$:
674, (1983).

17. Ramila, G., Studer, S., Mieschler, S., and Erb, P. J.
Immunol. $\underline{131}$: 2714, (1983).

18. Ramila, G., and Erb, P. Nature $\underline{304}$: 442, (1983).

19. Erb, P., Ramila, S., Studer, S., Loeffler, H., Cecka,
J.M., Conscience, J.F., and Feldmann, M. Immunobiology,
in press.

20. Inaba, K., Steinman, R.M., Van Voorhis, W.C., and
Muramatsu, S. Proc.Natl.Acad.Sci.USA. $\underline{80}$: 6041,
(1983).

21. Inaba, K., Granelli-Piperno, A., and Steinman, R.M.
J.Exp.Med. $\underline{158}$: 2040, (1983).

22. Keller, D.M., Swierkosz, J.E., Marrack, P., and
Kappler, J.W. J.Immunol. $\underline{124}$: 1350, (1980).

23. Sullivan, C.P., and Waldmann, H. Immunology. $\underline{51}$: 343,
(1984).

24. Malek, T.R., Clement, L.T., and Shevach, E.M.
Eur.J.Immunol. $\underline{13}$: 810, (1983).

25. Ziegler, H.K., and Unanue, E.R. Proc.Natl.Acad.Sci.USA.
$\underline{79}$: 175, (1982).

26. Lee, K.C., Wong, M., and Spitzer, D. Transplantation.
$\underline{34}$: 150, (1982).

27. Van Voorhis, W.C., Witmer, M.D., and Steinman, R.M.
Fed.Proc. $\underline{42}$: 3114, (1983).

28. Chesnut, R.W., Colon, S.M., and Grey, H.M. J.Immunol.
$\underline{129}$: 2382, (1982).

29. Grey, H.M., Colon, S.M., and Chesnut, R.W. J.Immunol.
$\underline{129}$: 2389, (1982).

30. Matis, L.A., Glimcher, L.H., Paul, W.E. and Schwartz,
R.H. Proc.Natl.Acad.Sci.USA $\underline{80}$: 6019, (1983).

31. Lamb, J.R., Skidmore, B.J., Green, N., Chiller, J.M.,
and Feldmann, M. J.Exp.Med. $\underline{157}$: 1434, (1983).

32. Lamb, J.R., and Feldmann, M. Nature $\underline{308}$: 72, (1984).

33. Stern, A.C., Erb, P., and Gisler, R.H. J. Immunol. $\underline{123}$
: 612, (1979)

34. Lamb, J.R., Zanders, E.D., Feldmann, M., Lake, P.,
    Eckels, D.D., Woody, J.N., and Beverley, P.C.L.
    Immunology. 50 : 2542, (1983).
35. Peterson, L.B., Wilner, G.D., and Thomas, D.W.
    J.Immunol. 130 : 2542, (1983).
36. Krzych, U., Fower, A.V., Miller, A., and Sercarz, E.E.
    J.Immunol. 128 : 1529, (1982).

CAN EPITHELIAL CELLS PRESENT SURFACE AUTOANTIGENS?

Ian Todd, Marco Londei, Ricardo Pujol-Borrell, Marc Feldmann and G. Franco Bottazzo

Dept. of Immunology, The Middlesex Hospital Medical School, London UK; and ICRF Tumour Immunology Unit, University College London, London, UK

INTRODUCTION

Organ-specific autoimmunity has been recognised in virtually all the defined endocrine glands, where it is the hormone-producing epithelial cells themselves which are destroyed. The mechanisms leading to this breakdown of self-tolerance are still unknown, although a variety of hypotheses have been proposed (reviewed in 1 and 2). Two requirements which may well be central to these mechanisms are the accessibility of autoantigens to cells of the immune system, and the presentation of such antigens in an immunogenic fashion. In recent years we have performed a variety of experiments relevant to these points, mainly in thyroid autoimmunity, in which there is marked lymphocytic infiltration of the gland, including activated T cells (3). Our results have led to a general model for the generation of organ-specific endocrine autoimmunity. Central to this hypothesis is the ability of endocrine epithelial cells to present their own surface molecules as autoantigens.

ACCESSIBILITY OF AUTOANTIGENS

Many potential autoantigens are found only on rare, specialized cells, such as most endocrine cells. It thus seems probable that autoreactive T cells will normally

323

be neither tolerized by, nor sensitized against, such autoantigens due to the minute amounts in the body and their usual inaccessibility to lymphocytes. An example of a 'hidden' autoantigen is the thyroid microsomal/microvillar antigen which is normally found only within the cytoplasm and on the apical border of thyroid follicular cells facing the colloid space: it is thus not exposed to lymphocytes at the basal vascular border of the follicles (4). However, examination of autoimmune thyroid follicles does show antibodies bound to the microvillar antigens at the apical border (4). A solution to this paradox may be provided by the observation that thyroid follicles cultured in relatively high serum concentrations can reverse their polarity such that microvillar antigens are exposed on the outer surface and, more significantly, spontaneous reversal is found in some autoimmune glands (5). This could permit an autoimmune response to the microvillar antigen with the resulting follicular damage permitting antibodies access to the apical surface of non-inverted follicles.

ABERRANT EXPRESSION OF HLA-D/DR IN AUTOIMMUNITY

Immunization against an antigen requires not only that it can be seen by lymphocytes, but that it is seen in an immunogenic form. The presentation of foreign antigen to helper T cells is usually accomplished in the context of major histocompatibility complex (MHC) Class II molecules (reviewed in 6). These molecules are of restricted tissue distribution, being mainly associated with cells of the immune system, of which the Class II$^+$ macrophages and dendritic cells have been principally implicated in antigen presentation. It might be assumed that these cell types must also function in the presentation of autoantigens. However, expression of Class II molecules has been noted on other cells not normally associated with immune functions, including capilliary endothelium and a variety of epithelia (eg. skin, gut, mammary gland) in circumstances such as graft versus host disease, dermatoses, parasitic infestation and lactation (5).

With respect to endocrine epithelia, we found that human thyroid follicular cells (thyrocytes), which are

normally HLA-D/DR negative, could be induced to express
HLA-D/DR antigens by culture with mitogenic plant lectins
(7). Yet more significant with regard to autoimmunity was
our observation that thyrocytes in sections or monolayers
of thyroid glands from patients with autoimmune thyroid
diseases (Graves' disease or Hashimoto's thyroiditis)
expressed HLA-D/DR antigens in the vast majority of cases
(3) and this has now been confirmed by others (8). The
HLA-D/DR positive cells in monolayers were identified as
thyrocytes by their reaction with anti-thyroid
microsomal/microvillar antibodies (3). These findings
raised the possibility that the Class II molecules
expressed by thyrocytes may play an active role in the
autoimmune process. We accordingly proposed that endocrine
epithelial cells can present their own surface autoantigens
in association with aberrantly expressed HLA-D/DR molecules
thus perpetuating, and possibly initiating, the T cell
activation which eventuates in autoimmune disease (9).

Inappropriate HLA-D/DR expression has been noted in
other tissues undergoing autoimmune attack, including bile
duct epithelium of liver biopsies from patients with
primary biliary cirrhosis (10), intestinal epithelium in
Crohn's and coeliac diseases (11) and autoimmune enteritis
(Mirakian, R., et al., in preparation), and in some
surviving Beta cells of a single pancreas obtained soon
after diagnosis of Type I diabetes (12). These
observations suggest that our hypothesis could be
applicable to a variety of organ specific autoimmune
diseases.

INDUCTION OF HLA-D/DR EXPRESSION

Since HLA-D/DR expression by endocrine epithelium
appears to be a common occurence in autoimmunity it was
important to determine the nature of the in vivo stimulus
for this expression. In view of the results with other
cell types (reviewed in 6) this was postulated to be
interferon (IFN) (9) which was tested in monolayer cultures
of normal human thyrocytes which are HLA-D/DR negative.
Addition of recombinant human IFN-gamma to the cultures
resulted in strong surface expression of HLA-D/DR antigens
by the thyrocytes as detected by indirect
immunofluorescence using monoclonal antibodies against non-

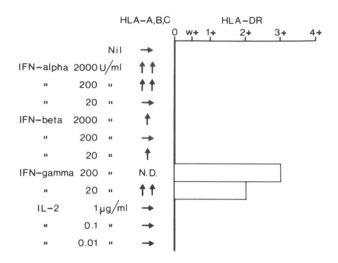

Figure 1 Induction of HLA-D/DR and HLA-A,B,C on human thyroid epithelium cultured with various stimulants for seven days. The surface MHC molecules were detected by indirect immunofluorescence using appropriate mouse monoclonal antibodies as the first layer (MID-3 for HLA-D/DR, W6/32 for HLA-A,B,C), followed by FITC-rabbit anti-mouse immunogloublin. For HLA-D/DR, the scale ranges from no positive cells (0) to most cells being very strongly positive (4+). For HLA-A,B,C, significant (↑) or very strong (↑↑) enhancement was scored relative to the basal control level (→). N.D. = not done.

polymorphic HLA-D/DR determinants (Fig.1) (13). Such expression was detectable within 24 hours of culture and doses of IFN-gamma as low as 1 U/ml were effective, thus being within the physiological range. The MHC Class II molecules appear to be synthesized by the thyrocytes themselves, as suggested by the observation that cytoplasmic vesicles bind anti-HLA-D/DR in IFN-gamma-induced cultures fixed prior to staining. Furthermore, use of Class II type-specific monoclonal antibodies indicated that both DR and DQ molecules are expressed.

In contrast to the activity of IFN-gamma, Namalva IFN-alpha, recombinant IFN-beta and recombinant interleukin-2

(IL-2) were unable to induce HLA-D/DR expression, even at very high doses (Fig.1). However, all three interferon species (but not IL-2) enhanced thyrocyte expression of HLA-A,B,C molecules (Fig. 1). This suggested that the expression of Class I and Class II MHC products by thyrocytes is regulated differently.

Since IFN-gamma is a T cell product, we investigated the effects of lymphocyte culture supernatants on normal thyrocytes. These were found to weakly induce expression of HLA-D/DR and this activity appeared to be inhibitable by IFN-gamma antiserum.

Our results suggest that IFN-gamma is the inducer of the HLA-D/DR expression by thyrocytes from patients with autoimmune thyroid diseases and, very probably, in other organ-specific autoimmune diseases. The production of IFN-gamma could result from local T cell activation by any one of a variety of environmental antigens. This initial sequence of events could trigger the immunological 'circuit' outlined in Fig.2 since the autoreactive T cell activation facilitated by the aberrant HLA-D/DR expression could result in further production of IFN-gamma and HLA-D/DR.

PRESENTATION OF ANTIGEN BY HLA-D/DR[+] THYROCYTES

Although essential for antigen presentation, the expression of HLA-D/DR molecules by endocrine epithelial cells does not of itself prove that these cells can effectively present antigen. However, it is worth noting

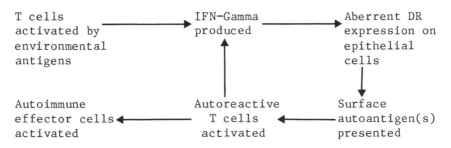

Figure 2. Possible events in the initiation and propogation of autoimmune activation.

that although antigen presenting function is usually
associated with macrophages, dendritic cells and, in
certain circumstances, B cells (reviewed in 6), other Class
II$^+$ cell types can perform this role. These
include murine L cells (fibroblasts) transfected with I-A
genes (14) and HLA-D/DR$^+$ human umbilical cord vein
endothelial cells (15). Since thyrocytes express Class II
molecules in Graves' disease (3) these were tested as a
source of potential antigen presenting cells (16). As
responding T cells, the cloned human T cell line HA1.7 was
used, which is specific for a defined peptide (p20,
residues 306-329) of the haemagglutinin molecule of
influenza virus strain A (17), and whose activation is
restricted by antigen presentation in the context of the

TABLE 1

PEPTIDE PRESENTATION BY DR$^+$ THYROCYTES

Cells		Antigen	Antibody	Response (cpm)
HA1.7		–	–	114
"		IL-2	–	40,813
"	thyrocytes	RB6B4	–	1,110
"	"	p20	–	75,041
"	"	"	Anti-HLA-DQ	3,460
"	–	"	–	1,112
–	"	–	–	142

Cloned T cells (5 x 10^4/ml) were cultured with MHC Class
II$^+$ irradiated (3000 Rad) thyrocytes (10^4/ml) in the
presence of p20 or RB6B4 (1 μg/ml). Anti-DQ ascites (HIG78)
was included at the initiation of the cultures at a
dilution of 1/200 and left in for the duration of the
experiments. The proliferative response was measured by
the incorporation of ^{3}H-thymidine. Control responses of
HA1.7 alone or with added IL-2 are shown.

HLA-DQ genes in linkage disequilibrium with HLA-DR1 (18).
Graves' Class II$^+$ thyrocytes of the appropriate HLA-DR type
were indeed able to effectively present p20 peptide to
HA1.7, but did not present an irrelevant peptide (RB6B4)
(Table 1). Moreover, the presentation of p20 was blocked
by an anti-HLA-DQ monoclonal antibody (Table 1). Various
control experiments made it very unlikely thatthis
presentation was actually effected by contaminating
macrophages, dendritic cells or lymphocytes. Thus, the
Class II$^+$ thyrocytes are capable of presenting antigen to a
T cell clone in an antigen-specific, MHC-restricted
fashion. However, as depicted in Fig 3, HLA-D/DR positive
thyrocytes were unable to present whole flu virus to HA1.7,
using either formalin inactivated virus, or even live,
infective virus. This was in contrast to peripheral blood
mononuclear cells (PBMC) from the same individual, which
efficiently presented both viral preparations as well as
p20. These findings suggest that thyrocytes are not

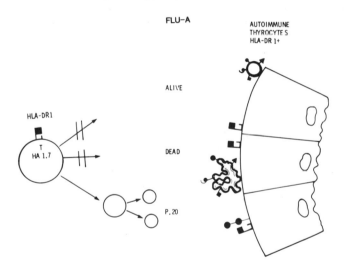

Figure 3   Presentation of antigen fragment, but not
whole virus, by thyroid epithelium.

capable of catabolising or 'processing' antigen for
presentation, which would not be required for an antigen
fragment like p20. This raises the possibility that in
vivo HLA-D/DR$^+$ epithelial cells may be restricted to
presenting autoantigens which require no modification, such

as their own surface molecules which are already inserted in the plasma membrane and may be presented in the context of membrane Class II molecules.

PRESENTATION OF SELF-ANTIGENS BY THYROCYTES

The ability of endocrine epithelial cells to present autoantigens was directly tested following the derivation of cloned T cell lines from the lymphocytic infiltrates of thyroid glands from Graves' disease patients (19). The mononuclear cells were initially expanded and cloned in the presence of mitogen-free IL-2, thus ensuring that only T cells already activated in vivo, and therefore possessing IL-2 receptors, were maintained. The specificity of each clone was then tested by examining their proliferation in response to autologous or allogeneic (HLA-mismatched) HLA-D/DR$^+$ thyrocytes, or autologous PBMC. Many of the clones responded to nothing other than IL-2. However, 10-15% of the clones were activated by autologous thyrocytes, but not

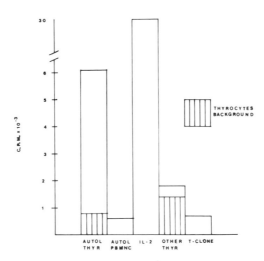

Figure 4   Cloned T cells (10^3 per well) were cultured with irradiated thyrocytes or PBMC (10^3 per well), or IL-2 (25% supernatant from PHA stimulated PBMC). Proliferation of the clones was determined by incorporation of tritiated -thymidine.

by autologous PBMC or allogeneic thyrocytes (Fig 4) and the
stimulation by autologous thyrocytes could be blocked by an
anti-HLA-D/DR monoclonal antibody.   These experiments thus
demonstrate, firstly, the presence in the lymphocytic
infiltrates of autoimmune diseased thyroids of activated,
autoreactive T cells whose stimulation occurs in an antigen
specific, MHC-restricted fashion.   Secondly, HLA-D/DR$^+$
thyrocytes are capable of mediating this stimulation by
presenting their own autoantigens.   This was visually
confirmed by autoreactive T cells strongly adhering to
autologous (but not allogeneic) thyrocytes with which they
were cultured.   The T cell clones were of the helper
subclass (T3$^+$, T4$^+$, T8$^-$).

A small number of the clones had a different response
pattern in that they were stimulated by autologous PBMC as
well as thyrocytes, but not by allogeneic thyrocytes (Fig
5).   This suggests that these cells recognize self-HLA-D/DR
determinants in a manner analogous to an autologous mixed

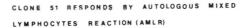

CLONE 51 RESPONDS BY AUTOLOGOUS MIXED
LYMPHOCYTES REACTION (AMLR)

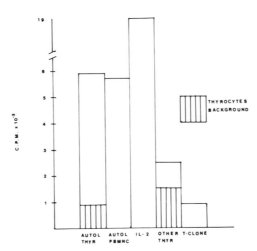

Fig. 5   Experimental details given in the legend to
Figure 4.

lymphocyte reaction.   They may play a role in the
autoimmune pathogenesis as has been similarly suggested in
certain animal models of autoimmunity (20,21).

SUMMARY

The results we have described clearly show that thyroid epithelial cells can be induced to express HLA-D/DR molecules and present antigen to T cells in a Class II-restricted fashion. More particularly, they can function as antigen presenting cells for auto-reactive T cells. The applicability of these findings to autoimmunity other than in the thyroid is suggested by the epithelial HLA-D/DR expression observed in autoimmune diseases of other organs as outlined above. The role we have put forward for epithelial HLA-D/DR expression in the induction and/or maintenance of autoimmunity is in accord with the relationship which others have proposed between inappropriate or excessive Class II expression and pathogenesis (20,22,23).

These processes would clearly operate in conjunction with other factors - environmental, genetic and somatic - in autoimmune pathogenesis. Thus, environmental factors (antigens) may play an important triggering role, as discussed above, while perturbations of normal suppressive mechanisms may permit the propogation of the autoimmune process (24). The initial autoactivation could occur long before disease symptoms are apparent (25) with somatic mutation of the T and/or B cell repertoires facilitating the increased tissue damage associated with the onset of overt disease (26).

ACKNOWLEDGEMENTS

We thank Professor D.Doniach and Professor I.M. Roitt for useful discussions, encouragement and support. I. Todd is supported by The Wellcome Trust Foundation and M.Londei and R. Pujol-Borrell by The Juvenile Diabetes Foundation International.

REFERENCES

1.   Roitt, I.M. Triangle, in press (1984).
2.   Smith, M.R. & Steinberg, A.D. Ann. Rev. Immunol. I, 175-210 (1983).

3.   Hanafusa, T., Pujol-Borrell, R., Chiovato, L.,
      Russell, R.C.G., Doniach, D. & Bottazzo, G.F. Lancet
      ii, 1111-1115 (1983).
4.   Khoury, E.L., Bottazzo, G.F. & Roitt, I.M. J. Exp.
      Med. 159, 577-591 (1984).
5.   Hanafusa, T., Pujol-Borrell, R., Chiovato, L.,
      Doniach, D. & Bottazo, G.F. Clin. exp. Immunol. 57,
      639-646 (1984).
6.   Unanue, E.R. Ann. Rev. Immunol. 2, 395-428 (1984).
7.   Pujol-Borrell, R., Hanafusa, T., Chiovato, L. &
      Bottazzo, G.F. Nature (Lond.) 303, 71-73 (1983).
8.   Jansson, R., Karlsson, A. & Forsum, U. Clin. exp.
      Immunol., in press (1984).
9.   Bottazzo, G.F., Pujol-Borrell, R., Hanafusa, T. &
      Feldmann, M. Lancet ii, 1115-1119 (1983).
10.   Ballardini, G., Bianchi, F.B., Mirakian, R., Pisi, E.,
      Doniach, D. & Bottazzo, G.F. Submitted for
      publication.
11.   Selby, W.S., Janossy, G., Mason, D.Y. & Jewell, D.P.
      Clin. exp. Immunol. 53, 614-618 (1983).
12.   Bottazzo, G.F. Diabetologia 26, 241-249 (1984).
13.   Todd, I., Pujol-Borrell, R., Hammond, L.J., Bottazzo,
      G.F. & Feldmann, M. (1984). Submitted for
      publication.
14.   Malissen, B., Price, M.P., Gaverman, J.M., McMillan,
      M.M., White, J., Kappler, J., Marrack, P., Pierres,
      A., Pierres, M. & Hood, L. Cell 36, 319-327 (1984).
15.   Nunez, G., Ball, E.J. & Stastny, P. J. Immunol. 131,
      666-673 (1983).
16.   Londei, M. Lamb, J.R., Bottazzo, G.F. & Feldmann, M.
      Submitted for publication.
17.   Lamb, J.R., Eckels, D.D., Lake, P., Woody, J.N. &
      Green, N. Nature (Lond.) 300, 66-67 (1982).
18.   Lamb, J.R. & Feldmann, M. Nature (Lond.) 308, 72-74
      (1983).
19.   Londei, M., Bottazzo, G.F. & Feldmann, M. Submitted
      for publication.
20.   Rosenberg, Y.J., Steinberg, A.D. & Santoro, T.J.
      Immunol. Today 5, 64-67 (1984).
21.   Wilson, D.B. Immunol. Today 5, 228-230 (1984)
22.   Unanue, E.R., Beller, D.I., Lu, C.Y. & Allen, P.M. J.
      Immunol. 132, 1-5 (1984).
23.   Janeway, C.A., Jr., Bottomly, K., Babich, J., Conrad,
      P., Conzen, S., Jones, B., Kaye, J., Katz, M., McVay,
      L., Murphy, D.B. & Tite, J. Immunol. Today 5, 99-
      105 (1984).

24. Topliss, D., How, J., Lewis, M., Row, V. & Volpe,R.
    J. Clin. Endocrinol. Metab. 57, 700-705 (1983).
25. Gorsuch, A. N., Spencer, K.M., Lister, J., McNally,
    J.M., Dean, B.M., Bottazzo, G.F. & Cudworth, A.G.
    Lancet ii, 1363-1365 (1981).
26. Bottazzo, G.F., Todd, I. & Pujol-Borrell, R. Immunol.
    Today 5, 230-231(1984).

ANTIGEN PROCESSING: A REEVALUATION

Jan Klein, Peter Walden, and Zoltan A. Nagy

Abteilung für Immungenetik, Max-Planck-Institut für Biologie, Corrensstr. 42, 7400 Tübingen, Federal Republic of
Germany

In immunology, like in many other sciences, there are
certain articles of faith in which we believe mostly
because they seem to make sense. Antigen processing, the
belief that antigen is taken up by cells, internalized,
degraded, and then reexpressed on the cell surfaces[1], is
one such article of faith. It makes sense because it is
known that things go into and come out of cells and because
the native antigen -- a bacterium, a virus, or a soluble
protein -- seems too large a morsel to wet the appetite of
a T cell. In addition, if one believes that antigen-presenting cells select, via their major histocompatibility
complex (Mhc) molecules, which antigenic determinant will
be recognized by the T cells, it makes sense that the
antigen is broken down into pieces and the fragments then
presented separately from each other by the antigen-presenting cell (APC). Yet, there is no direct evidence that
cells process antigen in this fashion. Nobody has ever seen
a protein globule disappear in a cell and then come out
again shattered into fragments that can associate with the
cell-surface Mhc molecules to be recognized by T lymphocytes. There is, to be sure, some circumstantial evidence
that such events occur and as long as there were no contradictory data, it seemed reasonable, indeed, to believe that
antigens need to be processed before they can be presented
to T cells. However, contradictory evidence has recently
been obtained and so it seems that the time has come to
evaluate critically the antigen processing hypothesis. This
article is a modest attempt to do just that.

ARGUMENTS FOR ANTIGEN PROCESSING

What, then, are the reasons why immunologists believe
in antigen processing? The reasons given by the proponents
of the processing hypothesis are these: First, there is a
lag between antigen uptake and antigen presentation.[2-4]
Second, T cells recognize denatured antigens just as well
as native proteins and small peptide fragments equally as
well as the whole protein.[5-6] Third, agents that raise
lysosomal pH, such as ammonia and chloroquine, inhibit
antigen presentation when present during the exposure of
APC to the antigen.[7-9] Fourth, paraformaldehyde- or glutaral-
dehyde-fixed APC are able to present peptides but neither
native nor denatured whole proteins.[10]

All these findings can be interpreted as supporting
the antigen-processing hypothesis, but can they also be
interpreted differently? We think that they can. Thus the
lag between antigen uptake and antigen presentation might
be the period when antigen is processed intracellularly.
But it could also be the period -- about one hour -- needed
for the antigen to bind to the cell surface in a sufficient
quantity and to distribute itself on the plasma membrane so
that enough of it occupies sites near the appropriate Mhc
molecules. Here we must distinguish between two processes
-- antigen uptake and antigen binding. Antigen uptake may
occur without an actual attachment of molecules to the cell
surface, by endocytosis of the fluid containing the soluble
protein. This process is probably rather rapid and occurs
within seconds of APC exposure to antigen. Antigen binding,
on the other hand, presumably requires interaction of the
soluble protein with the various membrane proteins. This
interaction may be totally nonspecific and therefore much
weaker than a true receptor-ligand interaction. It may
occur between any two proteins that show patches of charge
complementarity and may, therefore, be completely random.
The low affinity of these random interactions may mean that
a certain amount of time is needed before the right distribution and density of antigen on the cell surface is
achieved for antigen presentation.

Evidence that T lymphocytes do not recognize conformational determinants is not as convincing as it is sometimes
made to be. All that the data demonstrate is that you can
do things to an antigen and still have it recognized by T
cells which you cannot do to it and still retain its

ability to stimulate B cells. But such observation does not mean that the T-cell receptor recognizes primary structure of a protein. In fact, there is evidence that even T-cells recognize some kind of structural determinants. For example, the determinant recognized by mouse T cells on bovine insulin A chain is located in a disulfide-bonded loop -- an element of the tertiary structure[11]. When this loop is straightened out by oxidation, the T cells no longer recognize it. There is also other evidence that makes the same point[12]. However, the main objection is that this argument is largely irrelevant to the issue whether APC do or do not process antigen. Even if T cells recognized the sequence of amino acids rather than their spatial arrangement, there is nothing that would prevent them from recognizing the sequence on an intact protein. If determinants are located mostly on the surface of the antigenic molecule, as they seem to be, then T cells should have access to them in an intact protein just as well as on peptide fragments.

The argument based on the use of ammonia and chloroquine is not very convincing either. These experiments demonstrate only that chloroquine reduces the amount of antigen degraded intracellularly and then released by exocytosis, in comparison with the amount released in the absence of the agent. This finding is expected if the agent really does what it is supposed to do, but it constitutes no proof of antigen processing. The problem is that we know what chloroquine is doing to lysosomes but we do not know what it is doing to the rest of the cell, particularly to the plasma membrane and particularly during antigen presentation. The point has been made that chloroquine has no effect on antigen presentation because in its presence antigen uptake is normal and because after "processing" it does not disturb the interaction between T cells and APC. However, the measurements of antigen uptake were done on macrophages which are unsuitable for this kind of study. The cells that take up antigen most actively are the mature macrophages which cannot present antigen. In the macrophage population true antigen presenting cells constitute a small minority and it is therefore extremely unlikely that if chloroquine were to inhibit antigen uptake by these cells one would notice it. The observation that after a certain period of APC exposure to antigen chloroquine has no effect could in fact be interpreted as suggesting that this drug does interfere with antigen uptake. One must also consider

the possibility that the drug acts on antigen uptake
indirectly in a manner demonstrated for the mannose-specific receptors. It has been shown that chloroquine inhibits,
after a certain lag, uptake of glycoproteins with mannose,
fucose, or N-acetylglucosamine at the terminal position in
their glycans.[13] This uptake is mediated by mannose-specific
receptors expressed on the cell surface. In the presence of
chloroquine, recycling of these receptors is blocked so
that after the initial uptake, no additional binding of
glycoproteins can occur. If one would not know the mechanism of this process, one might be tempted to conclude that
chloroquine blocks processing of the glycoproteins. Therefore, the studies thus far carried out, and purportedly
demonstrating inhibition of antigen processing by chloroquine and similar agents, are simply too crude to allow one
to conclude where and how the inhibition occurs.

Finally, the evidence that there is a difference in
antigen presentation between live and fixed APC is also
ambiguous. One can interpret it as suggesting that fragmen-
ted but not native molecules are presented by fixed cells
because such cells fail to process the native antigen. But
one can also argue that the cause for this difference lies
at the cell surface and not inside the cell. For example,
the possibility has not been ruled out that the peptide
fragments are simply "stickier" than the whole proteins so
that they, but not the whole proteins, are taken up by
fixed cells in quantities sufficient for antigen presentation. Another possibility is that recycling of antigen-
binding proteins is needed for the bulky proteins but not
for the small peptide fragments so that a sufficient
quantity of antigen can be presented to the T cells. And
still another possibility is that membrane fluidity is necessary to bring bulky proteins in the vicinity of the Mhc
molecules and to orient them in a proper way; the small
peptides may have a higher probability then the proteins of
accomplishing both requirements in a rigid plasma membrane.
All these alternative explanations need to be excluded
before the experiments with fixed APC can be considered
proof for antigen processing.

Nonetheless, if there were no data to the contrary,
all these findings taken together would make a reasonably
good case for the antigen-processing hypothesis. But there
are data contradicting the hypothesis and because of them
one must entertain the possibility that the alternative

rather than the originally suggested explanations of these experiments might actually be right.

ARGUMENTS AGAINST ANTIGEN PROCESSING

As long as macrophages were thought to be the only antigen presenting cells, the antigen processing hypothesis made good sense. After all, phagocytosis was a kind of antigen processing and phagocytosis was a hallmark of macrophages. However, in recent years evidence has steadily accumulated that macrophages with pronounced ability to phagocytose particles probably do not present antigen and that many other cells that cannot phagocytose do present antigen. Antigen-presentation ability has been demonstrated for B-cell blasts[14, 15], B-cell lymphomas[16-19], dendritic cells[20], Langerhans cells[21], and astrocytes[22]. It appears, in fact, than any cell expressing class II Mhc molecules can present soluble antigens to T cells. These findings indicate that there is no special processing compartment in the cell and no special processing mechanism. Hence, if processing were to exist, it would have to be accomplished by the standard endowment of a cell and through a standard mechanism -- presumably through degradation in the lysosomal compartment. If so, one cannot expect much selectivity in the degradation process: Most of the internalized antigen would be degraded to the degree that it could no longer be immunogenic. This prediction could easily be tested by exposing proteins in vitro to the same conditions and to the same set of enzymes that exist in lysosomes. The experiments in which proteins were partially digested in vitro under carefully controlled conditions may not at all be pertinent to the events occurring in lysosomes in vivo.

One must also consider the fact that molecules recognized in the context of class I molecules, such as viral or minor histocompatibility antigens, can apparently be recognized in their native form. At least we are not aware of any evidence suggesting that they must be processed. And if they are not processed, why would a special processing mechanism be needed for antigens recognized in the context of class II Mhc molecules?

Also, conceptually it is difficult to imagine how many specific immunological cell-cell or factor-cell interactions would be possible if proteins were degraded to fragments each bearing only one antigenic determinant. How could then, for example, a helper T cell interact with a B cell or with a suppressor T cell?

In addition to these theoretical arguments, there is also experimental evidence indicating that processing is not needed for antigen presentation. First, Malek and his coworkers[23] demonstrated that the synthetic polymer GLT never leaves the cell surface during the period of antigen presentation and, therefore, has no opportunity to be processed inside the cell. The authors reach the conclusion that "the crucial events of MØ antigen handling of GLT may entirely be a cell surface phenomenon." Although this conclusion contradicts the one the authors reached in their earlier publication, the experiments, if confirmed, would strongly suggest that at least for this particular antigen, no intracellular processing of the antigen is needed.
Second, Lee and his coworkers[24] found no effect of chloroquine on the presentation of monomeric flagellin to T cells (although they found an effect on the presentation of the polymeric flagellin). They argue that only large antigens need to be processed, whereas small molecules can be presented in an unprocessed form. Obviously, it is a matter of opinion what one considers large and what small but it may be pertinent to remind ourselves that the "small" monomeric flagellin has a molecular weight of 40,000 and is therefore about the size of the Mhc class I polypeptide and far larger than either the α or ß class II polypeptides.

Third, in our own laboratory we were able to present antigen on artificial membranes (liposomes). A representative experiment in this series is shown in Table 1. In this study, we solubilized mouse class II Mhc molecules using the detergent ß-octylglucosid, isolated them, and mixed them with the activated lipid dipalmytoyl-L-α-glycerylphosphorylethanolamine (DPPE). The activation of the lipid was accomplished with N-succinimide-3(2-pyrodyldithio)propionate (SPDP) which produced an activated disulfide bond on the lipid. The mixture of the activated lipid and the solubilized Mhc molecules was then dialyzed against phosphate-buffered saline, and liposomes carrying integrated Mhc molecules were produced. To the activated lipid on the liposomes we then attached activated antigen via a disulfide bond. The activation of the antigen was achieved by treating it with SPDP and then reducing it with dithiothreitol (DTT) so that a free sulfhydryl group was

Table 1 Responses of OVA-primed T cells to OVA
presented on liposomes

Stimulator	Response (cpm $\pm$ S.E.)
SC[*] + OVA	81,237 $\pm$ 9,279
SC + Con A	74,790 $\pm$ 4,487
SC	1,533 $\pm$ 632
OVA	881 $\pm$ 287
A^b and KLH on liposome	1,413 $\pm$ 280
A^b and OVA on liposome	27,724 $\pm$ 4,325
OVA on liposome	6,472 $\pm$ 518
A^b on liposome	1,178 $\pm$ 39
A^b on liposome + OVA on different liposome	6,776 $\pm$ 978
A^b on liposome + free OVA	1,095 $\pm$ 289
---	1,546 $\pm$ 344

[*]Irradiated syngeneic spleen cells.

produced.

Liposomes with Mhc molecules inserted into the lipid
bilayer and antigen covalently attached to the lipid were
then used to restimulate primed T cells in vitro, and the
stimulation was measured in terms of T-cell proliferation
(incorporation of ^{3}H-thymidine). The T-cells were primed to
the same antigen as that coupled to the liposomes. Three
kinds of T cells were used: T-cell populations obtained
from animals immunized in vivo and restimulated twice in
vitro before the addition of liposomes, T-cell clones
maintained in culture for several months, and T-cell
hybridomas. All of them could be restimulated with liposomes carrying the proper antigen. Five antigens were
tested -- pig lactate dehydrogenase-B (LDH-B), ovalbumin
(OVA), key-hole limpet hemocyanin (KLH), insulin, and
pigeon cytochrome c -- and all of them, when attached to
liposomes, stimulated the appropriate T cells specifically. Liposomes with Mhc but without antigen or with antigen
but without Mhc molecules did not stimulate, nor did a
mixture of these two incomplete liposomes. Liposomes
carrying an inappropriate antigen or inappropriate Mhc
molecules also failed to stimulate the T cells. We conclude, therefore, that unprocessed antigen can stimulate

primed T cells, if presented together with the appropriate
Mhc molecules.

One possible objection to this kind of experiment is
that the liposomes might fuse with the plasma membranes of
cells in the culture (surviving APC, feeder cells, or even
T cells), the antigen might be processed by these cells,
and then presented in the context of the Mhc molecules
remaining in the membranes. Arguing against this explanation is the observation that when the antigen and the Mhc
molecules are on separate liposomes, the T cells fail to be
stimulated. If the antigen were presented by cells rather
than liposomes, stimulation should have occurred in this
control experiment.

One could also argue that antigen processing occurs on
the cell surface by enzymes present in the plasma membrane
and that the liposome-bound antigen is processed by the
membrane of the T cells. If this were the case, one would
expect that the T-cells should also be able to process free
antigen and then use the Mhc molecules of the liposomes for
the recognition of the fragments. However, in no case was
stimulation by free antigen observed in the presence or the
absence of liposome-bound Mhc molecules.

Finally, one must consider the possibility that
antigen-processing is required for primary but not for
secondary responses. If so, the determinants recognized on
the processed and unprocessed antigen would have to be the
same and the whole debate whether antigen is or is not
processed would become academic. In summary, we do not find
any plausible explanation of the liposome experiments other
than that T cells are able to recognize determinants on
unprocessed antigen. The selection of antigens used in
these experiments was sufficiently wide to support the
general validity of this conclusion (in fact, some of the
antigens used by us were those for which a requirement for
antigen processing has been claimed by other investigators).

A RECONCILIATION

It would be foolish to deny that antigen is picked up
by cells, degraded in lysosomes, and the degradation
products spit out again into the extracellular milieu.
After all, this is what endocytosis and exocytosis are all

about. It may even be that parts of the antigen survive the
harsh treatment in the lysosomes, reach the cell exterior
still in an immunogenic form, are picked up by the APC, and
are then recognized by T cells. This may particularly be
true for corpuscular antigens such as bacteria or erythro-
cytes. However, we wish to claim that antigen processing is
not a sine qua non for antigen presentation and that T
cells can recognize determinants on native, undegraded
antigen.

REFERENCES

1. Unanue, E. Adv. Immunol. 31, 1-136 (1981).
2. Waldron, J., Horn, R. & Rosenthal, A. J. Immunol. 112,
    746-755 (1974).
3. Calderon, J. & Unanue, E. J. Immunol. 112, 1804-1814
    (1974).
4. Ziegler, K. & Unanue, E. J. Immunol. 127, 1969-1875
    (1981).
5. Ishizaka, K., Okudaira, H. & King. T. J. Immunol. 114,
    110-115 (1975).
6. Chesnut, R., Endres, R. & Grey, H. Clin. Immunol.
    Immunopathol. 15, 397-408 (1980).
7. Ziegler, K. & Unanue, E. Proc. natn. Acad. Sci. U.S.A.
    79, 175-   (1982).
8. Lee, K.-C., Wong, M. & Spitzer, D. Transplantation 34,
    150-153 (1982).
9. Chesnut, R.S., Colon, S.M. & Grey, H.M. J. Immunol.
    129, 2382-2388 (1982).
10. Shimonkevitz, R., Kappler, J., Marrack, P. & Grey, H.
    J. Exp.Med. 158, 303-316 (1983).
11. Ishii, N., Klein, J. & Nagy, Z.A. Eur. J. Immunol. 13,
    658-662 (1983).
12. Glimcher, L.H., Schroer, J.A. Chan, C. & Shevach, E.M.
    J. Immunol. 131, 2868-2874 (1983).
13. Tietze, C., Schlesinger, P. & Stahl, P. Biochem.
    Biophys. Res.Commun. 93, 1-   (1980).
14. Chesnut, R. & Grey, H. J. Immunol. 126, 1075-1079
    (1981).
15. Kakiuchi, T., Chesnut, R.W. & Grey, H.M. J. Immunol.
    131, 109-114 (1983).
16. McKean, D.J., Infante, A.J., Nilson, A., Kimoto, M.,
    Fathman, C.G., Walker, E. & Warner, N. J. Exp. Med.
    154, 1419-1431 (1981).
17. Glimcher, L.H., Kim K.-J., Green, I. & Paul, W. J. Exp.
    Med. 155, 445-459 (1982).

18. Chesnut, R.W., Colon, S.M. & Grey, H.M. J. Immunol.
    128, 1764-1768 (1982).
19. Walker, E., Warner, N.L., Chesnut, R., Kappler, J. &
    Marrack, P. J. Immunol 128, 2164-2169 (1982).
20. Sunshine, G.H., Katz, D.R. & Feldman, M. J. Exp. Med.
    152, 1817-1822 (1980).
21. Stingl, G., Katz, S.I., Clement, L., Green, I. &
    Shevach, E.M. J. Immunol. 121, 2005-2013 (1978).
22. Fontana, A., Fierz, W. & Wekerle, H. Nature 307,
    273-276 (1984).
23. Malek, T.R., Clement, L.T. & Shevach, E.M. Eur. J.
    Immunol 13, 810-815 (1983).
24. Lee, K.C., Wong, M. & Spitzer, D. Transplantation 34,
    150-153 (1982).

THE NATURE AND FUNCTIONS OF FOLLICULAR DENDRITIC CELLS

G.G.B. Klaus* & J.H. Humphrey**

*National Institute for Medical Research,
Mill Hill, London NW7, UK.

**Royal Postgraduate Medical School,
Ducane Road, London W12, UK.

Recent years have seen remarkable progress in our understanding of the nature of the cell interactions involved in the induction of various types of immune response. In particular, the concept of accessory cells has become firmly entrenched in cellular immunology, with the realisation that there are several different types of accessory cell, mainly within the specialised architecture of the lymphoid system, but also elsewhere in other tissues in the body. Apart from macrophages, which perform several functions, each has a specialised role in immune induction.

In this review we will concentrate on one particular accessory cell, which although recognised some 20 years ago, has only recently been isolated (for reasons which will become obvious), and the function of which remains incompletely understood, although it is undoubtedly of major importance in various aspects of immunoregulation.

THE NATURE OF FOLLICULAR DENDRITIC CELLS (FDC)

The existence of a dendritic network of antigen-retaining cells amongst the densely packed B lymphocytes which comprise the follicles of spleen and lymph nodes was first clearly recognised by White[1]. The cells are difficult to distinguish by conventional light microscopic procedures.

345

By electron microscopy FDC are revealed as cells with highly
characteristic, lobed euchromatic nuclei, and cytoplasm
devoid of phagolysosomes[2]. The most striking features of
these cells, however, are their processes, which when fully
developed form an extraordinary labyrinth of dendritic
evaginations, typically covered with a layer of electron-
dense material, and ramifying extensively between the
surrounding lymphocytes[2,3]. This electron-dense layer
consists of deposits of antigen-antibody-complement
complexes (immune complexes, IC). It is this capacity of
FDC to retain IC on their processes which forms the crux of
their functional importance.

It should be stressed that, because these delicate
dendritic processes are intimately entangled with lymphocytes, the vast majority of FDC are torn apart and destroyed
during the conventional procedures used for the preparation
of lymphoid cell suspensions. However, recently several
groups have developed relatively atraumatic dispersion
methods, using various enzymes, which release FDC in
sufficient yields for the study of their morphology and
markers in vitro[4,5,6]. The strategy used in mice is to
inject the animals with fluorescent, or peroxidase-labelled
IC or aggregated Ig. After some 48 h the label initially
taken up by macrophages has been broken down and disappeared,
and only the FDC retain detectable amounts of IC[4]. In both
mouse and human tissues, even after extensive enzyme
digestion many of the cells are recovered in multinucleate
cell clusters, and those which emerge as single cells have
lost or withdrawn their dendrites. However, recently
Szakal et al.[6] have succeeded in recovering FDC from lymph
nodes which retain their dendritic morphology in isolation.
These authors have described FDC as consisting of two types
- the first having up to 6-10 rodlike, or filiform
dendritic processes, 6-11 um in length. The second are
similar in size, but their processes carry an array of
spherical, or ellipsoidal structures, giving the cells a
unique beaded appearance.

As a result of such studies, the markers carried by
FDC are gradually being catalogued. Table 1 compares the
known properties of various types of mouse dendritic cells
with macrophages[7]. The most distinctive features of FDC
are their lack of phagocytic activity, coupled with high
levels of both Fc and C3 receptors. The cells lack the
markers Mac 1, 2 and 3, which are characteristic of

macrophages, and in the case of the latter two, of
Langerhans and interdigitating cells as well. This marker
profile suggests that FDC are quite distinct from the
above-mentioned types of dendritic cells and from macrophages. This is supported by additional data (see below),
and also by the existence of monoclonal antibodies specific
for human[8] and rat[9] FDC, although none are yet available
for these cells in the mouse.

The expression of Class II MHC antigens by FDC is
still unresolved. Initial studies of isolated mouse FDC
indicated that the cells lack Ia antigens[4], although J.G.
Tew (pers. comm.) has been unable to confirm this finding.
Human FDC, on the other hand do apparently express low
levels of HLA-DR antigens[5,10]. However, since FDC are
often recovered in multinucleated clusters containing
entrapped B cells, the origins of Class II antigens in such
clusters can be difficult to ascertain with certainty.

Table 1. Markers of Mouse Dendritic Cells and Macrophages

Dendritic Cells:

Markers:	LC:	IDC:	FDC:	Macrophage:
Mac-1	−	−	−	+
Mac-2	+	+	−	+
Mac-3	+	+	−	+
Fc receptor	+	ND	+	+
C3 receptor	+	ND	+	+
ATPase	+	ND	+	+
Ia	+	+	−	+/−

Modified from ref. 7.
Key:
LC: Langerhans cell; IDC: Interdigitating cell; FDC:
Follicular dendritic cell.
The dendritic cells isolated by Steinman et al.[28] (which
may be equivalent to IDC) are Mac-1⁻, FcR⁻, C3R⁻, ATPase⁻
and Ia⁺.

THE ORIGINS OF FDC

It is firmly established that cells of the monocyte-macrophage axis, and other types of dendritic cells are all bone marrow derived[11,12]. Recently, the origins of FDC have been studied in mice using long-term $F_1 \longrightarrow P$ bone marrow chimaeras[13]. The results of these experiments showed that even after 12 months the FDC in the chimaeras were still of host phenotype (Fig.1). It is therefore highly unlikely that these cells are derived from a bone marrow-derived precursor cell. It has been suggested that FDC differentiate from reticulum cells in the follicular stroma[14]. If so, they must acquire Fc and C3 receptors, and the markers summarised above, which are not expressed by reticulum cells.

During ontogeny the capacity of lymphoid tissues to retain IC for long periods does not appear until there are recognisable follicles[15]. Furthermore, typical FDC are difficult to recognise in primary follicles (although they are undoubtedly there in some form). Following immunisation, and the appearance of germinal centres, FDC progressively develop their complex labyrinth of processes. From cytometric studies this appears to be due to an increase in cytoplasmic volume, rather than to cell recruitment[16]. This is manifested functionally as an increase in the capacity of germinal centres to trap IC, including those containing irrelevant antigens[17].

Taken together, these observations suggest that the microenvironment of the follicle stimulates the differentiation of FDC from a yet unidentified precursor cell, and that this process continues during the development of the germinal centre. There is a simultaneous increase in the number of associated B lymphocytes, some of which divide. Whether the FDC processes are stretched out by these additional lymphocytes, or the additional lymphocytes are trapped by the enlarged dendritic network is an open question.

THE MECHANISMS OF IMMUNE COMPLEX TRAPPING

It has been known for some time that FDC are quite radioresistant. However, irradiation or drugs which destroy lymphocytes abolish trapping of IC. Earlier

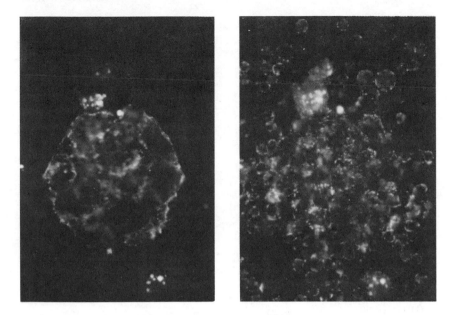

Figure 1. Host origin of FDC in long-term bone marrow
chimaeras. Eight week old C57BL/10 mice were lethally
irradiated and repopulated with bone marrow cells from (B10
X CBA)Fl mice. One year later they received FITC-labelled
aggregated human gamma globulin i.v. Follicular dendritic
cells were isolated 48 h later from the spleens. The
pictures show an FDC-containing cell cluster stained with
biotinylated anti-H2^k, followed by TRITC-labelled avidin.
The fluorescence filters reveal a) FITC, and b) TRITC.
Cells within the cluster, but not the FDC themselves, are
stained with the anti-donor H2 antibody (see ref. 13).

experiments of Brown et al.[18] showed that if the spleens of
mice were irradiated, but their bone marrow was shielded,
this temporarily prevented follicular localisation in the
spleen. They suggested that a radio-sensitive, sessile
cell was required for the transport of IC to the FDC. A
recent study by Gray et al.[19] in the rat supports this
concept, and provides evidence that IC are transported to
FDC by a relatively static population of IgM$^+$IgD$^-$ B cells
located in the marginal zone of the spleen, and which is
selectively destroyed by cyclophosphamide.

We have used a different approach to this problem in
the mouse. Development of either all B cells, or of IgD-
bearing cells only, was suppressed by treating mice from
birth with anti-IgM, or anti-IgD antibodies, respectively[20].
When the animals were 8 weeks old, radiolabelled IC were
injected i.v. As shown in Fig. 2, anti-IgM treated mice
totally failed to retain IC in their spleens. Histologically, the organs lacked recognisable follicular structures,
and may have lacked FDC as well (although this has not yet

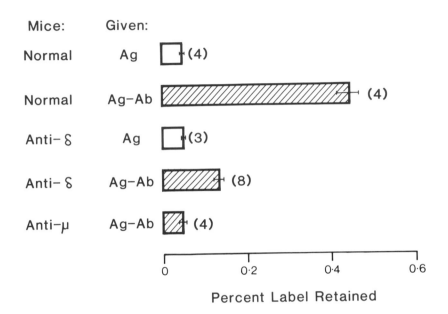

Fig. 2. Effects of suppression of B cell development on
trapping of IC in the spleen. Litters of C3H mice were
treated from birth with specific anti-u, or anti-δ
antibodies. When 8 w.o. they received ^{125}I-labelled antigen (Ag: DNP-KLH), either alone, or as complexes made with
a monoclonal anti-DNP antibody (Ag-Ab). After 24 h the
spleens were removed and counted for residual ^{125}I, and
processed for autoradiography. Spleens of normal mice
showed heavy labelling of FDC; those from anti-δ treated
mice showed light, but significant labelling, while those
from anti-u treated mice were totally negative (see ref.20).

been studied). Mice treated with anti-IgD trapped
significant, although much diminished amounts of IC when
compared to controls. Their spleens contained small
follicles, consisting of only IgM⁺IgD⁻ B cells.

These results confirm that B cells are required for
follicular trapping. In the mouse both IgD⁺ and IgD⁻ B
cells seem to be involved, perhaps not surprisingly, since
this species does not have the well-demarcated marginal
zones, consisting of IgM⁺IgD⁻ B cells, seen in the rat.

Follicular localisation of IC in vivo is known to be
strictly complement-dependent, and both pathways have been
shown to be effective[17]. The picture that has therefore
emerged within recent years is that B cells in the marginal
zone, which in the rat are known to carry both CR1 and CR2
receptors[19], somehow pick up and transport IC to FDC
within the mantle zone of the follicle. FDC have a very
high density of C3 receptors, and it seems likely that in
vivo IC are bound through these. Once bound the IC are not
released by subsequent treatment with cobra venom factor,
which implies that the receptors involved are covered and
protected by the IC. Although in vitro IC can apparently
bind to FDC via their Fc receptors[16], the function of the
Fc receptors in vivo remains a mystery.

Most studies on follicular localisation have employed
complexes containing protein antigens, or aggregated Ig.
Recently, we have shown that IC made with a particulate
antigen (TNP-sheep red blood cells, SRBC) and monoclonal
anti-DNP antibody also become localised on FDC, apparently
in an analogous fashion to those containing soluble
antigens[21]. The mechanisms involved here are not clear,
but we think it likely that macrophages (presumably those
in the marginal zone) first process the SRBC and release
soluble antigenic fragments. These then become complexed
with antibody dissociated from the original complexes,
activate C3, and finally find their way to FDC. Whatever
the detailed mechanisms may be, the results point to a
central role for FDC in the regulation of immune responses
to particulate as well as soluble antigens.

THE FUNCTIONS OF FOLLICULAR DENDRITIC CELLS

Follicular trapping of most antigens is both antibody,

and C-dependent. The role of the FDC in immune induction
therefore clearly depends on their capacity to retain
antigen, in the form of IC. The feature that distinguishes
these cells from all other accessory cells is this capacity
to retain detectable amounts of intact antigen on their
membranes for weeks, and even months[22]. This property,
coupled with their complex dendritic morphology, and the
traffic of B cells in their vicinity, makes them ideal
antigen-presenting cells for B lymphocytes. Studies on the
precise role of FDC in B cell activation have been hampered
by the difficulties involved in isolating the cells in a
functional state and in quantity. Nevertheless, in vivo
studies have produced two (overlapping) hypotheses, which
are supported by a wealth of data. These have been
extensively reviewed elsewhere, and are therefore only
summarised here.

The first model[17] proposes that following primary
immunisation, C-fixing IC are formed which become trapped
on FDC. Although the trapping phenomenon is not antigen-
specific, it is likely that antigen-specific B cells
themselves become trapped as they traverse the follicle, due
to binding to epitopes revealed on the surfaces of the FDC.
These B cells are stimulated to divide, and this is seen
histologically as the germinal centre response. In short,
this hypothesis envisages that FDC-associated antigen
stimulates virgin B cells to proliferate and to mature into
memory cells. In the absence of local T cell help these
cells differentiate no further but join the recirculating
pool. Germinal centres have long been suspected to be sites
of memory cell generation, and more direct support for this
concept has emerged recently. Germinal centre B cells
appear to represent a unique subpopulation since, unlike
resting B cells in primary follicles, they lack IgD, and
strongly bind peanut lectin (PNL)[24]. Recent studies have
shown that PNL-binding B cells are highly enriched in
functional memory cells (ref. 25; D.W. Dongworth & G.G.B.
Klaus, unpublished data). A second characteristic of
memory cells is that they have switched surface Ig isotype —
generally to IgG-bearing cells in spleen and lymph nodes.
There is now evidence that germinal centres are the sites
where this isotype switch occurs[26].

Many details of the above scheme remain to be filled
in. For instance, it is uncertain whether C3b is merely
involved in IC transport, or if it is also involved in

stimulating the germinal centre response. Secondly,
although B memory cell generation and germinal centre
formation are both T-cell dependent, the precise role of
T cells in the overall process remains ill-defined. This is
a particularly fascinating problem, since follicles and
germinal centres contain very few T cells.

The second hypothesis concerning the functions of FDC
concerns the role of the retained antigen in the long-term
maintenance and control of the humoral response[23]. This
concept emerged from attempts to explain two phenomena –
cyclical antibody responses, and 'spontaneous' antibody
production by fragment cultures of lymphoid tissues from
long-term immunised animals. Both effects are undoubtedly
due to retained antigen on FDC. In brief, Tew and his
collaborators[23] propose that IC on FDC will continue to
stimulate antibody production until epitopes on the
complexes are masked by rising levels of antibody.
Eventually, as antibody levels fall epitopes are again
exposed and stimulate a further wave of antibody synthesis.
This scheme readily accommodates the findings from earlier
experiments[27], which showed that if mice are immunised with
preformed IC, this leads to the rapid induction of memory to
both epitopes and (depending on the antigen-antibody ratio
of the complex) idiotopes in the IC. It is thus possible
that during the early phase of immune induction complexes
in antigen excess would favour the build-up of memory to
the antigen. As antibody levels rise, not only are epitopes
on the complexes masked, but increasing numbers of idiotypic
determinants on the antibodies would become available for
recognition.

In conclusion, it thus seems likely that retained
antigen on FDC plays a fundamental and central role in both
positive and negative aspects of the control of humoral
immunity. Hopefully, the methods currently being developed
for the isolation of these fascinating cells will yield
further details of their functions within the immune system.

REFERENCES

1. White, R.G. in The Immunologically Competent Cell, Ciba Foundation Study Group No. 16, ed. G.W. Wolstenholme & J. Knight, Churchill, London 1963, p.6.

2. Nossal, G.J.V. & Ada, G.L. Antigens, Lymphoid Cells and the Immune Response. Academic Press, New York 1971.

3. Szakal, A.K. & Hanna, M.G. Exp. Molec. Pathol. 8, 75 (1968).

4. Humphrey, J.H. & Grennan, D. in In Vivo Immunology, ed. P. Nieuwenhuis & A.A. van den Broek, Plenum, New York 1982, p. 823.

5. Heinen, E., Lilet-Leclercq, C., Mason, D.Y., Stein, H., Boniver, J., Radoux, D., Kinet-Denoel, C. & Simar, L.J. Eur. J. Immunol. 14, 267 (1984).

6. Szakal, A., Gieringer, R.L., Kosco, M.H. & Tew, J.G. (In the press).

7. Haines, K.A., Flotte, T.J., Springer, T.A., Gigli, I., & Thorbecke, G.J. Proc. Nat. Acad. Sci. USA 80, 3448 (1983).

8. Naiem, M., Gerdes, J., Abdulaziz, Z., Stein, H. & Mason D.Y. J. Clin. Pathol. 36, 167 (1983).

9. Barclay, A.N. Immunology 44, 727 (1981).

10. Gerdes, J., Stein, H., Mason, D.Y. & Ziegler, A. Virchows Arch B 42, 161 (1983).

11. Tamaki, K., Stingl, G. & Katz, S.I. J. Invest. Dermatol. 74, 309 (1980).

12. Van Furth, R. & Thompson, J. Ann. Inst. Pasteur 120, 337 (1971).

13. Humphrey, J.H., Grennan, D. & Sundaram, V. Eur. J. Immunol. (In the press).

14. Kamperdijk, E.W.A., Raaymakers, E.M., DeLeuw, J.H.S.
    & Hoefsmit, E.C.M. Cell Tissue Res. 192, 1 (1978).

15. Dijkstra, C.D., Van Tilburg, N.J. & Dopp, E.A.
    Cell Tissue Res. 223, 545 (1982).

16. Radoux, D. La Cellule Folliculaire Dendritique:
    Structure et Fonctions dans les Reactions immunitaire.
    Thesis, University of Liege, 1984.

17. Klaus, G.G.B., Humphrey, J.H., Kunkl, A. & Dongworth,
    D.W. Immunol. Rev. 53, 3 (1980).

18. Brown, J.C., Harris, G., Papamicail, M., Sljivic, V.S.,
    & Holborow, E.J. Immunology 24, 955 (1973).

19. Gray, D., McConnell, I., Kumararatne, D.S., Maclennan,
    I.C.M., Humphrey, J.H. & Bazin, H. Eur. J. Immunol.
    14, 47, 1984.

20. Enriquez-Rincon, F., Andrew, E., Parkhouse, R.M.E. &
    Klaus, G.G.B. Immunology (In the press).

21. Enriquez-Rincon, F. & Klaus, G.G.B. Immunology 52,
    107 (1984).

22. Mandel, T.E., Phipps, R.P., Abbot, A. & Tew, J.G.
    Immunol. Rev. 53, 29 (1980).

23. Tew, J.G., Phipps, R.P. & Mandel, T.E. Immunol. Rev.
    53, 175 (1980).

24. Rose, M.L., Birbeck, M.S.C., Wallis, V.J., Forrester,
    J.A. & Davies, A.J.S. Nature 284, 364 (1980).

25. Coico, R.F., Bhogal, B.S. & Thorbecke, G.J. J. Immunol.
    131, 2254 (1983).

26. Kraal, G., Weissman, I.L. & Butcher, E.C. Nature 298,
    377 (1982).

27. Klaus, G.G.B. Nature 272, 265 (1978).

28. Nussenzweig, M.C. & Steinman, R.M. Immunology Today 3,
    65 (1982).

MECHANISMS OF AUTOIMMUNITY

R. B. Taylor

and

A. Basten

The key issues in autoimmunity are concerned with the anti-self repertoire: how it is generated, how it is controlled and why these controls sometimes fail. The normal occurrence of "autoimmune" B cells is well documented. A striking confirmation of this was provided by making hybridomas with B cells from unimmunized mouse spleens and screening them for autoimmune specificities by immunofluorescence (Wassmer, Abstract 80). Significantly, up to 10% of these hybridomas secreted antibodies reacting with tissues commonly implicated in autoimmune disease including gastric mucosa, smooth muscle, cell nuclei, islets of Langerhans and anterior pituitary. It would be interesting to check whether these "autoimmune" B cells belong to the Ly-1 (T1) B cell subset reported previously and in Workshop A3 at this meeting (Herzenberg et. al., Abstract 58).

The status of autoimmune T cells is less clear. The early expectation that all autoimmune T-helper cells should be purged from the repertoire during ontogeny has already been eroded. For example, it is possible in susceptible strains of mice to induce autoimmune thyroiditis by injections of autologous thyroglobulin in adjuvant, implying that autoimmune helper cell precursors exist. T cells of the helper type have now been shown to proliferate in vitro both to mouse and human thyroglobulins (David et. al., Abstract 64). An even more direct demonstration of their

357

existence was provided by the isolation of partially cloned autoimmune T-helper cell lines derived from mice immunised with autologous red cell membranes in adjuvant.
These proliferated in vitro on exposure to mouse but not to
rat red cells (Kelly and Culbert, Abstract 69).   It is
possible that, rather than stimulating an existing pool of
T-helper cells, the adjuvant may have served to rescue
these cells from deletion during their differentiation -
possibly by an IL-2 dependant mechanism similar to that
responsible for prevention of neonatal tolerance to MHC
antigens (Workshop C2, Abstract 198).   Although this interpretation may weaken the argument for the existence of self
reactive T helper cells in the mature T cell pool, it does
provide one plausible explanation for the breakdown of self
tolerance.

      Deletion of at least some autoreactive cells occurs
during ontogeny of B cells, as well as helper cells and
cytotoxic cells, and serves to shape the mature repertoire.
However, it is not known whether suppressor T cells may also
be deleted.   This question was approached using an assay
in which T cells proliferated against either autologous or
allogeneic variants of the liver F antigen.   Spleen cells
from donors treated with large doses of soluble F antigen
were found to cause marked suppression of this proliferative
response (Lukić et. al., Abstract 73).   Since both allo-F
and self-F would induce suppressor activity it was evident
that self-F-specific suppressor cells had not been completely eliminated.   However, the fact that self-F induced
weaker suppression than did allo-F was consistent with partial elimination of suppressor cells.

      In the subsequent discussion suppressor cells were
brought into line with other types of lymphocytes by
Mitchison, who outlined a hypothetical scheme relating the
size of the "hole" in the anti-self repertoire to the effective concentration of an autoantigen.   In this scheme T
helper cells were considered to be most susceptible to deletion, followed by T suppressors, with B cells being the most
resistant.   These differences in susceptibility could
account for some observed differences in the anti-self repertoire (e.g. Simon and Kong, Abstract 78) and provide a
theoretical background for the concept of "suppressor determinants".

Suppressor cells are generally thought to function as a fail-safe mechanism which prevents responses to self antigens in postnatal life even in the presence of self-reactive helper and B cells. Their action in this regard is usually seen as being reversible. Not much thought has so far been given to the possibility that they may facilitate the irreversible inactivation of the cells they suppress, particularly during early differentiation in utero, and thus participate in the mechanism of deletion. To test this possibility embryo mice were subjected to transplacental treatment with anti-IJ antibodies by using IJ-immunised mothers. As young adults these mice made greatly enhanced responses to autologous red cells and DNA after immunisation with rat red cells and stimulation with LPS respectively (Gibson and Basten, Abstract 65). This result suggests that Ts are involved in the induction of self-tolerance. A possible mechanism for the effect was suggested in another workshop (E3): suppressor cell activity resulted in a decrease in the level of IL-2 which then allowed clonal inactivation to proceed more readily (Asherson et. al., Abstract 390) once again pointing to the potential importance of growth factors in the tolerance state.

Central to our consideration of autoimmunity is the question of how anti-self responses are triggered. Attention is now being focussed on the role of antigen presentation as the initiating stimulus. There is frequently an increase in expression of Ia in tissues affected by auto-immune disease, sometimes involving cells which were not previously known to be capable of expressing Ia, for example thyroid epithelial cells (thyrocytes). It was shown that such cells from patients with Graves' disease could effectively present irrelevant antigens like an influenza virus peptide (Londei et. al., Abstract 72) as well as thyroid specific microsomal antigens. Since Ia expression can be induced in thyrocytes by gamma interferon (Bottazzo, Workshop C1, Abstract 175) the autoimmune process could well be initiated by any viral infection which causes local release of gamma interferon. Subsequently, if the autoimmune response is not damped down by suppression, then the activity of self-reactive T cells themselves might suffice to maintain the aberrant expression of Ia. These findings therefore provide a neat explanation both for the organ specificity of certain autoimmune disorders and for the pathological changes seen in them.

     If the inflammatory process maintains a local focus of
autoimmunity in this way then the generation of effective
suppressor cells might only be able to occur outside of the
focus.   When the focus involves the whole organ, as
in thyroiditis, then only soluble antigen would be available to stimulate suppressor cells at sites distant from
the focus.   The importance of soluble antigen in this
regard was emphasised by the finding that a variety of
measures which increased the quantity and persistence of
circulating thyroglobulin would alleviate the severity of
thyroiditis (Lewis et. al., Abstract 70).   Such a conclusion was also supported by the demonstration of the suppressive effect of injections of soluble self-F antigen
(Lukić et. al., Abstract 73).   Taken together these findings emphasise the important role played by suppressor cells
in downregulating autoimmune responses.

     The increased susceptibility of some human individuals
and strains of mice to certain autoimmune diseases appears
to require both an MHC-related abnormality of presentation
and a defect in suppression - the latter possibly occurring
as a consequence of the former.   Such a defect in suppression was reported in multiple sclerosis patients, who maintained high proliferative responses to measles virus, together with high autologous mixed lymphocyte reactions, at
times when these were found to be suppressed in measles
patients who were not suffering from multiple sclerosis
(Greenstein et. al., Abstract 66).   It should, however,
be noted that the cells were obtained from peripheral blood;
thus enhanced responsiveness could have been due not to a
primary defect in suppression but rather to recruitment of
suppressor cells to sites involved in the disease process.
Alternatively the loss of suppression could have been an
indirect result of genetic anomalies in presentation, since
a number of immunological abnormalities (mitogen responses,
B cell numbers, helper/suppressor ratio) were found to be
associated with HLA-B8 in healthy subjects (McCombs et. al.,
Abstract 74).   These findings are consistent with the large
body of published work pointing to the strong associations
of the HLA-A1 B8, DR3 haplotype with hyperresponsiveness
and increased susceptibility to autoimmune disease.

     It now appears that T cells can recognise quantitative
changes in Ia expression and respond to an increase in Ia
expression by an autologous mixed lymphocyte reaction

(AMLR).   This may be an important factor in immunoregulation.   Such a hypothesis was supported by the isolation of
AMLR-reactive T cell clones (Saito and Rajewsky, no printed
abstract).   These could proliferate and help B cells in a
nonspecific fashion, suggesting that when Ia is increased,
e.g. by interferon, such cells contribute to the persistence of autoimmune reactions.

Finally, there was an interesting report that some
tumours (lymphomas) could be rejected solely because they
lacked a class 1 antigen which was present in the host
(Kärre et. al., Abstract 68).   This recognition of "absence of self" appeared to be mediated by NK cells.   Although
there is little evidence as yet to suggest that such a
mechanism could serve as a basis for autoimmune disease,
the findings are of considerable interest in the field of
tumour immunity where aberrant clones lacking normal class
1 antigens have been reported.

The data described in this Workshop provide a stimulus
for further investigations along several lines.   More work
is required with cloned cell lines to delineate precisely
the possible differences in the anti-self repertoire of
helper cells, suppressor cells and B cells, including the
Ly-1 (TI) B cell subset.   To be clearly interpretable these
experiments should be accompanied by characterisation of
self antigens which are the targets of autoimmune responses
- particularly with respect to the definition of suppressor
versus helper determinants.   The role of suppressor cells
as participants in deletion during ontogeny is also worthy
of further exploration, as is the precise significance of
the strong linkage of certain DR antigens with autoimmune
disease in the light of the recent findings with respect to
increase of Ia expression in disease affected tissues.

FUNCTION OF EFFECTOR T CELLS

Ben Bonavida and Elizabeth Simpson*

Dept Microbiology & Immunology, UCLA School of
Medicine, Centre for Health Sciences,
Los Angeles, CA 90024, USA.
*Clinical Research Centre, Watford Road
Harrow, Middlesex, HA1 3UJ, UK.

Effector T Cells

Effector T cells considered were Tc, either directed
toward class I (L3T4$^-$ Lyt2$^+$ in mouse, T4$^-$ T8$^+$ in man) or
class II (L3T4$^+$ Lyt1$^-$, T4$^+$ T8$^-$) MHC antigens and Th/TDTH
for which the majority are directed towards class II MHC
antigens with the L3T4$^+$ Lyt2, T4$^+$ T8$^-$ phenotype although
class I directed Th/T DTH cells exist, with the obverse
phenotype.

What do they recognise?

In addition to classic class I (K,D & L in mouse, A, B
& C in man) and class II (IA and IE in mouse, DR, DQ and DP
in man) MHC glycoproteins recognised as alloantigens or
restricting elements by T cells, the Qa/Tla region class I
antigens were discussed in the context of immune responses
to teratocarcinoma (TC) (Aspinall, Stern, Oxford).
Xenogeneic (rat anti mouse) *in vitro* secondary T cell responses are possibly directed against Qa/Tla antigens, as
may be certain *in vivo* responses in teratocarcinoma resistant mouse strains, since although in differentiated TC do
not express K, D or L class I antigens, they will react
with hetero anti TC antibodies which precipitate a molecule
of about 40 KD and it was reported that certain monoclonal
antibodies against public specificities on K and/or D

molecules crossreacted with determinants on Qa/Tla molecules, and that these antisera were cytotoxic to teratocarcinoma (Stern).

A cytotoxic Qa-1^b specific clone was used in a kinetic analysis of target cell killing of normal and leukaemic cells (Lefever, Milwaukee).   Unlike enzyme substrate complexes, it has been difficult to directly measure variables such as recycling, heterogeneity, and affinity within the cytotoxic system.   Dr Lefever has examined cytotoxicity using the Michaelis-Menten method and has been able to measure affinity, heterogeneity, and recycling of a clone CTL directed against Qa-1^b antigens.   Lefever has compared the results obtained from leukaemia target cells with those from normal peripheral blood cells.   Differences were noted, inferring that different targets express different density of surface antigens.

Cytotoxic T cells from AKR mice immunized with syngeneic thymomas are Gross Leukaemia specific and K^k restricted.   Schmidt (Giessen) discussed monoclonal antibodies raised against the 369 thymoma in AKR mice.   These antibodies reacted with 369 and other thymomas and with AKR PHA blasts but not with normal thymocytes or lymphocytes. They immunoprecipitated the same 45KD protein, identified as K^k from tumours and blasts.   It was proposed that the MAbs were directed against new epitopes on the K^k molecule induced by the association with it of Gross leukaemia virus. Thus they would represent H-2 restricted antibodies.

Plata (Paris) used transfected targets to show that MuLV specific cytotoxic T cells recognised the MuLV gag gene product, p30, expressed on the cell surface.

Induction of T Cell Responses

Albert (Marseille) discussed findings with attempts to induce T cell effectors _in vitro_ with a) membrane bound class I and II antigens, b) class I molecules in liposomes. Whilst it was possible to clone L3T4$^-$ Lyt2$^+$ cytotoxic T cells reactive with class I antigens from cultures initiated and maintained with allogeneic cells and growth factors, such clones could not be restimulated with liposomes containing class I molecules.   Cultures initiated by stimulation with such liposomes plus syngeneic feeder cells grew

as lines containing L3T4$^+$ Lyt2$^-$ and L3T4$^-$ Lyt2$^+$ subpopula-
tionsbut they could not be cloned and had a limited life
splan.

There was a general discussion about "non specificity"
of cytotoxic effectors   a) during the early induction
phase and   b) in lines or clones maintained for long
periods.   There was evidence that high concentrations of
growth factors early could induce nonspecificity (Braakman,
Amsterdam):   this might be due to NK activation or to an
"alternative pathway" whereby Tc could adhere to and
attack target cells not carrying the antigens used at
induction (Cerottini, Lausanne).   From early cultures
showing non specific cytotoxicity, specific effectors
could be subsequently cloned.   In lines and clones maintained long term, some find loss of specificity and original
function (Pawelec, Tübingen) whilst others are able to
maintain functional and specific clones, restimulated with
antigen and growth factors, for prolonged periods (Engers,
Cerottini, Simpson).

The cytotoxic hybridoma of Moscovitch (Rehovot) grows
autonomously *in vitro* in the absence of extrinsic growth
factors or antigen.   It is induced to kill after a 2 hour
lag period.   Cytotoxic hybridomas which are IL-2 dependent
have been reported from other labs (Nabholz) but are
unstable.   It was unclear whether the difficulty of producing autonomous cytotoxic hybridomas was due to their
instability.

In vivo Functions of Effector T Cells

The use of vitamin A in the diet of mice increased the
level of DTH responses to oxazalone (Miller, Carshalton).
These mice have increased T cell numbers and reactive lymph
nodes.   The increased function of the Lyt1$^+$2$^-$ cells could
account for the results, and this may be mediated via dendritic cells in lymph nodes.   Engers (Lausanne) reported
that selected cytotoxic T cell clones specific for MSV-MoMuLV
injected intravenously could prevent viral oncogenesis in
unirradiated, irradiated or "B" mice.   There was a discussion of the relative roles of Tc and Th/T$_{DTH}$ *in vivo*
under normal condition s, and while class I restricted Tc
clonescould act as antiviral and anti tumour effectors,
there was evidence that class II restricted cells played a

role in protection against Sendai and MSV since $H-2^b$ mutant mouse strains in which a cytotoxic response could not occur were still resistant to infection, although in some cases less resistent than the wild strain (quoted from the work of Melief, Amsterdam). Graft rejection of syngeneic male grafts by female mice is probably mediated entirely by class II restricted Th/T_{DTH} cells since it occurs in B10.A(5R) ($K^bI^bD^d$) mice as rapidly as in B10($K^bI^bD^b$) although since neither K^b nor D^d can act as restriction elements for anti H-Y Tc, B10.A(5R) do not make a Tc response to H-Y (Simpson).

$Ly1^+2^-$ T cell clones specific for PPD when injected into mice potentiated immunity to MC6A tumour cells following immunization with MC6A coupled with Con A PPD (Sia, Cambridge). The helper effect for the *in vivo* anti tumour response was thought to be mediated by linked recognition and in parallel these PPD specific clones were shown to provide help *in vitro* to hapten primed B cells.

How Do Effector Cells Function?

It has been recognized that CMC can be divided into three stages, namely: Mg++ dependent recognition taking place between the antigen specific receptor and class I H-2 or HLA antigens, Ca++ dependent programming for lysis and killer cell independent lysis of target cells. It has been hypothesized that these stages are mediated by distinct cell-cell interactions, and that it is possible to bypass the initial recognition event through the use of lectin in an antigen nonspecific, lectin dependent cellular cytotoxicity (LDCC) system.

In an effort to examine the role of class I MHC antigens in LDCC, Bonavida and colleagues have tested whether a class I deficient human target Daudi can serve as a target in LDCC. Their studies indicate that Daudi indeed serves as a target cell, and, based on this data, they postulate that other target antigens for cytotoxicity are papain sensitive and recover rapidly within two hours of incubation. The exact nature of the papain sensitive target cell structures involved in lysis is not known, but it is postulated that they may belong to the family of lymphocyte function antigens (LFA) described by Springer.

Berke has addressed the question of how a target cell is damaged by the cytotoxic lymphocyte.   Lysis appears to resemble a secretory system and it has been suggested that damage of the target membrane is the result of secretion and insertion of cytotoxins into the membrane.   These cytotoxins then form pores which lead to leakage and lysis. An alternative postulation by Berke is that lysis may be initiated by prelytic events inside the cell which lead to target membrane damage and lysis.   Berke reports that following contact of target and CTL, the target cell membrane depolarizes, which brings about a voltage dependent calcium influx.   The accumulation of calcium induces the stimulation of ATPase leading to depletion of high energy phosphate.   This results in sodium pumping being slowed down, and colloidal osmotic lysis.   These results are intriguing and warrant reconciliation with current models.

Tumour Immunity

The production of monoclonal antibodies to human tumours by *in vitro* immunization was described (Ho, Newton). A carbohydrate determinant appeared to be recognized by one MAb.

Dr Vanky has examined the proliferation to tumour associated HLA DR antigens *in vitro*.   He has demonstrated that there is no correlation between the expression of HLA DR antigen and syngeneic proliferation and these responses cannot be blocked by IA antibodies.   The syngeneic anti-tumour proliferative response appears to be different from that obtained in the autologous proliferative response or alloantigenic response.   Dr Vanky suggests that other mechanisms may be involved in the anti-tumour response. However, the question still remains as to whether the normal IA bearing host can process tumour antigens and present them to T cells.

Investigation of T cell subsets and IL-2 production in CLL patients showed that the T4/T8 ratio was not altered in 40 untreated patients, but that they produced more IL-2 than normal cells (Norris, Edinburgh).

ANTIGEN PRESENTING CELLS

Jay A. Berzofsky

Metabolism Branch, National Cancer Institute
National Institutes of Health
Bethesda, Maryland 20205 USA

and

Kozo Yokomuro

Department of Microbiology and Immunology
Nippon Medical School
Toyko 113, Japan

Three major issues were discussed in the workshop:
(1) the role of antigen processing in T-cell activation
and situations in which it may not be necessary for T-cell
stimulation, (2) the differences in antigen presenting
function of macrophages and dendritic cells and the ability of dendritic cells to process antigen, and (3) the
role of the type of antigen presenting cell in eliciting
preferentially different functional types of T cells such
as helpers and suppressors, and the role of presenting
cells in tolerance.

The first topic, antigen processing, was a source of
major controversy at the meeting in general as well as in
this workshop. It has been widely believed that native
protein antigens cannot be "seen" directly by T cells, but
must be first altered or "processed" in some way by the
antigen presenting cell, such as a macrophage. In his
plenary session talk, Emil Unanue (Boston) presented evidence that chloroquine, as an inhibitor of lysosomal function, or glutaraldehyde fixation, would prevent macrophage
presentation of native hen lysozyme, but not a peptide
fragment thereof, to two lysozyme-specific T-cell clones
specific for the same segment, residues 46-61, of lysozyme. This result was taken to imply that the native

369

molecule required some processing step not required by the
fragment. Moreover, these inhibitors did not inhibit presentation of reduced carboxymethylated lysozyme to one of
the clones. Similar results were presented in the workshop by Jay Berzofsky (Bethesda), who, with Howard
Streicher, Gail Buckenmeyer, and Ira Berkower, found that
chloroquine as well as a specific competitive protease
inhibitor, leupeptin, could inhibit the presentation of
native myoglobin but not of a peptide fragment (132-153)
bearing the same epitope to the same T-cell clone. Thus,
the native molecule required some step, prior to presentation, not required by the peptide, and this step appeared
to be proteolytic. An unfolded form of myoglobin,
S-methyl apomyoglobin, the same size as the native molecule but unfolded like the peptide, behaved like the peptide. Therefore, conformation rather than size was critical in determining the need for processing. It appeared
from both the lysozyme and the myoglobin work that processing was needed to unfold the native protein to expose
sites, such as hydrophobic residues, not normally exposed
in the native form, which might be necessary to interact
either with Ia or with the presenting cell membrane. Perhaps this served to convert the native, water-soluble protein into a form which could be stably associated with the
lipid plasma membrane of the macrophage.

Alex Miller (Los Angeles), with N. Shastri and E.E.
Sercarz, presented evidence that H-2^b T-cell clones
which responded to a tryptic peptide 74-96 of lysozyme,
shared by hen lysozyme and ring-necked pheasant lysozyme,
responded only to the pheasant and not the hen lysozyme
in native form. However, when the cyanogen bromide fragments from 13-105 or 16-105 of these lysozymes were used,
both species stimulated equally. The difference appeared
to be due to differences in the way the two native proteins were handled or processed by presenting cells, since
the T-cell site was the same. Surprisingly, this effect
depended on H-2, since H-2^k T cells showed the reverse
preference. Therefore, the critical step may be after Ia
becomes involved, or else differences in the T-cell repertoire between H-2^b and H-2^k may lead to requirements
for different sites of processing.

These studies were contrasted by two presentations
which suggested that processing was not necessary. First,
J.H. Robinson (Newcastle upon Tyne), with A.L. Bentley and

R.K. Jordan, reported that DNP-ovalbumin covalently coupled to spleen cells could be presented to T cells without
inhibition by chloroquine. Even Ia-negative EL-4 T-lym-
phoma cells, or nylon-purified thymocytes, could present
DNP-ovalbumin, but only if it was covalently coupled to
the cells. Thus, covalent coupling appeared to substitute
for processing. Another similar result arose from an
attempt by Peter Walden (Tübingen), with Z. Nagy and J.
Klein, to simplify antigen presentation to its minimal
components. They incorporated Ia molecules and antigen,
covalently bound to lipids, into liposomes and used these
to present antigen to polyclonal immune T cells as well
as T-cell clones and hybridomas. Only the hybridomas
could be rigorously shown to be free of other presenting
cells. Surprisingly, they observed presentation of several protein antigens, including lysozyme, KLH, lactic
dehydrogenase, cytochrome c, and ovalbumin, on liposomes
with appropriate Ia. They concluded that native proteins
could be presented without processing. Much discussion
ensued to try to resolve the conflicting conclusions of
these studies. One problem noted was that KLH-liposomes
could stimulate T cells without Ia, and that cytochrome
c-liposomes without Ia could stimulate a clearly Ia-
restricted T-cell hybridoma (from E. Heber-Katz and R.H.
Schwartz), resulting in 60% of the response obtained with
the appropriate Ia, albeit requiring higher antigen concentration. These results suggested reprocessing of liposomes by Ia-bearing cells, more likely than the alternative of T-cell stimulation without Ia. To test this,
Alison Finnegan (Bethesda) suggested blocking with anti-Ia
antibodies. If blocking were found it would imply reprocessing by Ia-positive cells.

A second issue in this study was the conformation of the
antigen after incorporation into liposomes. The studies
of Unanue and Berzofsky and coworkers cited above, which
supported the need for processing of native proteins,
agreed that peptide fragments or unfolded forms of the
intact protein did not require processing. Thus, all
agreed that not all forms of the antigen required processing. The issue, then, concerned only native antigen. Jay
Berzofsky (Bethesda) pointed out that globular proteins
assume a native conformation which gives the minimum
energy in water, with hydrophilic residues on the outside
and hydrophobic residues buried inside. Once covalently
incorporated into liposomes, these proteins are no longer

in a fully aqueous environment and the minimum energy conformation should be different, in some regions even inverted. Even disulfide-bonded lysozyme could be unfolded
because the method used to couple the proteins to lipid
via disulfide bonds required reduction with dithiothreitol. Thus, the proteins may have been artificially processed to a form not requiring further processing. If
unfolding is the goal of processing, it can be achieved by
several pathways, even though the cell chooses the short-
cut of proteolytic cleavage (analogous to Alexander's
approach to untying the Gordian knot). Dr. Walden indicated that the LDH retained enzyme activity and the cytochrome its spectrum, but since a small fraction of denatured protein may be sufficient to stimulate T cells, what
is needed is a positive test for denatured forms (such as
an antibody that does not crossreact with native) rather
than a test for native forms that may miss a small amount
of unfolded protein. A third possibility, if the purpose
of processing is to put a globular protein, designed to
be in aqueous solution, into a form in which it is stably
associated with the presenting cell membrane, is that both
covalent linkage to lipid for incorporation into liposomes
and covalent attachment to a presenting cell (Robinson)
would accomplish this end and bypass the need for processing. However, in that case, such results could not be
taken to imply that free, water-soluble, native protein
antigen would not require processing for presentation to
T cells.

The second topic discussed was a comparison of antigen presentation by dendritic cells and macrophages. M.L.
Kapsenberg (Amsterdam), with F. Stiekema, M. Teunissen,
and H. Keizer, found that dendritic cells presented ovalbumin as well as macrophages, but would not phagocytose
and present ovalbumin coupled to latex beads as macrophages could. However, a 1:4 mixture of macrophages:den-
dritic cells presented latex-ovalbumin much better than
either alone, suggesting that particulate antigen processed by macrophages could be presented by dendritic
cells. Surprisingly, presentation by dendritic cells was
not inhibited by chloroquine. In contrast, P.M. Kaye
(London), with B.M. Chain and M. Feldmann, working with a
particulate antigen, mycobacteria, found that nonphago-
cytic dendritic cells could take up and present the bacteria even better than phagocytic macrophages, so phagocytosis was not required. Moreover, with soluble KLH,

they found that presentation by dendritic cells was inhibited by the same concentration and time of treatment with
chloroquine as had been used by Kapsenberg et al. No
resolution of this inconsistency was found, so it could
not be stated whether dendritic cells process antigen or
not. Interestingly, Kaye et al. found that intracellular
bacterial infection suppressed Ia expression. This phenomenon may protect the bacterium from immune elimination
by preventing antigen presentation.

The third major topic was the ability of different
types of presenting cells to activate different functional
sets of T cells. E. Smet and P. de Baetselier (Brussels)
reported that antigen-pretreated B cells elicited helper
T cells whereas antigen-fed macrophages elicited suppressor T cells. Both types of presenting cells stimuated
proliferation. S.C. Knight (Harrow), with J. Krejci, A.
Gautam, and G. Asherson, reported that dendritic cells
from mice made tolerant by high-dose IV injection of
picrylsulphonic acid, were unable to present the antigen,
after skin painting, to T cells. Thus, a defect in antigen presentation may contribute to tolerance, although it
could not be excluded that reduced T-cell response led to
reduced activation of or Ia induction on dendritic cells
from these mice.

K. Yokomuro (Tokyo), with A. Mabuchi, O. Tsuchiya,
and Y. Kimura, found that presentation of antigen by Ia-
negative macrophage cell line SL4 and J774 cells induced
antigen-specific suppressor T cells, but this induction
of suppression was prevented by UV-irradiation of the presenting cells. Thus, two signals were necessary for induction of suppressor cells: (1) antigen in the relative
absence of Ia, and (2) a second signal produced by the
presenting cell and sensitive to UV irradiation. Immunization of recipients of UV-irradiated, antigen-pulsed J774
cells overcame the UV effect and induced suppression.
Thus, the second signal could be produced by the immunized
recipient when it could not be provided by the UV-irradiated presenting cells.

It is clear that much work remains to be done to
explain why as well as how T cells see antigen in association with Ia on presenting cells instead of free in solution, and how different types of presenting cells, with

different Ia levels and other differences, preferentially
activate different types of T cells. A few questions were
answered, but many more were raised. Perhaps, out of the
controversy is arising a consensus that processing serves
to alter antigen to a form which can be stably associated
with the antigen presenting cell surface, and alternative
maneuvers which accomplish this can bypass processing.

PROGRESS IN ANTIMICROBIAL IMMUNITY

Juraj Ivanyi[+] and Fernando Plata[°]

[+]Wellcome Research Laboratories, Beckenham,
Kent BR3 3BS, Great Britain; and [°]Institut
Pasteur, 75015 Paris, France.

The presented papers dealt with the interactions of
viral, bacterial and parasitic infectious agents with the
immune system in animal models and in man. Three main
approaches were undertaken : (a) immunogenetic control of
host resistance to infection; (b) the role of T cell-mediated
reactions in host protection and pathology; and (c) modulation of the host's immune functions by microbial infection.

A. IMMUNOGENETIC CONTROL OF RESISTANCE

The susceptibility to murine leukemia virus (MuLV)-
induced tumors in neonatal mice was reported to be under
genetic control by the *H-2* gene complex (Zijlstra *et al.*,
Abstract 345). The results suggested that the phenotype of
the developing lymphomas was determined by the *H-2* genotype
of the infected mouse, rather than by the type of MuLV
chosen for infection. Thus, resistant C57BL/10 mice developed high titers of anti-MuLV antibodies, produced very
little intrathymic MuLV, and only a proportion of these mice
developed B cell lymphomas late after infection. However,
mice from susceptible strains (*i.e.*, BALB/c and B10.D2) produced lower titers of anti-MuLV antibodies and large amounts
of intrathymic MuLV, and developed early T cell lymphomas.
In both susceptible and resistant strains of mice, tumor
induction by MuLV was controlled by genes mapping in the
IA/IE region of the *H-2* complex. The quality of the immune
response directed by these genes consequently determines the

phenotype (*i.e.*, T or B) of the induced lymphomas.

An immunogenetic analysis of resistance to infection
by *Trypanosoma congolense* was reported by Pinder and
Chassin (Abstract 328). Previous studies of infected cattle
had implicated at least one gene controlling resistance,
presumably by regulating anti-trypanosome antibody levels.
Infection of various inbred mouse strains with *T. congolense*
revealed that resistance to infection is controlled by a
recessive autosomal gene and correlates with temporal differences in the trypanosome-specific antibody response.
Thus, resistant C57BL/6 mice produced antibodies with an
early onset four days after infection, while susceptible
BALB/c mice showed comparable antibody titers only from the
tenth day after infection. The protective role of antibodies
was further proved in passive transfer experiments. Preliminary results indicate that the mechanisms which determine
the outcome of infection in this system probably involve
the generation of immune suppression by the trypanosome
infection in susceptible but not in resistant mouse strains.

B. T CELL-MEDIATED REACTIONS

A paradoxical deleterious effect on the course of infection with *Leishmania major* in BALB/c mice was observed upon
adoptive transfer of *L. major*-specific immune spleen T cells
or T cell clones (Louis *et al.*, Abstract 321). Cutaneous
lesions were exacerbated by helper/inducer T cells of the
Lyt-1$^+$2$^-$, L3T4$^+$ phenotype. The authors tentatively attributed
these observations to a T cell-enhanced migration of macrophages to the lesion site by secretion of macrophage-recruit-
ing factors. Since macrophages are the main susceptible
target cell for parasite infection and proliferation, an
increase in macrophage density amplifies the parasite load
in the lesion. It was particularly interesting that after
adoptive transfer, the same immune T cells also induced
L. major-specific delayed-type hypersensitivity reactions.

These observations should not be generalized towards
other systems. In the case of intestinal infection of mice
with another parasite, *Giardia muris*, deficiency in intestinal Lyt-1$^+$2$^-$ T cells correlated with impaired clearance of
the parasite (Heyworth and Owen, Abstract 319). Moreover,
Näher and colleagues (Abstract 323) reported that the

adoptive transfer of $H-2K$-restricted Lyt-1$^+$2$^+$ immune T cells
specific for *Listeria monocytogenes* led to granuloma formation, lower bacterial counts, and host protection. A subset
of $I-A$-restricted Lyt-1$^+$2$^-$ T cells was also detected in
granulomas but was less protective upon transfer.

The protective potential of T cell immunity towards
intracellular pathogens in man was implied from studies on
T cell clones directed to *Mycobacterium tuberculosis* (Rees
et al., Abstract 329). These T cells were specific for a
purified antigen defined by monoclonal antibody TB68, and
secreted a distinct macrophage-activating factor with an
apparent molecular weight of 25,000 daltons which could not
be neutralized with an antibody to gamma-interferon.

C. MODULATION OF IMMUNE FUNCTIONS

Antigen-specific modulation of T cell functions by
antibodies was reported by Celis and Chang (Abstract 332).
Monoclonal antibodies to hepatitis B surface antigen (HBsAg)
augmented specifically the proliferation of various human
T cell clones sensitized against HBsAg. The observed enhancement was higher with IgG than with IgM antibodies, and
required a functional Fc portion of the antibody molecule.
These results were attributed to a more efficient presentation of antigen by accessory cells due to binding of antigen-
antibody complexes to accessory cell Fc receptors. Mechanisms
of this nature could play important T cell regulatory roles
in infections by hepatitis B and other viruses.

The nonspecific immunosuppressive effects of various
infectious agents were also reported. Disruption of normal
macrophage functions resulting in the inhibition of T cell
proliferation and antibody responses was demonstrated with
porcine macrophages infected by African swine fever virus
(Enjuanes et al., Abstract 333). Likewise, infection of
human macrophages with human cytomegalovirus (HCMV) inhibited
IL-1 secretion and suppressed polyclonal T cell proliferative
responses *in vitro* (Rodgers et al., Abstract 339). Although
infectious HCMV was required, no virus replication or viral
antigens could be detected in the infected cells. Inhibition
of IL-1 secretion was restricted to HCMV and measles virus
when a panel of viruses was tested; this inhibitory effect
was ascribed to the production of a 95,000 dalton soluble

suppressor factor by HCMV-infected macrophages and monocytes.

Studies of suppressor macrophages produced in mice infected by *Trypanosoma cruzi* were reported by Harel-Bellan *et al.* (Abstract 318) and by Plata *et al.* (Abstract 327). The latter study also showed that infection by *T. cruzi* resulted in the enhanced growth of a syngeneic tumor, due to suppression of the host's anti-tumor immunity. Both macrophages and non-specific Lyt-2$^+$ suppressor T cells were shown to inhibit activation of tumor-specific Lyt-2$^+$ cytolytic T cell precursors. It is interesting to note that Lyt-1$^+$2$^-$ T cell-mediated delayed-type hypersensitivity reactions in the same mice were not suppressed.

CONCLUDING REMARKS

The three approaches reviewed in this Summary revealed new and interesting interactions between microbial agents and the immune system of the infected host. The molecular analysis of T cell- and macrophage-derived soluble mediators which contribute to the elimination of the infectious agents and which can modulate the immune response itself constituted a major topic of this Leucocyte Culture Conference.

MOLECULAR MEDIATORS OF LYMPHOCYTE

ACTIVATION AND PROLIFERATION

R. Callard and B.M. Vose

Institute of Child Health, London and

ICI Pharmaceuticals Division, Macclesfield

The pathway by which resting B cells differentiate into antibody-forming cells (AFC) may be divisible into three separate steps; namely, activation from G0 to G1, proliferation induced by binding of growth factors, and differentiation into AFC induced by maturation factors. The seven papers on B cell factors given at the workshop on 'molecular mediators of lymphocyte activation and proliferation' were mostly concerned with the molecular signals controlling the second and third steps of this pathway.

Assays for B cell factors can be divided into twobasic types: those using B cell lines or B cell tumours as targets, and those using T cell depleted B cells from normal tissues. The main disadvantage of the latter method is that it is virtually impossible in bulk cultures to distinguish between an effect of a factor binding directly to B cells, and activation via residual T cells, or other non-B cells, which are invariably present in T cell depleted mononuclear cell preparations. For example, Procopio and Ortaldo (NCI, Frederick) reported that large granular lymphocytes (LGL), which are invariably present in T cell depleted human mononuclear cell preparations, will secrete large amounts of B cell growth factors (BCGF) with molecular weights comparable with BCGF I and BCGF II (20K and 45K) when activated with mitogens. There was also much discussion about the problem of residual T cells present in the various B cell preparations, and the role played by IL-2 in B cell activation. This argument has certainly become more interesting with the reports of IL-2 receptors on activated normal, and malignant B cells (P. Beverley and I Ando, UCH Medical School (personal communication), and in two of the conference symposia by A. Fauci, NIH, and W. Leonard, NCI, Bethesda). This raises the possibility that IL-2 may act either indirectly via contaminating T cells, or directly on activated B cells. The first of these alternatives certainly does seem to occur. R. Sauerwein (Red Cross Blood Transfusion Service, Amsterdam) presented convincing evidence that IL-2 can induce IgM production by human mononuclear cells in the absence of any other mitogenic stimuli. Since both recombinant IL-2 (r-IL-2) and chromatographically purified material were equally effective, the effect could not have been due to contaminating B cell factors. The response was, however, dependent on the presence of significant numbers of T cells suggesting that the IL-2 was not acting directly on the B cells. Similar results were also reported by R. Callard (Institute of Child Health, London). In this system, T cell dependent antibody responses to influenza virus were obtained from human peripheral blood mononuclear cells (PBM). Addition of r-IL-2 significantly increased specific antibody formation, and also resulted in some non-specific IgM synthesis. As with Sauerweins experiments, the polyclonal IgM response depended on the presence of T cells, but unlike his system the presence of antigen was also required. This story was taken further by M. Melief (Red Cross Blood Transfusion Service, Amsterdam) who showed that the IL-2 induced IgM responses in human PBM required the presence of T4+ "T helper cells." Since pokeweed mitogen (PWM) induces IL-2 production by T4+ cells, it was argued that helper T cell function may be dissociated into two distinct activities: IL-2 production, and secretion of B cell growth and differentiation factors, with the second being contingent on the first. This contention was supported by experiments with neoplastic T4+ cells from a T-CLL patient which could not be made to secrete IL-2, and were unable to function as T helper cells in a PWM response unless exogenous IL-2 was added to the cultures.

There seems no doubt then that IL-2 can act indirectly through T cells to induce Ig synthesis. Whether it can also act directly on B cells is less certain. r-IL-2 was able to induce specific antibody formation in antigen stimulated cultures of T cell depleted PBM, but it was not possible to totally exclude a requirement for T cells (R. Callard, ICH, London). Other than resorting to the use of B cell lines, which would present yet another set of prblems, it seems that the only way to resolve this continuously vexatious question will be to develop techniques for culturing single B cells along the lines previously described by Nossal and Pike. In this way, the various activation and differentiation signals acting on antigen specific B cells may be studied without interference from other cell types.

The nature of B cell differentiation signals was explored further in two papers on T cell replacing factors (TRF). In the first of these, K. Takatsu (Institute for Medical Immunology, Kumamoto, Japan) presented some new data on the previously described TRF obtained from the B151K12 T cell hybridoma. The factor was assayed by the induction of IgM plaque forming cells (PFC) in the B cell leukaemic line, BCL1, and IgG anti-DNP responses in B cells from DNP-KLH primed mice. Chemical characterisation of B151K12 TRF showed it to be a hydrophobic glycoprotein which bound to lima bean agglutinin probably through residues of N-acetyl galactosamine. It has a molecular weight of 50-60K by gel-permeation chromatography, and 41K on SDS-PAGE under non-reducing conditions. Under reducing conditions, it migrated at about 20K. It could be distinguished from IL-1, IL-2, interferon and BCGF1, but the question remained open whether TRF defined by its functional activity is a single molecular species or a combination of, for example, BCGF and BCDF. Given the current three signal model (activation, proliferation, and differentiation) for antibody formation by B cells, this is not a trivial distinction. B151K12 TRF was able to induce B cell proliferation, but it was unclear whether this was necessary for antibody formation, and whether the mitogenic and differentiation signals came from the same molecule. Interestingly, it was found that free N-acetyl galactosamine was able to block TRF-mediated PFC responses suggesting a functional role for carbohydrate on the TRF glycoprotein. Could it be that the proliferation and differentiation signals come from different carbohydrate

determinants on the same molecule. Unfortunately, the
effect of N-acetyl galactosamine on B cell proliferative
responses to TRF was not tested.

A similar TRF, active in antibody responses to
influenza virus in man, was reported by R. Callard (ICH,
London). The factor was obtained from supernatants of
tonsil cells stimulated with PHA, or the Gibbon-Ape T cell
line, MLA-144, and was assayed on blood or tonsil T cell
depleted B cells. The TRF activity did not depend on the
presence of IL-2, and was shown by limiting dilution
experiments not to require the presence of T helper cells.
Preliminary purification on ACA-54 columns showed the
factor to have a molecular weight of between 35-45K which
distinguishes it from IL-1, IL-2 and BCGF1. A role for
gamma-interferon was also excluded by the fact that
recombinant gamma-interferon was quite inactive in this
system. However, as with the murine B151K12 TRF, it is
unknown whether this TRF activity is mediated by one or
more molecular species. Ultimately, the answer to this
quandary will depend on gene cloning of the various
factors. But in the meantime it may be possible to provide
some answers by raising monoclonal antibodies to cell
membrane receptors for the various B cell factors, and
testing them for selective inhibition of factor induced
responses. So far there has been little progress with this
approach for B cells although it is clear from recent
successes with the anti-TAC antibody, and the cloning of
the IL-2 receptor gene (reported in the symposium by W.
Leonard, NCI, Bethesda) that this approach is a viable one.
A start has perhaps been made by H. Yakura (Asahikawa
Medical College, Japan) who presented some evidence that
anti-Lyb2 antibody in the mouse may bind to or modulate the
receptor for BCGF1.

Finally, there were two papers on factors which
modulate isotype specific antibody responses. J. Revillard
(INSERM, Hopital E. Herriot, Lyon) described an IgA binding
factor, presumably an IgA specific FcR, which selectively
inhibited cytoplasmic IgA (cIgA) synthesis compared with
cIgM and cIgG in cultures of PWM activated PBM, and
non-specifically inhibited secretion of all Ig classes.
B. Vose (ICI, Macclesfield, UK) on the other hand,
described a factor in supernatants of mitogen activated
Peyer's patch T cells from mice, and tonsil T cells in man,

which selectively increased IgA formation by mitogen
activated B cells. The question which must always arise in
work of this nature is whether the factor is switching B
cells to IgA production, or selecting precommitted cells
from the total population. It was, therefore, of
considerable interest that the factor prepared from tonsil
T cells was able to induce IgA synthesis in the B cell
line, RAMOS. As this line does not normally synthesise
IgA, this finding suggests that the factor was inducing an
isotype switch.

In summary, it was clear from this workshop, and from
the conference as a whole, that our understanding of the
molecular signalling required for B cell activation and
maturation is far from complete. Moreover, with evidence
accumulating for functionally distinct B cell subsets,
which are likely to be subject to different sets of
regulatory molecules, it is likely that there will continue
to be significant growth in this area for some time to
come.

Interleukin-1 has a multiplicity of effects on a range
of different target cells. By definition IL-1 has the
capacity to act as a co-stimulator with mitogen for
thymocyte proliferation. It is also capable of inducing
proliferation of fibroblasts, is indistinguishable on
immunological and chemical grounds from endogenous pyrogen
and can induce collagenase secretion by chondrocytes. Four
papers were presented at the workshop on various aspects of
IL-1 biology.

The observation that IL-1-like activity might be cell
associated which was reported in the conference symposium
by E.R. Unanue (Harvard Medical School) gained further
support from A. Arnold (Cornell University Medical School,
New York). B lymphoblastoid cell lines were able to
support proliferation and IL-2 secretion by purified T
lymphocytes treated with sodium periodate and neuraminidase
galactose oxidise (NAGO) in the absence of accessory cells.
No soluble factor capable of inducing thymocyte
proliferation was found and cell-cell contact was
obligatory for this response. The accessory function and
production of soluble IL-1-like activity by B cell lines
and the premonocytic cell line U937 was reported in several
posters and Knudsen et al (Harvard Medical School)

described the purification of material from endotoxin
stimulated U937 cells by reverse phase and hydroxylapatite
HPLC. Further purification on TSK2000 SW HPLC yielded a
single species with IL-1 activity in the 15-20Kd range.
Activity of the purified molecule in the thymocyte
proliferation assay was neutralised by a rabbit antiserum
specific for endogeneous pyrogen and upon intravenous
injection into rabbits it induced low level pyrexia. These
two criteria suggest the close similarity between IL-1 and
endogeneous pyrogen (EP). However, the view that these two
activities invariably reside in the same molecule was
questioned by work reported by C. Damais (Institut Pasteur,
Paris). Muramyl dipeptide and non-pyrogenic analogues
(Murabutide) were shown to induce production of IL-1-like
activity by monocytes bearing receptors for C3 but only the
pyrogenic molecule (MDP) could elicit release of
endogeneous pyrogen. Thus, IL-1/EP could reside in
separate but closely similar molecules and may be produced
by different cells under different stimulation protocols.
The possibility that the different activities attributed to
IL-1 reside in a family of molecules necessarily implies
that specific receptors for these molecules also exist.
Further separation of activities of IL-1-like peptides was
described by J.L. Rossio (NCI-FCRF). Small molecular
weight peptides (2Kd) from human urine were shown to be
active in both thymocyte or dermal fibroblast
proliferation. The two activities could be separated by
anion exchange chromatography. Fibroblast activity was
focussed at pH7.9 while thymocyte activity focussed to two
peaks at pH5.3 and 6.3. These results indicate that
different portions of the IL-1 molecule may mediate
distinct biological effects although the definition of a
molecule devoid of thymocyte activity as IL-1 may be in
doubt. Clearly this question awaits sequencing and cloning
of the different active peptides and intact IL-1-studies
which are in progress in several centres.

INDEX

DE